STP 1229

Head and Neck Injuries in Sports

Earl F. Hoerner, Editor

ASTM Publication Code Number (PCN):
04-012290-47

ASTM
1916 Race Street
Philadelphia, PA 19103
Printed in the U.S.A.

Library of Congress Cataloging-in-Publication Data

ISBN: 0-8031-1886-4
PCN: 04-012290-47
LOC: 94-42668

Photocopy Rights

Peer Review Policy

Each paper published in this volume was evaluated by three peer reviewers. The authors addressed all of the reviewers' comments to the satisfaction of both the technical editor(s) and the ASTM Committee on Publications.

To make technical information available as quickly as possible, the peer-reviewed papers in this publication were printed "camera-ready" as submitted by the authors.

The quality of the papers in this publication reflects not only the obvious efforts of the authors and the technical editor(s), but also the work of these peer reviewers. The ASTM Committee on Publications acknowledges with appreciation their dedication and contribution to time and effort on behalf of ASTM.

Printed in Philadelphia, PA
December 1994

Foreword

This publication, *Head and Neck Injuries in Sports,* contains papers presented at the symposium of the same name, held in Atlanta, GA on 19–20 May, 1993. The symposium was sponsored by ASTM Committee F-8 on Sports Equipment and Facilities. Earl F. Hoerner, Chairman of Committee F-8, presided as symposium chairman and is the editor of the resulting publication.

Contents

PROTECTIVE EQUIPMENT APPLICATIONS

Overview

Conferences and symposiums on head and neck injuries in sports are not a recent development. It is noted in the many references to the papers authored in this special technical publication (STP) that they are dated over a 50- to 60-year span. The pioneers that have been evaluating and assessing the risk factors and equipment and facility protection include scientists and investigators such as Burstein, Patrick, Hodgson, Fenner, McElhaney, Schneider, and others. Although independent papers and publications appear on a sporadic basis in the literature, it has been a number of years since a group of scientists of various disciplines got together to review and present their research, clinical experiences, data collection, and the application of their accumulated experiences and knowledge.

In 1969, the American Society for Testing and Materials (ASTM) initiated a group composed of scientists, manufacturers of equipment, academicians, and other interested parties to prepare and write a standard for a helmet to be used in american football for head protection. To establish this standard, an ASTM Subcommittee, F08.53 on Headgear, was formed under the existing Committee F-8 on Sports Equipment and Facilities. As interest and scope broadened in the early 1970s, other subcommittees, including F08.51 on Medical Aspects and Biomechanics, as well as F08.91 on Biostatistics and Epidemiology, were established.

During this same time frame, basic and clinical Sciences, using the development of technology, established reference databases, as well as data collection and information sources for the study of motion, the application of physics, and the laws of natural science with special emphasis on the effects and results of forces and energy (kinetic) on the human body. In addition, scientific groups and associations began to evolve within the applied specialties of biomechanics, bioengineering, mechanical and electrical engineering, including as well, the clinical skills of human factors, ergonomics, and applied Physiology. These scientific groups and associations include the American Society of Biomechanics, the International Society of Biomechanics, the International Society of Sports Biomechanics, the American Academy of Orthopedic Surgery, the American College of Sports Medicine, Stapp Conferences, and others.

In 1992, ASTM Committee F-8, along with representatives from the other professional groups, initiated the planning to organize an international symposium on head and neck injuries in sports that would assemble a group of scientists in various disciplines to participate in this event. In May of 1993, the international symposium was conducted in Atlanta. However, it is extremely important that on a frequent and repetitive cycle, a review and summation of information and data be compiled by all personnel concerned with the topic of this symposium.

An important focus of the Symposium was on the epidemiology of head and neck injuries in sports. The article and presentation of Kenneth S. Clarke entitled, "The Critical Role of Epidemiological Studies in Assessing the Frequency and Causation Factors in Sports-Related Injuries," presented and published in *Safety in Ice Hockey, ASTM STP 1050*, had previously established the standard and parameters for the professional field of epidemiology. This standard was applied by such authors as Drs. Dick, Bixby-Hammett, Mueller, Clarke, and others in their excellent presentations and critical reviews published in the epidemiology section of this STP, *Head and Neck Injuries in Sports*.

In addition to epidemiology and the critical review of the data and information in this reservoir of information, the symposium also had these objectives:

1. Review and evaluate the effectiveness of factors related to safety, "Risk Factors."
2. Determine whether these safety factors could be modified/improved to reduce injury rates, while in the process, not adversely modifying or affecting the basic nature of the physical activity or sport in which the injuries occurred.

In the symposium, high priority and consideration was also given to presentations concerning the "Mechanism of Injury," with emphasis on the application of biophysics, mechanical engineering, biomechanics, and bioengineering. The role of the medical clinician, both on-field and within the laboratory, is considered to be an integral aspect in correlating, integrating, and establishing the factors involved in the "Mechanism of Injury." This is true for both the anatomical areas addressed in this symposium, the head and the neck, or both.

The presentations published cover a broad spectrum of sporting activities including ice hockey, football, baseball, swimming and diving, equestrian, soccer, gymnastics, and others. Topics such as playing facilities, playing, and protective equipment were also addressed. Other relevant and associated factors (for example, in the sport of equestrian, the Horse) are also reviewed, analyzed, and assessed by the various authors and symposium presenters. Examined as a whole, it can be seen that these articles serve to reveal the very complex nature of the subject of head and neck injuries in sports.

Although the views expressed within the articles and presentations generated by this symposium are those of the authors of the various papers, and while their readers may or may not agree with the methods used in their analysis or the conclusions drawn, such presentations will undoubtedly foster additional investigation and application, thereby ultimately improving safety in the field of physical activity. It is the resolution of these differing views coupled with new findings that will inevitably emerge in the future, which forms the basis of ASTM consensus standard philosophy and its review process.

Despite the broad spectrum of topics covered in this international symposium, it is important to note that there are areas in the applied sciences that are not included in this volume but that need to be further explored, expanded, and applied. The head and neck deserve attention, and the protection of these areas should continue to be a prime subject for the on-going evaluation and application of new data and information, including the application of data concerning newer products and materials for head protection. For example, research regarding the unresolved problem of trying to protect for both linear as well as angular acceleration in head protection needs to be continued. Another area that needs further study is the question of whether neck rolls, shoulder pads, or some other method of neck protection can be of value or even considered in the cervical/neck area. The application of technology is a dynamic process that needs to be constantly reassessed and evaluated.

It is the steering committee and the leadership of ASTM Committee F-8 on Sports Equipment and Facilities' recommendation that this volume will serve as a significant catalyst and stimulate the scientific aspects of data and information on this important subject from interdisciplinary groups. This will continue to promote safety and decrease risk factors through better equipment, facilities, and knowledge of the mechanism of injury. The on-going evaluation of the constant changes that occur with the playing and participating in a physical activity, whether it be leisure, recreational, wellness/fitness, or a competitive athletic contest, is a major factor in the success of protection in head and neck injuries in sports.

Earl F. Hoerner, M.D.

Chairman, Subcommittee F08.51 on Medical Aspects
and Biomechanics, ASTM

Keynote Paper

Kenneth S. Clarke*

CORNERSTONES FOR FUTURE DIRECTIONS IN HEAD/NECK INJURY PREVENTION IN SPORTS

REFERENCE: Clarke, K. S., **"Cornerstones for Future Directions in Head/Neck Injury Prevention in Sports,"** Head and Neck Injuries in Sports, ASTM STP 1229, Earl F. Hoerner, Ed., American Society for Testing and Materials, Philadelphia, 1994

ABSTRACT: Much progress has been made in the last two decades in the effort to minimize serious head and neck injuries in football. More importantly, much has been transferred to the attentions given the threat of catastrophic injuries in other sports. Issues arise, however, as to the need for, and nature of, further attentions. It is timely for this forum to address and update for future collective attentions what is known and acceptable as to each cornerstone supporting these attentions -- Awareness, Mechanism, Guidelines & Standards, and Shared Responsibility expectations.

KEYWORDS: Sports Injury, epidemiology, quadriplegia, football, risk.

The dollar cost to a new young quadriplegic has been estimated as up to $100,000 in one-time medical and living adaptation costs, about $150,000 annually in continuing medical and living adaptation expenses, and up to $2 million in lifetime lost income. How accurate these estimates may be with respect to a given individual...or for a person with permanent loss from brain trauma...or how much of these costs may be assumed by accident insurance, catastrophic medical insurance, endless charity benefits, family assets, or law suits...are not the topics of this paper. The topic of this paper and this symposium is the preventability of permanent neurological brain or spinal cord injury in sport, brain or spinal cord. Of all that can go wrong to human beings in sport, neurotrauma must remain the priority of our

---

*Senior Vice President/Risk Analysis, K&K Insurance Group, Inc., Fort Wayne, IN 48604.

attention. It is the profundity of such injury, not its dollar cost, that is at stake.

And so it has been. By the late 1960s, the annual football fatality tally, mostly from head injuries, had reached the high 20s. Today, with far more playing the game, the annual fatal injury count is no more than a handful. As for non-fatal quadriplegia from football, we were experiencing at least 30 annually when the rules for blocking and tackling were changed in 1976 at both the high school and college level. Since then, we have been within one or two handfuls annually. Not only has football gained, much of what was learned has been transferred to the threat of catastrophic injuries in other sports.

CORNERSTONES

I will be emphasizing four cornerstones for linking the past with the future in this presentation: Awareness, Mechanism, Standards, and Shared Responsibility--plus the common theme underlying all, that of "Calculated Risk".

What is meant by Calculated Risk? It is not safety or injury control that justifies sport participation; it is the various values one can attain from participation that makes the serious risks worth it. If not, then instead of Calculated Risk, we have Russian Roulette in which the goal is only to survive the taking of risk.

The simplest way to minimize sports neurotrauma is to minimize participation in sport. In selected cases, this is justified, such as when the individual still shows signs or symptoms of prior brain trauma. In the general, however, "to avoid risk" is impossible in sport. The goal is to avoid <u>unnecessary</u> foreseeable risk in a given sport and then to try to control that which is understood to be <u>necessary</u> or inherent to the sport. It <u>follows</u> then that Calculated Risk requires an understanding of what safeguards are relevant to the necessary and unnecessary risks involved.

Cornerstone #1: Awareness

Without meaningful data, one cannot be truly aware of the extent and nature of the risk of the rare but persistent catastrophic injury in sport. In 1931, the annual football fatality report began. By 1962, its findings had caused the American Medical Association (AMA) to appoint an expert Committee on Medical Aspects of Sports and to host a National Conference on Head Protection for Athletes. This Conference convened the principal authorities of that era to discuss the evident rising frequency of fatalities that were associated with the advent of the new protective helmet and facemask and the style of play enabled by them.

The Conference reached consensus that the new protective gear was good for the football player, provided that "spearing" was condemned, and that research was needed to lead to the development of universally acceptable impact test standards for the new hard-shell helmet. During that era, very limited research had accompanied the declaration of cause and solution. It took awhile, therefore, for things to happen, most pointedly being the acceptance of Gurdgian's work at Wayne State on cadavers for arriving at impact tolerance levels and the in-game telemetry work by Reed at Northwestern for helmet configuration.

ASTM F-8 was created in 1968, but football created NOCSAE in 1969-70 as the means of implementing this particular goal. Interestingly, the downward slope of the annual football fatality report started before the eventual standards emerged from the process, probably from the industry's awareness from the annual fatality report of the need for a commitment to quality control while awaiting those standards.

But while the focus of awareness and attention was identified as head/neck neurotrauma, it in fact was confined in football to the cerebral injury. Even Schneider's classic work in this regard of the early 60s only gave brief attention to the cervical cord injury problem and then to advance a contention of cause and solution that proved later to be incorrect. It was not until the mid-1970s that the national prevalence of quadriplegia in football was first obtained, concurrently by Torg through his medical colleagues and me through the NCAA and the NFSHSA. Both of us were able to document virtually the same results, which in tandem provided the awareness needed to support profound changes in the method of teaching blocking and tackling in football. Further, Torg continued his documentation of football neurotrauma prospectively which affirmed the value of those 1976 rule changes via an immediate dramatic drop in the incidence of this injury and over the years an ever lowering plateau. Head fatalities entered another downward trend with these same rule changes that had forced coaches and officials to minimize the helmeted head receiving the brunt of the initial impact. In fact, this was the first time in recorded history that the trendlines of head and neck injuries were following the same pattern. Which leads us nicely into the second cornerstone.

Cornerstone #2: Mechanism

It is one thing to know the frequency. The other is to know the essential force at work. For only then can rifles instead of shotguns be used in the effort to control that force. For head injuries in football, need for minimum standards of engineering quality was a relatively easy discernment. For neck injuries, the problem and the solution was much more subtle and long-coming in acceptance.

In 1967, a joint statement of the AMA and the National Federation brought attention to the "inadvertent spear" as the probable cause of serious neck injuries in football. Very few coaches identified with the warnings against spearing, the intentional malicious striking of the opponent with the helmet. "Face in the numbers", however, was rapidly becoming the accepted way to teach blocking and tackling. With head up, eyes forward, and neck bulled, it was considered the antithesis of spearing as well as the ideal football position for contact. Hitting as taught, it did not break necks and was not associated with malicious intentions. But in the attempt to do so as taught, by whatever reason within the mix of a football collision, the athlete who was sighting on the other's numbers sometimes was unable or unwilling to hit as taught and made contact with the head lowered. Sometimes as a result the other guy was hurt by that helmet, at the sternum or forearm, for example, but until the biomechanical explanation called "axial loading" came into the picture along with the abrupt drop in frequency data following the 1976 rule changes, few had an awareness and appreciation that it was the person who was doing the hitting under such conditions who was the one at risk of serious injury.

The 1976 rule changes were for the purpose of protecting the spearer, whether inadvertent or intentional, from neurotrauma. The effect of those rules was at least to require coaches to teach shoulder-blocking and tackling, i.e., controlling the risks present so that should the player drop his head inadvertently at the moment of impact, it was less apt to receive the brunt of that impact. While championing NOCSAE standards for the helmet to minimize head injuries, football had to rely on technique, not external protection, to minimize neck injuries. It turned out to be a most satisfying reliance on scholarly faith.

Axial-loading, requiring a very specific posture and angle of impact, provided a welcome explanation of what careful review of the frequency data was showing. The helmet was not the cause or the solution. First, the relatively infrequent number of quadriplegic injuries despite an estimated two billion helmet-to-person contacts per season reflected that the cause could not be common-place, i.e., the back of the helmet or any commonly utilized design characteristic of an helmet was an unlikely mechanism from an epidemiological persepctive. Something much more unique was happening. Second, by separating the neck-related fatality data from the head-related through the 60s, one could see that the neck death frequency remained flat during the rise and decline of the head deaths. Further, as the head deaths continued to decline, non-fatal quadriplegia was found to be rising. Lastly, with nothing else changing overnight but technique as defined by rules and ethics, it was more than gratifying, it was amazing to learn how dramatic a drop in the frequency of this serious contact injury was to occur.

As for catastrophic cerebral damage, an awareness of the mechanism behind its frequency count led to football's appreciation of engineering standards. With the effectiveness of the modern helmet, players no longer suffered life-threatening skull fractures and epidural hemorrhaging and became accustomed to an approved return to play that day or the next when experiencing the so-called minor concussion. With time, however, it became apparent to those involved with these concerns that invariably the sudden awareness of extensive intercranial bleeding was still occurring, with either fatal or non-fatal neurological impairment, or with good fortune a full recovery from prompt surgical intervention. These were not coming from the "hit" of that moment but from an earlier "hit", typically many days earlier, from which more minor cerebral trauma had not yet healed, as evidenced by retrospective awareness that the athlete had complained of headache, nausea, or the like, but not to the coach because of the motivation to play. Which takes us into the third Cornerstone.

Cornerstone #3:   Standards & Guidelines

A guideline is a direction we want to take. A standard measures the minimum distance we must take in that direction. However, whenever consensus arrives by guideline or standard that a particular level of quality of care is important and reasonable to expect for the protection of the athlete, "standards" exist. Whether it is in the form of rule of play, an administrative guideline, a coaching technique, or a laboratory measurement, consensus standards are there to provide consistency within the calculated risk equation and to receive continuous evaluation. Reliability or reproducibility in compliance is one factor to look for in arriving at consensus. Validity, the confidence that the standard is effective for the stated purpose, however, is another.

One issue of personal concern on the validity side of our workshop's focus is the tendency to extrapolate from laboratory test results to the field that which was not tested in the laboratory. Whether it be the hardness of a baseball or softball or the protectiveness of a helmet, some measurable index for some purpose must gain consensus as reasonably valid and acceptable as the determinant for that important purpose. In football, for example, in the mid-to-late 1970s, epidemiological surveillance of concussions by brand & type of helmet being worn at the time having met the NOCSAE standard, validated the laboratory impact test acceptance threshold to the extent that all helmets had equivalent rates of association with concussion by degree of exposure or opportunity for such. The corrollary was that this does not necessarily mean that the better the results of a helmet beyond that threshold, the better would be the injury rate. Until tested in a design to explore that contention, extrapolation is conjecture, not fact.

Cornerstone #4:   Shared Responsibility

Everyone is an expert in sport, including the injury problem. The experts in football injury control therefore do indeed share a responsibility for maintaining while evaluating the progress to date. The calculated risk of sport, moreover, warrants a reasonable awareness on the part of the participant that fatal and permanently disabling injuries can happen and that preventive measures have been taken via rules, equipment standards, and coaching practices -- and why -- and that the athlete whether of minor age or older has by his/her behavior and acceptance of the calculated risk a shared responsibility as well. I recall helping in the development over ten years ago of an Athletic Institute film on catastrophic injuries in football, now out-of-date in detail but not in principle, that my son's high school showed at the August pre-season meeting of coaches, parents, and athletes. At the film's conclusion, the parents actually applauded it and then signed their waivers.

This is the ideal informed consent, one that can be fostered in a variety of ways, but one that enables the athlete and their family to understand, appreciate, and share responsibility for balancing the risks to be taken in the pursuit of the fun and other benefits to be gained from participation. Placing warning labels on helmets is a prudent effort on the part of manufacturers, but human factors' research consistently reminds us to remind others who share responsibility for minimizing head and neck injuries in sport that reliance on warning labels for influencing their behavior would not be prudent. Which takes me into the projection of this historical review into future directions.

COMMENT

It is indeed fortunate for the athlete and those who enable sport experiences to exist that the catastrophic injury is rare. Its rareness, however, paradoxically works against the awareness of its presence and an appreciation of the mechanisms that lie in readiness. Even with football fatalities nearing 30 a year in the 60s, actuarially this was much lower a serious threat to the teen male player by hour exposure than the alternative activity of riding in an auto. Even with quadriplegia from football going to 30 a year by the mid-70s, only a few of the 20,000 teams who played football experienced it. And with nearly 30 years now behind me of opportunistic inquiry when I had the occasion, I have heard of only one instance in which a player left the team after seeing a teammate suffer a catastrophic injury.

It remains very important, however, to try to keep the awareness of what is happening alive and as widespread as possible, and combining new thoughts on blunting the mechanisms at work with current realities. Fortunately, Mueller and Cantu have since the early 1980s broadened the annual football fatality report to a registry and annual report of all school/college sport-related catastrophic injuries coming to their attention. Through that source it was discernible that only a few years ago, quadriplegia occurrences from high school & college football re-entered double figures for the first time for a decade for three years in a row. It is now apparent that this regression, so common when years of success tend to dull sensitivity to the problem and what turned it around many years earlier, is responsive to new action. The NCAA has since edited its rules and points of emphasis to explicitly confirm that the facemask is part of the helmet (and thereby precluding the return of face-into-the-numbers as a coached technique). In addition, the NCAA as well as the NFSHSA, whose rules already were explicit against this technique, cooperated with Riddell, Inc., produced a conscious re-heightening of national appreciation of this mechanism of injury via widespread distribution of Torg's new film. These combined efforts resulted in two consecutive years now of the lowest ever combined headcount of both fatalities and quadriplegia from football.

The fatality and quadriplegia threats in sport remain, as does the nagging persistence of non-fatal cerebral trauma that cries for athlete self-reporting of continuing symptoms that suggest the brain is not yet ready for more. But to tinker with what obviously is working, in which the numbers have a lot more opportunity to go back up than go down, must be a major consideration in charting progress for the future.

I have used the many convenient illustrations from the calculated risk in football. Fortunately, much has been transferred to the attentions given the threat of catastrophic injuries in other sports. A deliberate transfer in association of the football mechanism of axial loading to that in hockey, the inadvertent spear of the boards by the sliding hockey player when checked from behind, led rapidly to tougher rules against that technique, to published and filmed warnings to coach and athlete as to the why, and in the States to a distinct drop in quadriplegic hockey accidents. In rugby, the mechanism is different and is responding to the control of the scrum when it begins to break down. In swimming, another mechanism of neck injury is now respected and better controlled in the effort to gain those important milliseconds at the start of the race. In boxing, it is the repeated blow, not merely the knockout blow, that now receives studied attention. In whatever sport, continuous awareness of the nature and frequency of the catastrophic injury must be encouraged, not feared, so that contentions of mechanism can be shared for plausibility, implementation, and study, and so that the shared responsibility of all involved, including the participant, can be sorted, understood, and merged for the sake of the participant.

Epidemiology

Randall W. Dick [1]

A SUMMARY OF HEAD AND NECK INJURIES IN COLLEGIATE ATHLETICS
USING THE NCAA INJURY SURVEILLANCE SYSTEM.

REFERENCE: Dick, R. W., "A Summary of Head and Neck Injuries in
Collegiate Athletics Using the NCAA Surveillance System," Head
and Neck Injuries in Sports, ASTM STP 1229, Earl F. Hoerner, Ed.,
American Society for Testing and Materials, Philadelphia, 1994.

ABSTRACT: The NCAA Injury Surveillance System (ISS) was used to evaluate head and neck injuries in twelve intercollegiate sports for 3-6
years through the 1990 season. Sports were categorized as those with
and without mandated head protection. Prevalence of head and neck
injuries were expressed as both a percentage of all reported injuries
in a specific sport (%) as well as an injury rate (IR). In addition
the primary injury mechanism was noted. Concussions were also listed
as a percentage of all reported injuries in a sport and as an injury
rate. Of the sports with no head protection, field hockey, men's
soccer and women's soccer had the highest prevalence of head injuries
and concussions expressed as both % or IR. Ice hockey and football had
the highest head injury values of the sports with head protection.
Wrestling and football showed the highest % and IR for neck injury.

KEYWORDS: head injury, neck injury, concussion, intercollegiate
athletics, NCAA Injury Surveillance System

Head and neck injuries in football have received increased attention in the last few years with most of the literature focusing on
those injuries that result in permanent brain damage, quadriplegia or
fatalities in the sport of football (1,2,3). However, head and neck
injuries are not unique to football and many of these injuries, while
serious in nature, are not severe enough to be classified as
catastrophic. Systems currently exist that monitor the catastrophic
head and neck injuries in football (4,5) and multiple sports (5). Less
attention however, has been devoted to monitoring the prevalence of
less severe head and neck injuries, such as concussions, in a variety
of sports. The purpose of this study is to review head and neck
injuries in twelve intercollegiate sports using data collected from the
NCAA Injury Surveillance System (ISS).

[1] Assistant Director of Sports Sciences, National Collegiate
Athletics Association, 6201 College Boulevard, Overland Park, Kansas
66211.

METHODS

The NCAA Injury Surveillance System (ISS)

The ISS was developed in 1982 to provide current and reliable data on injury trends in intercollegiate athletics. Injury data are collected annually from a representative sample of NCAA member institutions in sixteen sports, and the resulting data summaries are reviewed by the NCAA Committee on Competitive Safeguards and Medical Aspects of Sports. The committee's goal continues to be to reduce injury rates through suggested changes in rules, protective equipment or coaching techniques based on data provided by the ISS.

Sampling

Participation in the ISS is voluntary and limited to the 847 member institutions (as of September 1991). ISS participants are selected from the population of institutions sponsoring a given sport. Selections are random within the constraints of having a minimum 10 percent representation of each NCAA division (I, II, and III) and region (East, South, Midwest, West).

It is important to emphasize that this system does not identify every injury that occurs at NCAA institutions in a particular sport. Rather, it collects a sampling that is representative of a national cross-section of NCAA institutions.

Data Reporting

Injury and exposure data are recorded by certified and student athletics trainers from participating institutions. Information is collected from the first official day of preseason practice to the final tournament contest.

Injury Definition

A reportable injury in the NCAA Injury Surveillance System is defined as one that:

1. Occurs as a result of participation in an organized intercollegiate practice or game;

2. Requires medical attention by a team athletics trainer or physician, and

3. Results in any restriction of the student-athlete's athletics participation or performance for one or more days beyond the day of injury.

Each injury is described in detail including body part injured, type of injury, injury mechanism, severity, field condition and special equipment worn.

Exposure Definition

An athlete exposure (A-E), the unit of risk in the ISS, is defined as one athlete participating in one practice or game where he or she is exposed to the possibility of athletic injury.

Injury Rate Definition

An injury rate (IR) is a ratio of the number of injuries in a particular category to the number of athlete exposures in that category. In the ISS, this value is expressed as injuries per 1,000 athlete exposures.

Concussion Definition

In this study, concussion was defined as a traumatically induced alteration in mental state with confusion or amnesia common, and loss of consciousness in Grade 3 (6,7).

RESULTS

Head and Neck

Head and neck injuries from practices and games were reviewed for a three to six year period (1984-1990) for twelve intercollegiate sports. Values are expressed as a percentage of all reported injuries (%) and as injuries per 1000 A-E (IR). The primary injury mechanism for head injuries is also reported. It should be noted that eyes, ears, nose, face, chin, jaw, mouth, teeth, and tongue are separate ISS body part categories and are distinct from the head. In other words, head injuries as defined in this study, do not include injuries to the body parts mentioned above. Information from seven collegiate sports with no mandatory head protection is shown in Table 1. Table 2 shows the same information for five collegiate sports that require head protection.

TABLE 1--Head and neck injuries - sports with no head protection

| Sport | Head | | Neck | | Primary Injury |
	(%)	(IR)	(%)	(IR)	Mechanism
Field Hockey	4.5	(0.23)	1.0	(0.05)	Contact w. stick
Women's Lacrosse	4.1	(0.17)	0.7	(0.03)	Contact w. ball
Men's Soccer	4.0	(0.31)	0.4	(0.03)	Contact w. player
Women's Soccer	3.7	(0.29)	1.0	(0.08)	Contact w. player
Women Basketball	3.1	(0.16)	0.9	(0.05)	Contact w. player
Men's Basketball	2.5	(0.14)	0.8	(0.04)	Contact w. player
Wrestling	2.9	(0.28)	5.4	(0.51)	Contact w. player

TABLE 2--Head and neck injuries - sports with head protection

| Sport | Head | | Neck | | Primary Injury |
	(%)	(IR)	(%)	(IR)	Mechanism
Ice Hockey	5.4	(0.30)	1.7	(0.09)	Contact w. player
Football	4.5	(0.29)	4.2	(0.28)	Contact w. player
Men's Lacrosse	3.2	(0.22)	1.7	(0.12)	Contact w. player
Women's Softball	2.9	(0.11)	1.6	(0.06)	Contact w. ball (non-pitch)
Baseball	2.8	(0.09)	0.3	(0.01)	Contact w. ball (non-pitch)

<u>Head Injuries</u> -- Data indicate that ice hockey had the highest percentage of head injuries of the sports monitored (5.4%), followed by football and field hockey (4.5%), women's lacrosse (4.1%) and men's soccer (4.0%).   Injury rates in sports with no head protection such as men's soccer, women's soccer and field hockey were comparable to the helmeted sports of ice hockey, football and men's lacrosse, respectively.

<u>Neck Injuries</u> -- Wrestling had almost double the neck injury rate (0.51) as football (0.28) and more than four times higher than that of men's lacrosse (0.12). Neck injury rates in the nine remaining sports were significantly lower than these three activities. Most of the neck injuries were muscle-tendon strains.

<u>Head Injury Mechanism</u> -- Player contact was the primary injury mechanism for all but four sports monitored. Contact with the stick was the primary head injury mechanism in field hockey while contact with the ball was the chief mechanism in women's lacrosse. Contact with a non-pitched ball was the primary head injury mechanism in both softball and baseball.

<u>Concussions</u>

Concussions, a subset of head injuries, are listed as a percentage of all reported injuries (%) and as injuries per 1000 A-E (IR) for sports with mandatory head protection (Table 3) and sports with no required head protection (Table 4). Concussions accounted for at least 60% of head injuries in each of the sports monitored.

TABLE 3--Concussions - sports with no head protection

Sport	Concussion	
	(%)	(IR)
Women's Lacrosse	3.9	(0.16)
Field Hockey	3.8	(0.20)
Men's Soccer	3.2	(0.25)
Women Basketball	3.0	(0.15)
Women's Soccer	2.8	(0.24)
Men's Basketball	2.1	(0.12)
Wrestling	1.8	(0.20)

TABLE 4--Concussions - sports with head protection

Sport	Concussion	
	(%)	(IR)
Ice Hockey	4.5 %	(0.25)
Football	4.1 %	(0.27)
Men's Lacrosse	3.0 %	(0.19)
Women's Softball	2.9 %	(0.11)
Baseball	2.1 %	(0.07)

DISCUSSION

This study has shown that head and neck injuries are not unique to the sport of football. Ice hockey, wrestling, and soccer have been shown to exhibit head injury rates rivaling those of football, while men's lacrosse and field hockey have rates of slightly smaller magnitude. Most of these injuries are not catastrophic in nature. Neck injuries are less frequent except in the sports of wrestling and football.

The activities analyzed in this study were grouped by whether they required head protection. Both categories included similar ranges of head injury data, expressed either as a percentage of all injuries or as an injury rate. This finding should not be interpreted as questioning the efficacy of head protection; most would agree that protective helmets reduce head injuries in the sports in which they are worn. Instead, these data present a baseline that can be used to evaluate effectiveness of future rules or equipment changes in the monitored sports. For example, the effectiveness of a mandatory helmet rule in women's lacrosse could be monitored by comparing injury data collected following the rule implementation with the data reported here.

With regard to injury mechanism, it is interesting to note that player contact was the primary cause of head injuries in the "non-contact" sports of basketball and soccer. Such injuries may be best controlled by a more stringent enforcement of playing rules by game officials. The ball and the stick were the primary cause of head injuries in women's lacrosse and field hockey, respectively. Such mechanisms may not be as easily controlled by playing rules. Interestingly, these sports have been opposed to the introduction of head protection (8). In baseball and softball, contact with a non-pitched ball was the primary head injury mechanism. This category translates into errantly thrown balls by fielders or contact with a batted ball. Prevention may include better field maintenance and an evaluation of ball liveliness.

Concussion make up the majority of head injuries in the twelve sports examined. With the recent focus on multiple impact syndrome, an evaluation of concussions may be a first step in the prevention of severe injuries (7). Without protective headgear, the rate of concussions in sports requiring this equipment would be even higher.

Mouth guards have also been shown to be an effective means of prevention of concussions in sport (9). Currently mouth guards are required in the sports of NCAA ice hockey, football, men's lacrosse, women's lacrosse and field hockey. Mouth guards are also worn by many men's and women's soccer and basketball players, although they are not currently mandatory equipment in these sports.

In summary, non-catastrophic head injuries have been shown to account for three to five percent of the injuries in twelve intercollegiate sports while neck injuries were much less frequent. Concussions made up the bulk of the reported head injuries. Medical personnel should be educated on the diagnosis and treatment of such injuries in all sports and rules protecting the head and neck should be enforced. The rules against butting, ramming and spearing are for the protection of both the player initiating the blow as well as the receiver of the blow. A player who does not comply with these rules in any sport is a candidate for a serious head or neck injury.

REFERENCES

(1) Fine, K.M., Vesgo, J.J., Sennett, B., and Torg, J.S., "Prevention of Cervical Spine Injuries in Football: A Model for Other Sports," The Physician and Sportsmedicine, Vol.19, No. 10, 1991, pp 55-64.

(2) "Football-Related Spinal Cord Injuries among High-School Players - Louisiana, 1989," Morbidity and Mortality Weekly Report, Vol. 39, No.24, 1990, pp 586-587.

(3) Henderson, J.M., "Head Injuries in Sports," Sports Medicine Digest, Vol. 15, No. 9, 1993, pp 1-2.

(4) Torg, J.S., Vesgo, J.J., Sennett, B., and Das, M., "The National Football Head and Neck Injury Registry: 14 Year Report on Cervical Quadriplegia, 1971-1984," Journal of the American Medical Association, Vol. 254, 1985, pp 3439-3443.

(5) Cantu, R.C. and Mueller, F.O., National Center for Catastrophic Injury Research Annual Reports. (University of North Carolina, Chapel Hill, North Carolina 27514).

(6) Kelley, J.P., Nichols, J.S., Filley, C.M., et. al., "Concussion in Sports: Guidelines for the Prevention of Catastrophic Outcome," Journal of the American Medical Association, Vol. 266, No. 20, 1991, pp 2867-2869.

(7) Cantu, R.C., "Second Impact Syndrome Immediate Management," The Physician in Sportsmedicine, Vol. 20, No. 9, 1992, pp 55-58.

(8) Hawthorne, P., "Don't Rush to Force Helmets on Women's Lacrosse," Lacrosse Magazine, May/June 1993, pp 13-17.

(9) Kerr, I.L., "Mouth Guards for the Prevention of Injuries in Contact Sports", Sports Medicine, Vol. 5, 1986, pp 415-427.

Frederick O. Mueller,[1] Ph.D. and Robert C. Cantu,[2] M.D.

Annual Survey of Catastrophic Football Injuries: 1977–1992

REFERENCE: Mueller, Frederick O. and Cantu, Robert C.; **"Annual Survey of Catastrophic Football Injuries: 1977–1992,"** *Head and Neck Injuries in Sports, ASTM STP 1229,* Earl F. Hoerner, Ed., Amerian Society for Testing and Materials, Philadelphia, 1994.

ABSTRACT: Football catastrophic injuries may never be totally eliminated, but continued research has resulted in rule changes, equipment standards, improved medical care both on and off the playing field, and changes in teaching the fundamental techniques of the game. These changes were the results of a united effort by coaches, administrators, researchers, equipment manufacturers, physicians, trainers and players.

Research based on reliable data is essential if progress is to be made. Research provides data that indicate the problems and reveal the adequacy of preventive measures.

KEYWORDS: sports injuries, catastrophic, head, neck, registry, database, risk factors, prevention

In 1977 the National Collegiate Athletic Association initiated funding for the First Annual Survey of Catastrophic Football Injuries. Frederick O. Mueller, Ph.D., and Carl S. Blyth, Ph.D., both professors in the Department of Physical Education at the University of North Carolina at Chapel Hill were selected to conduct the research. The research is now being conducted as part of the National Center for Catastrophic Sports Injury Research, University of North Carolina at Chapel Hill, Frederick O. Mueller, Director.

The Annual Survey of Catastrophic Football Injuries was part of a concerted effort put forth by many individuals and research organizations to reduce the steady increase of football head and neck injuries taking place during the 1960's and 1970's. The primary purpose of the research was and is to make the game of football a safer sport.

Data Collection

Since 1977 and the initiation of this research, catastrophic injuries were defined as football injuries which resulted in brain or spinal cord injury or skull or spine fracture. It should be noted that all cases involved some disability at the time of the injury. Neurological recovery is either complete or incomplete (quadriplegia or quadriparesis). Yearly follow-up is not done, thus neurological status (complete or incomplete recovery) refers to when the athlete is entered into the registry which is usually two to three months after injury. Injuries which result in death are not included in this report.

[1] CB# 8605, 311 Woollen; University of North Carolina; Chapel Hill, NC 27599-8605.
[2] Chairman, Department of Surgery; Chief, Neurosurgical Service; Emerson Hospital; Concord, MA 01742.
Research Funded by a Grant from the National Collegiate Athletic Association.

Data were compiled with the assistance of high school and college coaches, athletic directors, school administrators, physicians, athletic trainers, executive officers of state and national athletic organizations, sporting goods dealers and manufacturers' representatives, a national newspaper clipping service, and professional associates of the researchers. Data collection would have been impossible without the help of the National Federation of State High School Associations and the National Collegiate Athletic Association. The research was funded by a grant provided by the National Collegiate Athletic Association.

Upon receiving information concerning a possible catastrophic football injury, contact by telephone, personal letter, and questionnaire is made with the injured player's coach, physician and athletic director. The questionnaire provides background data on the athlete (age, height, weight, experience, previous injury, etc.), accident information, immediate and post-accident treatment, and equipment data. After reviewing the 1977 data, a telephone follow-up, which provided valuable information, was added to the study protocol to ascertain the status and prognosis of the injured player.

In 1987, a joint endeavor was initiated with the section on Sports Medicine of the American Association of Neurological Surgeons. The purpose of this collaboration was to enhance the collection of medical data. Dr. Robert C. Cantu, Chairman, Department of Surgery and Chief, Neurosurgery Service, Emerson Hospital, in Concord, MA, and the Medical Director of the National Center for Catastrophic Sports Injury Research has been responsible for collecting the medical data.

Background

An early investigation into serious head and neck football injuries was conducted by Schneider [1]. He reported 30 permanent cervical spinal cord injuries in high school and college football during the period from 1959–1963. A later study by Torg indicated a total of 99 permanent cervical spinal cord injuries in high school and college football from 1971 to 1975 [3]. Torg has discontinued his research, but his data show a decline in permanent cervical cord injuries in high school and college from 34 cases in 1976 to 5 cases in 1984. A study published in 1976 reported the incidence of neck injuries based on roentgenorgraphic evidence was as high as 32% in a sample of 104 high school students and 75 college freshman in Iowa [2].

In order to help alleviate this problem the National Collegiate Athletic Association and the National Federation of State High School Associations implemented rule changes in 1976 to prohibit using the head as the initial contact point when blocking and tackling. Furthermore, the American Football Coaches Association Ethics Committee went on record opposing this type of blocking and tackling. Emphasis on complete physical examinations and improved physical conditioning programs have also been recommended to mitigate the injury issue.

Summary

1. During the 1992 football season there was a total of five cervical cord injuries with incomplete neurological recovery. Four of the injuries occurred in high school, none at the college level and one at the professional level (Table 1).
2. The incidence of catastrophic injuries is very low on a 100,000 player exposure basis. For the approximately 1,800,000 participants in 1992 the number of injuries with incomplete neurological recovery was 0.28 participants per 100,000 players.

TABLE 1—*Cervical cord injuries 1977–1992.*[a]

Year	Sandlot	Pro and semi-pro	High School	College	Total
1977	0	0	10	2	12
1978	0	1	13	0	14
1979	0	0	8	3	11
1980	0	0	11	2	13
1981	1	0	6	2	9
1982	1	1	7	2	11
1983	0	0	11	1	12
1984	1	0	5	0	6
1985	0	0	6	3	9
1986	0	0	3	0	3
1987	0	0	9	0	9
1988	0	0	10	1	11
1989	0	1	12	2	15
1990	0	0	11	2	13
1991	0	1	1	0	2
1992	0	1	4	0	5
Total	3	5	127	20	155

[a] Figures are updated annually due to new cases investigated after publication.

3. The incidence of injuries with incomplete neurological recovery in high school football was 0.27 per 100,000 players and the incidence at the college level was 0.00 (Table 2).
4. A majority of catastrophic spinal cord injuries occur in games. During the 1992 season three of the injuries occurred in games and two in practice.

TABLE 2—*Incidence per 100,000 participants 1977–1992.*[a]

Year	High School	College
1977	0.77	2.67
1978	1.00	0.00
1979	0.62	4.00
1980	0.85	2.67
1981	0.46	2.67
1982	0.54	2.67
1983	0.85	1.33
1984	0.38	0.00
1985	0.46	4.00
1986	0.23	0.00
1987	0.69	0.00
1988	0.77	1.33
1989	0.80	2.66
1990	0.73	2.66
1991	0.07	0.00
1992	0.27	0.00

[a] From 1977–1988 based on 1,300,000 high school—junior high school players and 75,000 college players. In 1989 high school and junior high school figure increased to 1,500,000.

TABLE 3—*Offensive vs. defensive football 1977–1992[a]*

Year	Offense	Defense	Unknown	Total
1977	0	7	5	12
1978	2	11	1	14
1979	1	5	5	11
1980	3	8	2	13
1981	3	5	1	9
1982	3	8	0	11
1983	2	10	0	12
1984	1	4	1	6
1985	1	8	0	9
1986	0	3	0	3
1987	1	6	2	9
1988	2	9	0	11
1989	0	14	1	15
1990	2	11	0	13
1991	1	1	0	2
1992	2	3	0	5
Total	24	113	18	155

[a] Figures updated with availability of new information.

5. Tackling and blocking have been associated with the majority of catastrophic football injuries. In 1992 three of the injuries were caused by tackling, one by being tackled in a tackling drill, and one by being tackled on a kick-off return. As shown in Table 4 tackling has been associated with 71.6% of the catastrophic injuries since 1977. It should be noted that two of the spinal cord injuries in 1992 were associated with running backs lowering their heads during contact with the tackler.
6. As indicated in Table 3 a majority of the catastrophic injuries occur while playing defensive football. In 1992, three of the five spinal cord injured players were playing defense.
7. During the 1992 football season there were three subdural hematoma injuries that resulted in incomplete recovery. All three were at the high school level (Table 6).

TABLE 4—*Catastrophic injuries 1977–1992 type of activity.*

Activity	Number	Percent
Tackling	56	36.1
Tackling head down	43	27.7
Tackling on punt	4	2.6
Tackling on kick-off	8	5.2
Tackled	12	7.7
Tackled on kick-off	2	1.3
Collision	3	1.9
Blocking on kick	3	1.9
Blocking	2	1.3
Contact after interception	2	1.3
Blocked	2	1.3
Hitting tacklematic machine	1	0.7
Unknown	17	11.0
Total	155	100.0

TABLE 5—*Catastrophic injuries 1977–1992 position played.*

Position	Number	Percent
Defensive back	56	36.1
Kick-off team	16	10.3
Defensive line	8	5.2
Linebacker	15	9.7
Kick-off return	6	3.9
Defensive end	6	3.9
Offensive back	7	4.5
Quarterback	4	2.6
Flanker	2	1.3
Wide receiver	2	1.3
Punt coverage	3	1.9
Punt return	1	0.6
Drill	2	1.3
Offensive lineman	1	0.6
Unknown	26	16.8
Total	155	100.0

8. In 1992 there were also twelve injuries that involved either a head or neck injury but the athlete had full neurological recovery. High school athletes were associated with six cervical vertebra fractures and two serious head injuries. College athletes were associated with four fractured cervical vertebra injuries (Table 7).
9. The 1991 data has been updated to include new cases.

Discussion

For the past 16 years there have been a total of 155 football players with incomplete neurologial recovery from cervical cord injuries. A total of 127 of these injuries have been to high school players, 20 to college players, three to sandlot players and five to professionals. This data indicate a reduction in the number of cervical cord injuries with incomplete neurological recovery when compared to data published in the early 1970s. While the 1988,

TABLE 6—*Cerebral injuries 1984–1992[a] incomplete recovery.*

Year	Sandlot	Pro and Semi-pro	High School	College	Total
1984	0	0	5	2	7
1985	0	0	4	1	5
1986	0	0	2	0	2
1987	0	0	2	0	2
1988	0	0	4	0	4
1989	0	0	6	0	6
1990	0	0	2	0	2
1991	0	0	3	1	4
1992	0	0	3	0	3
Total	0	0	31	4	35

[a] Figures are updated annually due to new cases investigated after publication.

TABLE 7—*Catastrophic injuries 1992[a] complete recovery.*

Injury	High School	College	Total
Subdural hematoma	2	0	2
Transient cord symptoms	2	1	3
Cervical spine fracture	4	3	7
Total	8	4	12

[a] Researchers realize that this data may not be complete due to the difficulty of receiving non-disability injury information.

1989, and 1990 data suggested a gradual increase in these type of injuries, the 1991 data shows the most dramatic reduction since the beginning of the study in 1977. In 1991 there was only one high school cervical cord injury with incomplete neurological recovery, one at the professional level and none at the college level. Coaches, players, trainers, physicians and administrators should be congratulated and continue the emphasis on eliminating paralyzing injuries to football players.

The latest participation figures show 1,500,000 players participating in junior and senior high school football and 75,000 in college football. Table 2 illustrates the incidence of spinal cord injuries for both high school and college participants. The incidence rates per 100,000 participants are low in both high school and college. In looking at the incidence rates for the past 16 years, the high school incidence is 0.59 per 100,000 participants and the college incidence is 1.66 per 100,000 participants.

As indicated in past reports a majority of the permanent cervical cord injuries are taking place in games. In 1992 three of the five injuries took place in games.

Table 3 indicates that when comparing cervical cord injuries to offensive and defensive players, it is safer playing offensive football. During the 16 year period from 1977 to 1992, 113 of the 155 players with cervical cord injuries were playing defense. A majority of the defensive players were tackling when injured. In 1992, three of the injured players were tackling, one was tackled in a tackling drill, and one was tackled on a kick off. Coaches have indicated that their players have been taught to tackle with the head up, but for some reason many of the players are lowering their heads before making contact. In 1992, all three players injured while tackling had their heads in a down position (chin to chest and contact with the top or crown of the helmet).

Past reports (Table 5) have revealed that defensive backs were injured at a higher rate than other positions. In 1992, one of the five injured players was a defensive back, one a linebacker, one a defensive end, one a ball carrier in a tackling drill and one a ball carrier tackled on a kick-off return.

In 1992 there were three subdural hematoma injuries with incomplete neurological recovery. All three injuries were at the high school level. There were also two players at the high school level with subdural hematoma injuries and complete neurological recovery.

Recommendations

As stated in earlier reports, there has been a reduction of permanent cervical cord injuries when compared to data from the early 1970s. The 1990 data continued to show a reduction from the early 1970s, but for the period from 1987 to 1990 there has been a gradual increase to 15 in 1989 and thirteen in 1990. The 1991 data show a dramatic reduction to one permanent cervical cord injury in high school football and one at the professional level. This is a great accomplishment and every effort should be made to continue this trend. The 1992 data show an increase to five. For the past ten years, including 1992, there has been an average of 8.5 cervical cord injuries with incomplete neurological recovery in football.

The initial reduction was the result of efforts put forth by the total athletic community concerned with safety to football participants. Major areas of emphasis that once again should be emphasized are the 1976 rule change that eliminated the head as the initial point of contact during blocking and tackling, improved medical care both at the game site and in medical facilities, improved coaching techniques in teaching the fundamentals of tackling and blocking, and the increased concern and awareness of football coaches.

A concerted effort must be made to continue the reduction of cervical spine injuries and to aim for the elimination of both cervical and cerebral catastrophic injuries. Following are several suggestions for reducing these catastrophic injuries:

1. Rule changes initiated for the 1976 football season which eliminated the head as a primary and initial contact area for blocking and tackling are of utmost importance. Coaches should drill the players in the proper execution of the fundamentals of football—particularly blocking and tackling. *SHOULDER BLOCK AND TACKLE WITH THE HEAD UP—KEEP THE HEAD OUT OF FOOTBALL*
2. Athletes must be given proper conditioning exercises which will strengthen their necks in order to be able to hold their heads firmly erect while making contact during a tackle or block. Strengthening of the neck muscles may also protect the neck from injury.
3. Coaches and officials should discourage the players from using their heads as battering rams when blocking and tackling. The rules prohibiting spearing should be enforced in practice and games. The players should be taught to respect the helmet as a protective device and that the helmet should not be used as a weapon. Ball carriers should also be taught not to lower their heads when making contact with the tackler.
4. Football officials can play a major role in reducing catastrophic football injuries. The use of the helmet-face mask in making initial contact while blocking and tackling is illegal and should be called for a penalty. Officials should concentrate on helmet-face mask contact and call the penalty. If more of these penalties are called there is no doubt that both players and coaches will get the message and discontinue this type of play. A reduction in helmet-face mask contact will result in a reduction of catastrophic football injuries.
5. All coaches, physicians and trainers should take special care to see that the players' equipment is properly fitted, particularly the helmet.
6. It is important, whenever possible, for a physician to be on the field of play during game and practice. When this is not possible, arrangements must be made in advance to obtain a physician's immediate services when emergencies arise. Each institution should have a team trainer who is a regular member of the institution's staff and who is qualified in the emergency care of both treating and preventing injuries.
7. Coaches must be prepared for a possible catastrophic head or neck injury. Everyone involved must know what to do. Being prepared and knowing what to do may be the difference that prevents permanent disability.
8. When a player has experienced or shown signs of head trauma (loss of consciousness, visual disturbances, headache, inability to walk correctly, obvious disorientation, memory loss), he should receive immediate medical attention and should not be allowed to return to practice or game without permission from the proper medical authorities.
9. Both past and present data show that the football helmet does not cause cervical spine injuries but that poorly executed tackling and blocking technique is the major problem.

Catastrophic football injuries may never be totally eliminated, but continued research has resulted in rule changes, equipment standards, improved medical care both on and off the playing field, and changes in teaching the fundamental techniques of the game. These changes were the result of a united effort by coaches, administrators, researchers, equipment manufacturers, physicians, trainers and players.

Research based on reliable data is essential if progress is to be made. Research provides data that indicate the problems and reveal the adequacy of preventive measures.

References

[1] Schneider, R. C., *Head and Neck Injuries in Football,* Baltimore, William and Wilkins Co., 1973.

[2] Albright, J. P., Moses, J. M., Feldick, H. G., et al. "Nonfatal Cervical Spine Injuries in Interscholastic Football," *Journal of the American Medical Association,* Vol. 236, 1976, pp. 1243–1245.

[3] Torg, J. S., Trues, R., Quedenfeld, T. C., et al. "The National Football Head and Neck Injury Registry," *Journal of the American Medical Association,* Vol. 241, 1979, pp. 1477–1479.

[4] Mueller, F. O. and Schindler, R. D., *Annual Survey of Football Injury Research 1931–1992,* National Collegiate Athletic Association, National Federation of State High School Associations and the American Football Coaches Association, 1993.

Doris M. Bixby-Hammett[1]

HEAD AND NECK INJURIES IN EQUESTRIAN SPORTS

REFERENCE: Bixby-Hammett, D. M., **"Head and Neck Injuries in Equestrian Sports,"** Head and Neck Injuries in Sports, ASTM STP 1229, Earl F. Hoerner, Ed., American Society for Testing and Materials, Philadelphia, 1994.

ABSTRACT: Horse activities have a large number of participants in the United States. Most accident occur in leisure activities making record keeping difficult. Horse activities are relatively safety ranking 67 in the number of admissions to hospital emergency rooms in the USA. Injuries when they occur to equestrians tends to be severe. Statistics from Medical Examiners in the United States and morbidity studies from Australia and New Zealand are given as well as statistics from four sources: the National Electronic Surveillance System (NEISS), the Justin Sportsmedicine Program, the National Park System visitor and employee injuries and the United States Pony Clubs. The figures show head/face/neck injuries in horseback riding are frequent and severe and can be prevented or reduced in severity by wearing secured ASTM SEI protective helmet. The horse and academic community by communication and cooperation should design studies which can provide information needed to prevent these injuries.

KEYWORDS: horse related injuries, horse related deaths, protective headgear

---

Activities involving horses occupy a prominent place in modern day sports world. There are 6.6 million equine in the United States. Horse sports draw more than 110 million spectators annually. Persons riding horses in the National Parks number 1.73 million a year. Youth were involved in 219,488 in horse projects through 4-H programs in 1989.[1] Horses have been an integral part of America's

---

[1] Pediatrician, Secretary/Treasurer, Newsletter Editor, American Medical Equestrian Association, 103 Surrey Road, Waynesville, NC, 28786.

heritage and continue to play a vital role in the recreational activities of America.

Most horseback riding is not in organized events making record keeping difficult. Over 99% of horse related accidents occur in leisure activities[2]. This paper will report on morbidity studies and records from National Electronic Injury Surveillance System, the National Park System, the Justin Sportsmedicine Program, and the United States Pony Clubs.

MORBIDITY STUDIES

South Australia reported 18 horse related deaths for the 11 years from 1973 to 1983, of which two deaths were sudden natural deaths. Of the 18 deaths, 14 (77.8%) were the result of head injuries[3]. Sweden reported on 53 deaths from 1969 to 1982, of which 72% were from head injuries[4]. In 28% of the deaths, the victim was not riding. New Zealand reported on 54 fatal falls from horses, in which 64% were from head injury[5].

Medical Examiner records are available for 208 horse related deaths in the United States[6]. Females have a little over a fourth of all the horse related deaths.

TABLE 1--Horse related deaths by gender and age

AGE	MALE	%ofAge	FEMALE	% ofAge	TOTAL	%ofTotal
0-4	6	85.7%	1	14.3%	7	3.4%
5-14	14	40.0%	21	60.0%	35	16.8%
15-24	26	72.2%	10	27.8%	36	17.3%
25-44	47	72.3%	18	27.7%	65	31.3%
45-64	36	81.8%	8	18.2%	44	21.2%
65+	20	95.2%	1	4.8%	21	10.1%
TOTAL	149	71.6%	59	28.4%	208	

Head injuries were the cause of over 60% of these deaths. Studying the medical examiner head injuries by age and gender, males and females are equally divided, but more females below the age of 15 years have head injury deaths, and more males over the age of 44 have head injury deaths(TABLE 2).

TABLE 2--Medical Examiner horse related deaths from head
            injury by gender and age

AGE	MALE	%ofAge_	FEMALE	%OFAge	TOTAL
0-4	0		0		0
5-14	3	18.8%	13	81.3%	16
15-24	7	50.0%	7	50.0%	14
25-44	14	46.7%	16	53.3%	30
45-64	7	58.3%	5	41.7%	12
65+	8	88.9%	1	11.1%	9
TOTAL	39	48.2%	42	51.9%	81

NATIONAL ELECTRONIC INJURY SURVEILLANCE SYSTEM

The National Electronic Injury Surveillance System
(NEISS)[7] estimates the injuries which go to the
emergency rooms of hospitals across the nation. From time
to time, NEISS changes its figures from which projections
are made. Although the base figures can not be compared,
the figures made from these projections can be compared.
The figures do not include injuries that were not treated,
injuries treated in physicians offices or free standing
clinics, or who went directly to the morgue.

NEISS figures have been broken down into the years
1979 to 1982 during which knowledge concerning safety and
accident prevention was just appearing in the horse press.
NEISS did not record horse related injuries in the years
1983 to 1986, but restarted in 1987. The years 1987 to
1991 have been separated to see if increased knowledge of
safety and accident prevention may have made a difference
in the emergency room admissions (TABLE 3).

TABLE 3-National Electronic Injury Surveillance System
        horse related emergency room admissions estimates

BODY PART	%1979-82	%1987-91	%All Years
Head	11.3%	9.9%	10.5%
Face*	7.2%	8.9%	8.37%
Neck	1.9%	0.9%	1.1%
TOTAL	20.4%	19.8%	

* (Includes:ear/eye/mouth)

Head injuries (including face, neck, ear, eye, and mouth) have decreased from 20.4% for 1979-82 to 19.8% in 1987-91. Concussion decreased from 3.7% to 3.3%.

TABLE 4--NEISS estimates in head injuries by age

AGE	1979-82	1987-90	%CHANGE
AGE 5-14	29.2%	20.6%	Decrease 29.19%
AGE 15-24	33.5%	25.3%	Decrease 24.58%
AGE 25-44	29.5%	40.8%	Increase 38.11%
AGE 45-64	6.8%	9.6%	Increase 41.06%
AGE 65+	1.0%	1.7%	Increase 69.31%

The ages below 25 years have had a decrease in head and neck injuries but the ages above 24 years have increased(TABLE 4).

JUSTIN PRO RODEO[8]

The JUSTIN SPORTSMEDICINE PROGRAM compiled statistical data at rodeos officially designated a JUSTIN SPORTSMEDICINE RODEO. For the purpose of this study an evaluation was considered any question/answer session with an athlete that pertains to a specific injury during a JUSTIN SPORTSMEDICINE RODEO. A treatment is considered as being any exercise where a therapeutic modality is used on or with an athlete. An injury report was submitted for each athlete each time a modality was used in the treatment of a rodeo athletic injury.

During this period, 11,154 persons were evaluated, with 2,593 or 14.2% treated. Of the 2,593 with injuries sufficient for treatment, head/face injuries occurred in 113 or 4.4% of those injured. Comparing the first five years of head/face injuries with the second five years there was an increase of 125%. Cervical spine injuries were slightly increased during this period. There was a total of 150 (5.8%) cervical spine injuries. Comparing the first five years with the second five years there was a increase of 13.3% (TABLE 5).

TABLE 5--Justin Sportsmedicine Program athletes treated

TOTAL	%ofTotal	Body Part	1981-85		1986-90		Change	
113	4.4%	Head/Face injury	25	2.5%	88	5.6%	Increase	125%
150	5.8%	Cerv Spine	54	5.4%	96	6.1%	Increase	13%

There were 5.8% major injuries (defined as one that requires the transportation by qualified medical technicians to a treatment facility and/or the confinement in a treatment facility for approximately twelve {12} hours or longer)(TABLE 6).

TABLE 6 --Justin Sportsmedicine Program major injuries

Injury	Total	%ofTotal	1981-1985	1986-1990	Change
Concussion	66	33.3%	23	21.70%	43	46.7%	Increase 115.4%
Facial Fx/Jaw	6	3.1%	2	1.89%	4	4.3%	Increase 130.4%
CSpine Fx	14	7.1%	11	10.38%	3	3.3%	Decrease 68.6%

The definition of concussion in this program was "an alteration of consciousness which followed trauma but cleared within 60 minutes." Although concussions were listed under major injuries, they had a specific definition.

NATIONAL PARK SERVICE[9]

The National Park Service kept records of horse related injuries to the employees and visitors during the years 1983 to 1987[10] (TABLE 7).

TABLE 7--National Park Service horse related injuries

Body Part	Multiple	Head	Face	Neck	Total
Employees	15.8%	4.2%	5.0%	1.7%	120
Visitors	23.0%	8.0%	4.4%	0	113
				TOTAL	223

Concussion was listed as the type of injury in 1.7% of National Park employees and 3.5% of visitors. From these numbers it is not possible to make conclusions, but it can be suggested the NPS employees who are more likely to be conditioned, trained, and experienced will have less injuries, less severe injuries, and fewer head injuries. The NPS employee figures do not include the young and the old as does the age spread of the visitors.

UNITED STATES PONY CLUBS[11]

The United States Pony Clubs study is unique in that:
1. It involves only youth up to the age of 22 years.
2. It records accidents (defining an accident as any incident of concern to the rider, parent, instructor, or leader, whether or not an injury occurred).
3. It considers a concussion as any momentary "seeing stars", temporary confusion, loss of memory, as well as the usual definition of concussion.
4. It is a continuing study now in its 12th year.

These figures cover 10 years from 1982 to 1991. The total membership for the USPC for the years 1982-1991 was 96464, giving an average of 9,646 members a year. A total of 399 accident forms were returned, 6 (1.5%) were not completed, 20 (5.0%) had no injury, with 373 (93.5%) reporting an injury.

Of these 373 accident reports, 500 injuries occurred. Of those accidents in which injuries occurred, 25.6% of the injuries were to the head, face and neck. The persons who had head injuries had a greater percent of hospitalization (TABLE 8).

TABLE 8--United States Pony Club accident study 1982-91

Treatment Required	Total		Head	
No treatment	52	13.8%	5	8.1%
Rx grounds returned	27	9.2%	5	8.1%
Rx Grounds not Return	18	6.1%	1	3.2%
Rx Hosp/Dr returned	42	14.3%	6	9.7%
RX Hosp/Dr not return	170	57.8%	34	43.5%
Hospitalized	37	9.3%	14	27.4%
TOTAL	399		74	
Known	294		62	

Form not complete on 53 total and 12 head injuries

In the accident forms reporting head injuries (74), 66.2% reported concussions, 8.1% lacerations with sutures, 6.8% bruise/abrasion, 6.8% "Shook Up", 4.1% a closed fracture and 8.1% reported no injury.

In an effort to determine if changes have occurred in the area of the body injured in USPC over the most recent 10 years two time spans were compared. The years of 1982-1989 were compared with the years 1990-1991. The new protective ASTM standard helmet was mandated early in 1990.

This hat replaced the USPC standard mandated hat. This helmet is an estimated 4 times more protective and comes with a non-removable harness.

TABLE 9--United States Pony Club head injury

Body Injury	82-89	%ofInj	90-91	% ofInj	Decrease
Head	53	15.7%	19	11.4%	27.2%
Face	33	9.8%	6	3.6%	63.1%
Neck	12	3.6%	5	3.0%	15.4%
TOTAL		29.1%		18.0%	38.1%
Concussion	33	10.3%	11	7.4%	27.9%

During this same two year period of 1990-1991, the severity of the injuries decreased, resulting in a decrease percent of those injured requiring hospitalization and being treated but not able to return to the activity. There was a corresponding increase in the percent who could be treated and return to the activity or be treated on the grounds(TABLE 10).

TABLE 10--United States Pony Clubs treatment

Treatment	1982-89	%ofRX	1990-91	%ofRX	Change	
NO TREATMENT	19	7.3%	33	23.9%		
RX GROUND RETURN RIDE	14	7.4%	13	12.5%	Increase	69.6%
RX GROUND NOT RETURN	6	3.2%	12	11.5%	Increase	265.4%
RX MD/HOSP RETURN	27	14.2%	35	33.7%	Increase	136.8%
RX MD/HOSP NOT RETURN	115	60.5%	35	33.7%	Decrease	44.4%
HOSPITALIZED	28	14.7%	9	8.7%	Decrease	41.3%
REPORTS	261		138			
INJURY REQUIRING RX	190		104			

NEEDED RESEARCH:

Accidents are the number one cause of death between the ages of 1 and 44 years. If we are to make changes in these figures, we must address the various factors involved in the numerous activities causing these deaths. Horse sports are one of these activities. The horse community is increasingly concerned about safety of their activities.

As demonstrated by their studies, horse activities need the involvement of the academic community to develop studies that will give sufficient numbers in a manner to give the results sought. I implore both to communicate and establish such studies.

CONCLUSIONS:

Horseback riding has a large number of participants in the United States. Horseback riding is a safe sport, but when accidents occur they are more likely to have a greater mortality and morbidity and to leave a greater residual disability. Head and neck injuries are frequent and are the most severe type of injury. Youth and young adults are more likely to have horse related accidents, but when an older rider has an accident it tends to be more severe. Females are more likely to have horse related accidents than males, but head injuries cause an equal percentage of deaths in males and females. Head, face, and neck injuries can be prevented, their frequency decreased and the severity of the injury reduced by wearing ASTM SEI protective headgear at all times when mounted or preparing to mount.

REFERENCES

[1] American Horse Council, Horse Industry Directory 1991-1992, pp 3.

[2] Phillips, G. H. and Stuckey, W. E., Accidents to Rural Ohio People Occurring During Recreational Activities Extension Bulletin MM-295, Research Circular 166, Cooperative Extension Service, Ohio State University, 1969.

[3] Ponder, D. J., "The Grave Yawns for the Horseman," Medical Journal of Australia, 141:632-635, 1984.

[4] Ingemarson, H., Grevsten, S and Thorlan, L., "Lethal Horse-riding Injuries", Journal of Trauma, Vol. 20, No. 1, pp 25-30.

[5] Buckley, S., Chalmers, D. and Landley, J., "Falls from Horses Resulting in Death and Hospitalization," Medical School, University of Otago, PO Box 913, Dunedin, NZ.

[6] Bixby-Hammett, D. M., and Brooks, W. H., "Common Injuries In Horseback Riding", Sports Medicine Vol. 9, No.1, pp 36-47, 1990.

[7] National Electronic Injury Surveillance System (NEISS),
    Consumer Product Safety Commission, 5401 Westbard Avenue,
    Washington, DC, 20297.

[8] Andrews, D. M., Program Director, Mobile Sports Medicine
    Systems, Inc., 411 N. Washington, Suite 2000, Dallas,
    TX, 75127.

[9] Branch of Safety Management, National Park Service,
    Washington, DC, 20013-7127.

[10] United States Pony Clubs, Inc., 4071 Iron Works Pike,
     Lexington, KY, 40511.

Charles H. Tator,[1] Virginia E. Edmonds,[1] and Lillian Lapczak[1]

Spinal Injuries in Ice Hockey: Review of 182 North American Cases and Analysis of Etiological Factors

REFERENCE: Tator, Charles H., Edmonds, Virginia E., and Lapczak, Lillian, **"Spinal Injuries in Ice Hockey: Review of 182 North American Cases and Analysis of Etiological Factors,"** *Head and Neck Injuries in Sports, ASTM STP 1229,* Earl F. Hoerner, Ed., Amerian Society for Testing and Materials, Philadelphia, 1994.

ABSTRACT: This paper describes 182 cases of spinal injuries in North American ice hockey players occurring between 1966 and 1991. One hundred and seventy-three injuries occurred in Canada, 8 in the United States, and one Canadian player was injured in a game in Germany. The median age of the players was 18 and 96% were males. One hundred and thirty-eight had neck injuries. The majority of the injuries occurred in games in organized leagues. Spinal cord injury occurred in 106 cases, 51 of whom had complete spinal cord injuries. Collision of the helmeted head with the boards, especially following a check or push from behind, was the most common mechanism of injury. It is felt that most of these injuries are preventable.

KEYWORDS: Ice hockey, spinal injuries, demography, prevention

The Committee on Prevention of Spinal Cord Injuries Due to Hockey of SportSmart Canada has been collecting data on major injuries to the spine or spinal cord sustained while playing ice hockey since 1981. To date the database contains 182 cases with injuries reported from January, 1966 to April, 1991. It is distressing that the number of hockey related major spinal injuries reported per year is not decreasing. More than half the injuries occurred in players under 20 years of age. The most frequent mode of injury was a push or check from behind which usually caused the player to hit the boards head first. This paper describes the method of data collection, the demographic details of the 182 injuries and various prevention programs that have been implemented.

Methods

The Committee on Prevention of Spinal Cord Injuries Due to Hockey conducted national surveys of the incidence of spinal injuries in hockey in Canada in 1981, 1985, 1987, 1989, and 1991. Bilingual questionnaires were sent to approximately 1000 neurosurgeons, orthopaedic surgeons, and physical medicine and rehabilitation specialists practicing in Canada. Injuries published in the media were added to the database though eventually nearly all such cases were verified by physicians. In addition, the Committee has received reports of spinal injuries in the United States and some other countries. The Committee has also conducted

---

[1] Director, Associate Director and Programmer/Analyst, respectively, SportSmart Canada, Toronto Hospital and University of Toronto, Toronto, Ontario, Canada.

periodic searches of the worldwide literature to obtain information on spinal injuries in hockey in other countries. The present report contains the information on the 182 North American cases.

Information was obtained on all patients with hockey related major injuries to the spine, with or without injuries to the nerve roots or spinal cord. Not included were patients with minor spinal injuries such as sprains, strains, flexion-extension injuries and whiplash. The questionnaire asked for the date, location of injury, initials, age and sex of the player. Thus, duplicated reports were detected. The survey also obtained information about the circumstances of the accident, the protective equipment worn by the player, and the nature of the bony and neurologic injury.

The data were processed at SportSmart Canada at the Toronto Hospital, which is the research facility of the Committee on Prevention of Spinal and Head Injuries Due to Hockey.

Results

Geographic Location

Nearly all (94%) the injuries reported occurred in Canada. Those accidents which happened in the United States were reported by US physicians aware of our registry. The patient injured in Germany was a Canadian player treated at the Toronto Hospital. Ontario had the highest number of injuries (52%), and Quebec had only 19 cases (10%). The remainder of the Canadian cases were proportionally distributed across the country (Table 1).

Annual Incidence

Prior to 1980, major injuries in hockey were rare. Starting in 1980 the number of cases occurring annually increased, and between 1982 and 1991 they numbered about 15 per year (Table 2).

TABLE 1—*Geographic location of hockey related spinal injuries sustained by 182 patients between January, 1966 and April, 1991.*

Location	Frequency (%)
Ontario	94 (52)
Quebec	19 (10)
Alberta	14 (8)
British Columbia	12 (7)
Saskatchewan	9 (5)
Nova Scotia	7 (4)
Manitoba	5 (3)
New Brunswick	4 (2)
Prince Edward Island	4 (2)
Newfoundland	2 (1)
Yukon	1 (0.5)
United States	8 (4)
Germany	1 (0.5)
Unknown	2 (1)
Total	182

TABLE 2—*The number of spinal injuries occurring annually,[a]*
reported to the Committee on Prevention of Spinal Injuries Due
to Hockey, from January, 1966 to April, 1991.

Year	Number of Injuries
1966	1
1975	1
1976	2
1977	2
1978	4
1979	2
1980	8
1981	12
1982	15
1983	15
1984	15
1985	12
1986	15
1987	9
1988	16
1989	13
1990	19
1991	14

[a] The injuries are recorded for the year in which they occurred
rather than the year when they were reported to the committee.
Data are missing for 7 injuries.

Sex and Age

The majority of players injured were male (96%). Though membership in girls' hockey
is on the rise there was not a corresponding increase in injuries. Fifty-five percent of the
players were between 15 and 19 years old. The median age was 18 years and the range was
from 11 to 47 years (Tables 3, 9, 12).

Level of Injury

Injuries involving the cervical spine were the most common (75.8%) and 18.6% of the
cases affected C5-6. Thoracic, thoracolumbar and lumbosacral injuries were much less common (Table 4).

TABLE 3—*Age of injured players.*

Age	Frequency (%)
11–20	119 (65)
21–30	35 (19)
31–40	13 (7)
41–50	3 (2)

Data are missing for 12 cases (7%).
Age range 11 to 47 yr., mean 20.4 yr., median 18 yr.

TABLE 4—*Vertebral level of spinal injury.*

	Frequency	Percent
Cervical		
C1–C7/T1	138	75.8
Thoracic		
T1–T11	3	1.6
Thoracic-Lumbar		4.4
T11/12–L1/2	8	
Lumbo-Sacral		3.8
L2–S5	7	

Data are missing for 26 cases (14.3%)

Neurologic Deficit

Minor injuries such as vertebral strain were excluded, but fractures or dislocations of the spine were included even if they did not cause neurologic injuries. The spinal cord was affected in 58.2% of the injuries and damage to one or more roots occurred in 8.8% of the cases. Forty-one (22.5%) players sustained complete permanent spinal cord injuries with no preservation of motor or sensory function below the level of injury. Twenty-eight of these players with complete spinal cord injuries were 20 years of age or younger. There was a higher percentage of severe spinal cord injuries in the patients with cervical injuries as compared with injuries at the other levels of the vertebral column. There were six known fatalities in the 182 reports. Cases with transient sensory loss and transient paralysis were collected only after 1987 (Tables 5, 10).

Type of Athletic Event

The majority of injuries (72%) happened in supervised games with in an organized hockey league. Only twelve players were injured during practices or unstructured events (shinny) (Table 6).

TABLE 5—*Neurological injuries.*

	Frequency	Percent
1. Spinal Cord Injury:		
Complete Motor and Complete Sensory Loss	41	22.5
Complete Motor and Incomplete Sensory Loss	10	5.5
Incomplete Motor Loss and Incomplete Sensory Loss	34	18.7
Incomplete Sensory Loss	4	2.2
Transient Sensory Loss and/or Transient Paralysis[a]	17	9.3
Sub-totals		
	106	58.2
2. Root Injury Only	16	8.8
3. No Neurological Injury	38	20.9
4. Missing Data/Incomplete Data	22	12.1
Sub-totals		
	76	41.8
Overall totals		
	182	100.0

[a] This information collected only after March/87.

TABLE 6—*Type of hockey played when spinal injury occurred.*

Type of Play	Frequency (%)
Organized games	131 (72)
Practices	8 (4)
Unstructured play (shinny)	4 (2)
Unknown	39 (21)
Total	182

Mechanism of Injury

Axial loading was found to be the most common mechanism causing cervical-spine and cervical cord injury [1]. Axial loading was applied to the head when the helmeted head struck another object, usually the boards. This most commonly occurred when the player was pushed or checked from behind (53 injuries, 29%). Impact with the boards accounted for 109 injuries (59.9%), and this impact produced the spinal cord injury (Tables 7, 11). Unfortunately, the incidence of players being pushed and/or checked from behind is not on the decline, and in these cases the impact that produced the spinal injuries was with the boards.

Discussion

Since the results of the first national survey were reported, the number of hockey related spinal cord injuries per year has not diminished. The Committee received reports of 12 to 15 injuries per year occurring in Canada between 1981 and 1991. Even though the Canadian Amateur Hockey Association put a rule in effect in 1985 prohibiting pushing or checking from behind, a push or check from behind has remained the most common mechanism of injury. Young men in their teens playing organized hockey were at the greatest risk of spinal injury. Similarly, Gerberich and colleagues [2] in their Minnesota study found that the majority of all types of hockey injuries happened during organized games.

An interesting point surfaced in the Minnesota study. Players were asked to rank their reasons for participating in the game. Players, who for their first or second choice, put down that playing hockey was a means of ridding tension and aggression, ran a fourfold increased

TABLE 7—*Type of collision.*

	Frequency	Percent
Boards	109	59.9
Other players	18	9.9
Boards and players[a]	9	4.9
Ice	8	4.4
Goal post	2	1.1
Boards and ice[a]	1	0.5
Boards and goal post[a]	1	0.5
Players and ice[a]	1	0.5
Players and goal post[a]	1	0.5
Incomplete/missing	32	17.6
Total	182	100.0

[a] More than one type of collision.

TABLE 8—*Mode of injury.*

	Frequency	Percent
Single mechanisms		
Pushed/checked from behind	48	26.4
Pushed/checked	26	14.3
Tripped on ice	24	13.2
Slide	12	6.6
Tripped by player	5	2.7
Multiple mechanisms		
Slide + pushed/checked from behind	5	2.7
Tripped on ice + slide	5	2.7
Slide + pushed/checked	4	2.2
Slide + tripped by player	1	0.5
Tripped on ice + slide with player	1	0.5
Tripped on ice + pushed/checked	1	0.5
Incomplete/missing	50	27.5
Totals		
	182	100.0

risk of concussion. It is this aggressive attitude that must be taken into account when preventive programs are being developed.

Analysis of Etiologic Factors

No one factor is responsible for these tragic hockey related spinal injuries. SportSmart Canada has identified several causal factors. The most common factor, pushing and/or checking from behind caused about the same percentage of cervical spinal injuries as injuries at the other levels of the spine. Also, there were no major differences in the mechanisms involved in the etiology of spinal injuries alone as compared with those involving the spinal cord as well, and thus the conclusions and recommendations apply to both groups. Prior to the introduction of face masks and helmets, head injuries, including face, scalp and brain injuries, accounted for 40% to 50% of all serious injuries in hockey [3–6]. With the use of helmets, head injuries comprise about 25% of hockey injuries [7]. Most of the remaining injuries are to the limbs, specifically the lower limbs [8].

1. *Physical factors related to current players.* Hockey players today are generally taller and heavier. Due to the advances in technology, players can skate at higher speeds than in previous years. This increased weight and speed raise the forces generated by collisions.
2. *Social and psychological factors among young hockey players.* Young players now wear a considerable amount of protective equipment including helmets, and consequently, play an aggressive game believing they will not be hurt. Many of the injured players

TABLE 9—*Sex of players.*

Sex	Frequency (%)
Male	175 (96.2)
Female	7 (3.8)

TABLE 10—*Survival.*

	Frequency (%)
Survivors	167 (91,8)
Fatalities	6 (3.3)

Data are missing in 9 cases (4.9%).

were not aware of the fact that spinal injuries can occur in hockey. The aggressive style of professional players is copied by many younger players. However, most of these teenagers have neither the physical fitness nor the conditioning of the professionals.

3. *Rules and Refereeing.* Injuries occurred when rules were not enforced, and thus many of the injuries occurred during illegal play, especially pushing or checking from behind.

4. *Coaching.* The players were often not told about the risks of hockey and the methods of protecting the spine. There was not enough stress placed on physical conditioning, especially the neck muscles.

5. *Hockey rinks and equipment.* Small rinks 30.5 m by 60.9 m (85 ft. by 185 ft.), have been considered a possible factor because in smaller rinks collisions may be more frequent. The lack of shock absorption of the boards in most rinks has been queried as a possible etiologic factor. Players started to wear helmets in the 1970's, and a few years later there was a marked increase in neck injuries. However, biomechanical studies have not supported the hypothesis that the helmet is an important factor [9]. In fact, the helmets have been effective in reducing the number of brain injuries in hockey players. As noted above, helmets contributed to the feeling of invincibility and may have indirectly altered behavior.

TABLE 11—*Year by mode of injury.*

Year	Slide	Pushed Checked	Pushed Checked from behind	Tripped by player	Tripped on Ice	Unknown
			Frequency of Mode of Injury			
1966	...	...	...	...	...	...
1975	...	...	1	...	...	...
1976	1	...	...	...	1	...
1977	...	...	1	...	...	...
1978	...	...	...	...	1	...
1979	...	1	...	...	...	...
1980	2	2	3	...	1	...
1981	2	2	2	...	4	2
1982	2	2	5	1	1	...
1983	2	3	6	...	2	1
1984	3	3	...	1	...	1
1985	2	3	5	...	1	2
1986	1	4	6	...	2	1
1987	...	...	2	1	3	...
1988	2	3	7	...	4	...
1989	3	1	6	...	4	1
1990	3	5	5	1	5	...
1991	1	4	4	1	1	...
Total	24	33	53	5	30	8

Eye and dental injuries were drastically reduced by regular use of face masks [10,11]. It has been suggested that face masks are related to the increase in spinal cord injuries, but we have found no evidence to corroborate that finding [12].

Prevention Programs

The Committee on Prevention of Spinal Injuries Due to Hockey has developed several programs to reduce the number of spinal injuries.

1. *Players education and conditioning.* A videotape, *Smart Hockey with Mike Bossy* was produced in 1988 by the Committee and has been distributed to leagues and schools. The video stresses the risks of certain aspects of play, especially going into the boards face first and *blindly.* Several defensive tactics for avoiding spinal injuries are shown, specifically avoiding impact of the head with the boards, the ice surface, or other players.

   Since 1984 a brochure entitled *Neck and Spine Conditioning for Hockey Players* has been made available to all hockey players by the Committee. It contains specific exercises to strengthen the neck muscles.

   We strongly urge players to do neck conditioning exercises. A neck protector is no

TABLE 12—*Age distribution of injured players.*

Age	Frequency	%	Cum Freq	Cum %
11	2	1.2	2	1.2
12	1	0.6	3	1.8
13	1	0.6	4	2.4
14	8	4.7	12	7.1
15	16	9.4	28	16.5
16	25	14.7	53	31.2
17	30	17.6	83	48.8
18	13	7.6	96	56.5
19	16	9.4	112	65.9
20	7	4.1	119	70.0
21	3	1.8	122	71.8
22	5	2.9	127	74.7
23	3	1.8	130	76.5
24	3	1.8	133	78.2
25	4	2.4	137	80.6
26	4	2.4	141	82.9
28	2	1.2	143	84.1
29	6	3.5	149	87.6
30	5	2.9	154	90.6
31	1	0.6	155	91.2
32	2	1.2	157	92.4
33	2	1.2	159	93.5
34	2	1.2	161	94.7
35	2	1.2	163	95.9
36	1	0.6	164	96.5
37	2	1.2	166	97.6
38	1	0.6	167	98.2
41	1	0.6	168	98.8
45	1	0.6	169	99.4
47	1	0.6	170	100.0

Data are missing for 12 cases.

substitute for these exercises and there is no evidence that such a protector will prevent spinal injuries.

2. *Rules and refereeing.* In 1985, as a result of the data made available by the Committee, the Canadian Amateur Hockey Association introduced specific rules against pushing or checking from behind. The Association is determined to reduce violence in the game by enforcing these rules.

3. *Equipment manufacturers and rink contractors.* There exists excellent research on the safety of hockey equipment, but further work needs to be done [9,13]. More research should be carried out on the shape, friction and shock absorption of helmets, and on the shock absorption of the boards. Placing inflexible backing, such as concrete blocks, behind the boards should be discouraged. The rink size should be increased to international standards. With smaller rinks the goal lines should be moved forward to reduce the incidence of collisions with the end boards.

4. *Sports medicine research.* Specialists and researchers in sports medicine should be encouraged to do further research into spinal injuries caused by sports and recreational activities. To develop and assess preventive programs it is imperative to continue to collect data on sports/recreational injuries.

In the U.S., the number of major spinal cord football related injuries was reduced by improving awareness and attitude and by effecting rule changes [1,14–17]. It should be possible to produce similar results in hockey.

Summary

During the 1980s there was an increase in the number of spinal injuries in hockey players. Many factors contribute to these injuries. The increased weight, speed and aggressiveness of players are important factors. Lack of awareness of the risks, such as a push or check from behind are also factors. Physical conditioning and player attitude are important. Once these factors were identified, specific actions were taken to correct them and a registry was established to assess the effectiveness of prevention programs. Greater awareness of all the risk factors by players, coaches, league officials, referees, and parents is essential for reducing these tragic injuries.

Acknowledgments

This research was supported by the Rick Hansen Man-in-Motion Legacy Fund, the Dr. Tom Pashby Sports Safety Fund, and the Canadian Amateur Hockey Association.

References

[1] Torg, J. S., Vegso, J. J., O'Neill, J., and Sennett, B., "The Epidemiologic, Pathologic, Biomechanical, and Cinematographic Analysis of Football Induced Cervical Spine Trauma," *American Journal of Sports Medicine,* Vol. 18, No. 1, 1990, pp. 50–57.

[2] Gerberich, S. G., Finke, R., Madden, M. et al., "An Epidemiological Study of High School Ice Hockey Injuries," *Childs Nervous System,* Vol. 3, 1978, pp. 59–64.

[3] Biener, K. and Muller, P., "Les Accidents du Hockey Sur Glace," *Cahiers de Medecine,* Vol. 14, 1975, pp. 959–962.

[4] Hayes, D., "Hockey Injuries: How, Why, Where, and When?," *The Physician and Sportsmedicine,* Vol. 3, 1975, pp. 61–65.

[5] Hornof, Z. and Napravnik, C., "Analysis of Various Accident Rate Factors in Ice Hockey," *Medicine and Science in Sports,* Vol. 5, 1973, pp. 283–286.

[6] Sutherland, G. W., "Fire on Ice," *American Journal of Sports Medicine,* Vol. 4, 1976, pp. 264–268.

[7] Jorgensen, U. and Schmidt-Olsen, S., "The Epidemiology of Ice Hockey Injuries," *British Journal of Sports Medicine,* Vol. 20, 1986, pp. 7–9.

[8] Sim, F. H. and Somonet, W. T., "Ice Hockey Injuries," *The Physician and Sportsmedicine,* Vol. 16, 1988, pp. 92–105.

[9] Bishop, P. J., Norman, R. W., Wells, R. et al., "Changes in the Centre of Mass and Moment of Inertia of a Headform Induced by a Hockey Helmet and Face Shield," *Canadian Journal of Applied Sports Science,* Vol. 8, 1983, pp. 19–25.

[10] Pashby, T. J., Pashby, R. C., Chisholm, L. J., et al., "Eye Injuries in Canadian Hockey," *Canadian Medical Association Journal,* Vol. 113, 1975, pp. 663–666.

[11] Pashby, T. J., "Eye Injuries in Canadian Hockey. Phase III: Older Players Now at Most Risk," *Canadian Medical Association Journal,* Vol. 121, 1979, pp. 643–644.

[12] Sim, F. H., Simonet, W. T., MeHong, L. J. et al., "Ice Hockey Injuries," *American Journal of Sports Medicine,* Vol. 15, 1987, pp. 30–40.

[13] Wells, R. P., Bishop, P. J. and Stephens, M., "Neck Loads During Head-First Collisions in Ice Hockey: Experimental and Simulation Results," *International Journal of Sport Biomechanics,* Vol. 3, 1987, pp. 432–442.

[14] Clarke, K. S. and Powell, J. W., "Football Helmets and Neurotrauma—An Epidemiological Overview of Three Seasons," *Medicine and Science in Sports,* Vol. 11, 1979, pp. 138–145.

[15] Clarke, K. S., "An Epidemiologic View," *Athletic Injuries to the Head and Face,* J. C. Torg, Ed., Lea & Febiger, Philadelphia, 1982, pp. 15–25.

[16] Hodgson, V. R., "Reducing Serious Injury in Sports," Interscholastic Athletic Administration, Vol. 7, 1980, pp. 11–14.

[17] Torg, J. S., Truex, R., Jr., Quedenfeld, T. C. et al., "National Football Head and Neck Injury Registry, Report and Conclusions, 1978," *Journal of the American Medical Association,* Vol. 241, 1979, pp. 1477–1479.

Robert E. Frye[1]

THE NATIONAL ELECTRONIC INJURY SURVEILLANCE SYSTEM (NEISS) AND HAZARD ANALYSIS

REFERENCE: Frye, Robert E.; "The National Electronic Injury Surveillance System (NEISS) and Hazard Analysis," Head and Neck Injuries in Sports. ASTM STP 1229, Earl F. Hoerner, Ed., American Society for Testing and Materials, Philadelphia, 1994.

ABSTRACT: This paper describes the design and operation of the U.S. Consumer Product Safety Commission's National Electronic Injury Surveillance System (NEISS), the development of national estimates and data on injuries, associated with products used in recreational and residential settings, and the identification of reasonable approaches to reducing the frequency and severity of injuries and deaths. The NEISS is a national probability sample of 91 hospitals which provide data on over 280,000 case reports each year. It is a multi-level data collection system, including extracts from hospital emergency room records, telephone follow-ups to injured persons, and on-site in-depth investigations of specific cases of interest. Examples are given on the development of national estimates and trends in injuries for such products as fireworks, playground equipment, and all-terrain vehicles. The identification of incident hazard patterns for specific sports activities or product types and the development of remedial efforts are discussed. These efforts may involve new product safety standards, public information and educational activities, or other steps to reduce unreasonable risks of injury. A description of how to obtain NEISS data and copies of CPSC reports from the National Injury Information Clearinghouse is included.

KEYWORDS: hazard analysis, NEISS, surveillance, sports injuries, emergency room, database, follow-up, assessment - national program, biostatistics.

---

[1] Director, Hazard Analysis Division, Directorate for Epidemiology, U.S. Consumer Product Safety Commission, Bethesda, MD, USA.

I.   Introduction

The U.S. Consumer Product Safety Commission's (CPSC) mission is to protect the public from unreasonable risks of injury and death associated with consumer products. The Commission's objective is to reduce the estimated 28.6 million injuries and 21,700 deaths associated with the 15,000 different types of consumer products under CPSC's jurisdiction.

Since 1973, the epidemiological research group at CPSC has operated the National Electronic Injury Surveillance System (NEISS). It collects injury and incident data from a national probability sample of 91 hospital emergency rooms (ERs) from across the U.S. (Figure 1 shows the general locations of the participating hospitals.) Current NEISS hospitals in the State of Georgia are Rockdale County in Conyers, Southern Regional Medical in Riverdale, and Martin Army at Fort Benning.

One of CPSC's concerns is the severity of product-related injuries, and head and neck injuries can be among the most severe. The latest CPSC staff analysis of data on head injuries[†] was completed in 1990, using 1988 NEISS data. The primary findings show the relative frequencies of hospital ER treated, sports-related head injuries and illustrate some of the NEISS system's capabilities. Highlights from these data are presented in this paper for the ASTM Committee F-8 on Sports Equipment and Facilities Symposium on Head and Neck Injuries.

It should be noted that although this paper was prepared by the author in his official capacity, the views expressed concerning CPSC programs and policy are personal and do not necessarily reflect the views of the Commission.

[†]   For this presentation, head injuries include those to the face but not the neck.

U.S. Consumer Product Safety Commission NEISS Hospitals

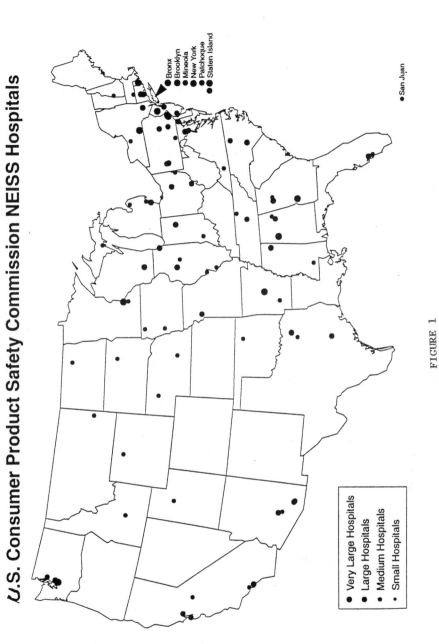

Bronx
Brooklyn
Mineola
New York
Patchoque
Staten Island

San Juan

Very Large Hospitals
Large Hospitals
Medium Hospitals
Small Hospitals

FIGURE 1

II.   NEISS Capabilities

The NEISS sample was selected from a list of all U.S. hospitals with at least six (6) beds and 24 hour service. Under contract with CPSC, each hospital in the sample provides such information as the age and sex of the victim, injury diagnosis (including the body parts involved), product codes, and a brief narrative comment with information from the ER record. This is done by a "NEISS Coder" (a hospital or other staff person) who briefs hospital emergency room staff on NEISS requirements, reviews daily ER records for in scope cases, codes reportable cases, and enters the data in a personal computer (PC) provided by CPSC. Each night, a CPSC PC polls the local PCs and collects their cases. In a year, NEISS collects over 280,000 case reports.

The NEISS is a versatile system with some powerful attributes. First, large numbers of consumer product-related injuries are treated in ERs (about 20 percent of ER treatments, as shown in Figure 2). Much of the data needed for hazard identification efforts have already been recorded in ER records. Second, the information is timely. The ER records are generally reviewed by the NEISS Coder within a day of the treatment. This facilitates NEISS operations as a multi-level data collection system with the capability to perform telephone call backs and on-site investigations for more detailed case information, photographs, and product sample collection. Because these case follow-ups can be conducted within the statistical framework of the basic sample design and in a timely manner before human memory decay and product availability become problems, NEISS can provide national estimates with statistical confidence intervals on a large array of factors related to injury incidents.

NEISS initial surveillance and case follow-up data are used by CPSC (for monitoring trends in product-related injuries, Figure 3); other Federal agencies (a list of Federal agencies which have used NEISS data is shown in Figure 4); and the media (an excerpt from the February 2, 1993 "Health" section of The Washington Post is shown in Figure 5).

III.   NEISS Head Injury Data

Overall, there were an estimated total of 2.9 million product-related head injuries treated in U.S. Hospital ERs in 1988. They were about 30 percent of all consumer product-related hospital ER treated injuries in 1988. Of the 2.9 million injuries, an estimated 341,400 (about 12 percent) were related to sports. [This estimate does not include injuries related to bicycles (169,000), skateboards (21,800), or all terrain vehicles (12,200).] For comparison purposes, it is interesting to note that 735,000 and 602,000 head injuries were related to household structures and contents, respectively.

Percent ER Treatments
by Reason for Visit

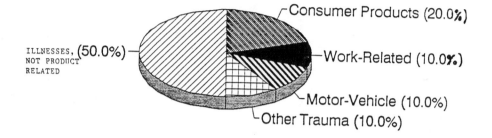

Consumer Products (20.0%)

ILLNESSES, (50.0%)
NOT PRODUCT
RELATED

Work-Related (10.0%)

Motor-Vehicle (10.0%)
Other Trauma (10.0%)

FIGURE 2

By age of victim, 16,800 (5 percent) of the sports-related head injuries were to children under age 5, 101,600 (30 percent) to children ages 5 to 14, and 222,600 (65 percent) to ages 15 and above. While young and older adults may be aware of much of the risk of injury associated with their participation in sports, this cannot be said about younger age groups. Therefore, sports rule setting groups, sports equipment manufacturers, safety specialists, and others have a special obligation to find ways to reduce the frequency and severity of these injuries.

Of the 341,400 sports-related head injuries, 67,100 (about 20 percent) were concussions, fractures, and internal head injuries, with 23,500 (35 percent) of these serious injuries to children ages 5 to 14. It is worth noting, from a product safety point of view, many of these injuries might be prevented or reduced in severity by increased use of helmets or other head and eye protection devices.

NEISS Estimates 1980-1991
Chain Saws and ATVs

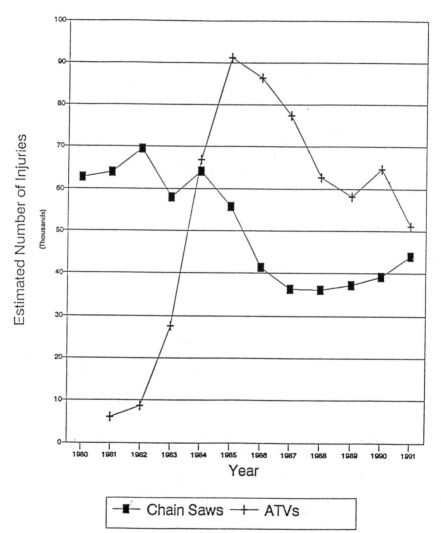

FIGURE 3

Inter-Agency Data Sharing

- *National Highway Traffic Safety Administration*
- *National Institute for Occupational Safety and Health*
- *Food and Drug Administration*
- *Environmental Protection Agency*
- *Housing and Urban Development*
- *Bureau of Justice Statistics*
- *Center for Injury Control*
- *Coast Guard*

FIGURE 4

Following are NEISS estimates* for specific sports-related activities in 1988.

Activity	Estimated Head Injuries**	Percent Ages 5 to 14
Baseball	95,200	46
Basketball	60,900	19
Swimming	44,500	5
Football	39,200	36
Fishing	13,200	30
Soccer	12,000	28
Skiing, Snow	10,000	21
Golf	9,200	42
Ice Hockey	9,100	13
Horseback Riding	8,400	30
Roller Skating	7,800	61
Ice Skating	7,400	51
Hockey, other or unknown	6,600	35
Paddle Ball	6,600	6
Skiing, Water	6,000	10
Wrestling	5,400	25

NEISS Data are Used by the Media

February 2, 1993 "Health" section of the Washington Post

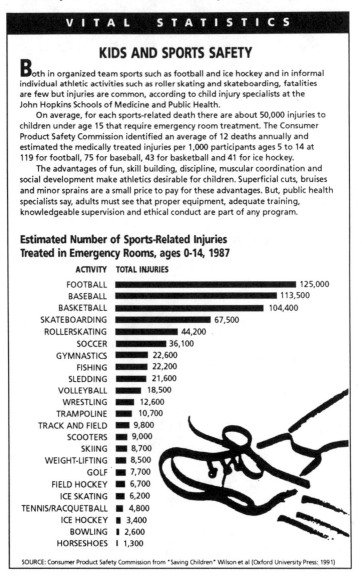

VITAL   STATISTICS

KIDS AND SPORTS SAFETY

Both in organized team sports such as football and ice hockey and in informal individual athletic activities such as roller skating and skateboarding, fatalities are few but injuries are common, according to child injury specialists at the John Hopkins Schools of Medicine and Public Health.

On average, for each sports-related death there are about 50,000 injuries to children under age 15 that require emergency room treatment. The Consumer Product Safety Commission identified an average of 12 deaths annually and estimated the medically treated injuries per 1,000 participants ages 5 to 14 at 119 for football, 75 for baseball, 43 for basketball and 41 for ice hockey.

The advantages of fun, skill building, discipline, muscular coordination and social development make athletics desirable for children. Superficial cuts, bruises and minor sprains are a small price to pay for these advantages. But, public health specialists say, adults must see that proper equipment, adequate training, knowledgeable supervision and ethical conduct are part of any program.

**Estimated Number of Sports-Related Injuries
Treated in Emergency Rooms, ages 0-14, 1987**

ACTIVITY	TOTAL INJURIES
FOOTBALL	125,000
BASEBALL	113,500
BASKETBALL	104,400
SKATEBOARDING	67,500
ROLLERSKATING	44,200
SOCCER	36,100
GYMNASTICS	22,600
FISHING	22,200
SLEDDING	21,600
VOLLEYBALL	18,500
WRESTLING	12,600
TRAMPOLINE	10,700
TRACK AND FIELD	9,800
SCOOTERS	9,000
SKIING	8,700
WEIGHT-LIFTING	8,500
GOLF	7,700
FIELD HOCKEY	6,700
ICE SKATING	6,200
TENNIS/RACQUETBALL	4,800
ICE HOCKEY	3,400
BOWLING	2,600
HORSESHOES	1,300

SOURCE: Consumer Product Safety Commission from "Saving Children" Wilson et al (Oxford University Press: 1991)

FIGURE 5

Clearly from these data, it is easy to conclude that baseball, basketball, swimming, and football were major sources of sports-related head injuries. Of these, CPSC has had a major project on swimming pool diving hazards. In addition, CPSC has participated in voluntary safety standards development efforts related to many of the other sports.

In reviewing these data for the percentages of children ages 5 to 14 treated in hospital ERs for head injuries related to specific sports, it is also clear that much remains to be done to protect this vulnerable group of sports participants (and some bystanders) from potentially life altering injuries. Particularly, where relatively large proportions of children were treated for head injuries in sports such as various forms of hockey (48 percent), baseball (46 percent), golf (42 percent), football (36 percent), soccer (28 percent), and wrestling (25 percent) and activities such as roller skating (30 percent), "the development of new information, including research on the application of technology to safe and effective use of sports equipment and to safety in participation in sports" (which is from this Symposium's theme) should be encouraged.

Most (97 percent) of the 341,400 cases were treated and released, not hospitalized. Among the more serious hospitalized injuries (involving concussions, fractures, and internal head injuries including some DOAs), it is worth noting that the following were the head injury estimates[*] for the sports-related activities with the highest frequencies.

Activity	Estimated Head Injuries[**]
Horseback Riding	2,200
Football	1,500
Baseball	1,400
Skiing, Snow	1,100
Basketball	500

---

[*]   Because comparative data on the number of participants (or number of hours of participation) were not available, these estimates should not be considered as measures of the relative risks of injury for each of these activities.

[**]   Though these estimates are given in the order of descending frequencies, relatively small differences between estimates may not be statistically significant.

IV.   Closing Comments

Hopefully, this Symposium will assist in developing new ideas on reducing both the frequency and severity of sports-related head injuries. As noted earlier in this paper, many of these injuries might be prevented or reduced in severity by increased use of helmets or other head and eye protection devices.

In creating the CPSC in 1973, the Congress emphasized widespread sharing of injury incident information and data by the Agency. To carry out this mandate, the National Injury Information Clearinghouse was established. The Clearinghouse maintains computerized files including millions of NEISS surveillance and other case reports for public access. It responds to over 6,000 requests each year (see Figure 6). Requesters typically include lawyers, researchers, manufacturers, and consumers. Many Clearinghouse reports and services are available free of charge and most of the others involve only a nominal charge. To request injury information from CPSC, interested persons should call (301) 504-0424 or write:

National Injury Information Clearinghouse
U.S. Consumer Product Safety Commission
5401 Westbard Avenue, Room 625
Washington, D.C.   20207

Clearinghouse Support

- *Established to provide product-related injury data to interested parties*

- *Annually responds to over 6,000 information requests*

- *Data users include researchers, lawyers, manufacturers, and consumers*

- *Many reports are available free of charge and most others involve only a nominal charge*

- *Call (301/504-0424) or write for information*

FIGURE 6

Milton Gabrielsen,[1] Ph.D. and Arthur H. Mittelstaedt, Jr.[1] Ed.D.

Causes of Pool Diving Accidents

REFERENCE: Gabrielsen, M. and Mittelstaedt, A. H., **"Causes of Pool Diving Accidents,"** *Head and Neck Injuries in Sports, ASTM STP 1229,* Earl F. Hoerner, Ed., American Society for Testing and Materials, Philadelphia, 1994.

ABSTRACT: Increasing research into diving injuries and fatalities as revealed in litigation over the years, can provide an insight into prevention and correction of the causes.

KEYWORDS: diving, pools, accidents, injuries, head, neck

Increasing research into diving injuries and fatalities as revealed in litigation over the years, can provide an insight into prevention and correction of the causes. These causes have been divided into the following categories.

Victim Performance

The following identifies what untrained divers are apt to do:

1. The person, while in the process of executing a dive into the pool, runs on the board rather than walks to the point where he/she hurdles to the end of the board.
2. The person's hurdle to the end of the board is usually too long, which then causes too much forward momentum, resulting in a low forward take-off rather than an upward high take off.
3. The person makes the take-off dangerous by causing too much forward momentum.
4. The person's height of the hurdle is too low, causing late adjustment of the body.
5. The person's take-off is from one foot in a running dive rather than both feet, causing a lack of control.
6. The person's angle of take-off is too low (such as 40° or less instead of near the vertical), propelling the diver too far out into the pool.
7. The person's head is in a flexed position on entry into the water, rather than being aligned with the body, with eyes looking at the water.
8. The person's arms are not in the correct overhead position, which would absorb any shock of contact with the bottom and prevent head contact.
9. The person does not anticipate striking the bottom, thus when the hands come in contact with the bottom, collapse the arms, exposing the head.
10. The person's dive is not properly "programmed" in the mind of the diver to ensure a safe dive under the conditions that exist in the pool.

[1]Recreational Safety Institute, 39 Shady Side Ave., Port Washington, NY 11050.

Victim Unawareness

The following identifies what untrained divers are apt to not be aware of.

1. The person, once leaving the board, is unaware that the laws of physics apply and will determine entry speed, distance traveled in the air and underwater speed.
2. The person is unaware that it is possible to reach the bottom of the pool on any dive.
3. The person is unaware of the fact that it takes very little force to break one's neck when diving.
4. The person is unaware of the precise configuration of the pool's bottom into which the dive is being done.
5. The person is unaware of the depth of water where he or she is apt to enter and make contact with the bottom.
6. The person is unaware of the performance efficiency of the board he/she is about to dive from.
7. The person is unaware that the angle with which they enter the water may project him/her forward underwater from the entry point as much as 5 to 8 feet, depending upon the trajectory.
8. The person is unaware that the arms are not likely to be able to absorb the force generated by the dive if the diver comes into contact with the bottom at a perpendicular angle.
9. The person is unaware of the degree of flexibility of the board and its affect on the dive.
10. The person is unaware of the short time one has for taking or making moves to alter the course once under water.

Pool Facility's Non-Compliance

The following identifies what untrained divers are apt to not be aware of.

1. A pool with a diving board is an invitation to dive and signals to the user that diving is safe even when the depth and bottom configuration are inadequate.
2. A pool of older design has a potential landing area that is designed to accommodate divers, which is too small and thus unsafe for diving.
3. A pool surface area creates an illusion of safety because it implies a safer envelope of water than might actually be underwater, such as the hopper bottom type pool.
4. A pool bottom's upslope or start of the transition from the bottom of the pool pitching from the deep end to the shallow portion of the pool is too close to the end of the board, which can result in the diver striking the slope at a perpendicular angle.
5. A pool depth of water in the diver's potential landing area is too shallow to provide a safe diving envelope, as it is often as shallow as 4 foot.
6. A pool's absence of depth markers, and signs warning against diving, provides no signal of hazards.
7. A pool's breakpoint with no lifeline indicating the start of slope from shallow portion of pool down to deep end provides no signal of any hazard.
8. A pool's absence of markings, including lines or targets on bottom, does not provide divers with a visual reference point.
9. A pool's inadequate lighting of the interior and deck area for safe diving at night creates shadows and deception.

10. A pool's width which is usually narrow, does not provide any recovery space or distance.
11. A pool board's efficiency in relation to the pool's depth of water.

Board Fixture's Non-Compliance

The following identifies what untrained divers are apt to not be aware of.

1. A board's length, including jumpboards which range in length from 3' to 6', and springboards from 8' to 16', creates inherent conflicts.
2. A board's flexibility and efficiency and the relative "quickness" of the board creates insecurity or unsureness.
3. A board's height above the water requires more depth.
4. A board's position of the fulcrum alters the board's performance.
5. A board's stand or mounting is placed improperly.
6. A board's angle or slope should be horizontal to the water.
7. A board's placement, overhand and center alignment affects its performance.
8. A board's condition, such as slippery surface or cracks. can alter performance.
9. A board on coil springs and other devices which are often created by manufacturers in an attempt to achieve more spring in the board produces an unstable condition.
10. A board's manufacturer fails to adequately and scientifically test the performance level of their board in relation to dives of different physical characteristics and pools of different dimensions and depths.

Operator Failures

The following identifies what untrained divers are apt to not be aware of.

1. Failure to provide lifeguards at all public pools (city, county, school, as well as motels, hotels, apartments, condominiums) and other properties.
2. Failure to supervise swimmers and divers, and tend to ignore the fact that people often use motel/hotel and apartment pools when the pool is supposedly closed.
3. Failure to prohibit swimming and diving at night when the lighting is often below acceptable standards.
4. Failure to have a means of securing the pool when it is not intended to be open.
5. Failure to maintain pool water so that it does not become turbid or cloudy, thus reducing visibility.
6. Failure to use known methods to secure springboard from use when pool is closed.
7. Failure to post warning signs and rules governing use of board.
8. Failure to maintain signs, depth markers, lights, diving boards and other equipment.
9. Failure to install a board that corresponds to a safe diving envelope, for example, a 16' long competitive type board in a pool whose diving envelope cannot safely accommodate it.

Every pool designer, manufacturer, fabricator, installer, and owner must recognize these causes, foresee that they can happen, and provide remedies to correct these failures.

The Estimated Incidence of Diving Injuries

The only reliable statistics are those coming from The National Spinal Cord Injury Data Research Center located at the Good Samaritan Hospital in Phoenix, Arizona and The National Spinal Cord Injury Statistical Center's data base located at the University of Alabama at Birmingham, AL. In 1979 the Phoenix Center indicated that there were approximately 8000 spinal cord injuries and 10.6% were the result of diving injuries, which would come out to an annual rate of over 800.

The University of Alabama Center in 1985 published a book entitled *Spinal Injury—The Facts and Figures.* Table 1, which is from that source indicates the relationship between diving injuries and other sports. It is shocking to realize that diving accounts for 66% of all sport related injuries. Although no breakdown was given as to the number that occurred in swimming pools it has been estimated by some that as many as 25 to 30% took place in pools.

Since 1975 I have collected data on 339 diving and sliding injuries which occurred in swimming pools. A summary of the data follows.

Summary of Data

1. What Is the Profile of the Individual That Is Injured?

- He was a male between 18–31 years of age.
- He was close to 6 feet in height and weighed over 175 pounds.
- He was not intoxicated, but in 40 to 50 percent of the cases had consumed some alcoholic beverage, mostly beer.
- He had little or no formal training in diving.
- He was visiting the pool for the first time and the dive he made was the first one in that pool.
- He was not warned, either verbally or by any signs, that he should not dive at the place where he made his fateful dive.
- He had witnessed other people diving before he made his dive.
- He was removed from the pool by friends who were not aware that he had fractured his neck. No spine board was used.
- He was not aware that he could break his neck by making a dive where he did.

TABLE 1—*Distribution of sports-related accidents.*

Sport	Percent
Diving	66.0
Football	6.1
Snow Skiing	3.8
Surfing	3.1
Trampoline	2.6
Other Winter Sports	2.3
Wrestling	2.3
Gymnastics	2.2
Horseback Riding	2.0
Other	9.6

2. How Serious Are the Diving Injuries?

Of the 339 victims 94 percent were partial or quadraplegics. 4 percent ended up with some neurological impairment and two percent had other injuries to the neck, shoulders, face and arms.

3. What Is the Cost of Maintaining a Quadraplegic?

The annual cost for maintaining a quadraplegic has been estimated to exceed $100,000.

4. Who Are the People Most at Risk?

The people at greatest risk are adult males between 18 and 25 years of age.

5. Who Are the Owners of the Pools Where the Injuries Occurred?

Table 2 shows who the owners were of the 339 pools where the injuries occurred.

6. What Was the Comparison Between Sexes?

Of the 339 diving accident victims 88 percent were males. However, only 4 of the 22 springboard accident victims were females, and only 2 of those struck the bottom of the pool.

7. How Many of the Pools Had Depth Markers?

Only 142 of the 339 pools had any depth markers on the pool or deck of the pool.

8. How Many of the Pools Had Bottom Markings?

Thirty-two of the pools had some type of bottom markings.

9. To What Extent Were There Warnings Against Diving?

In only 24 of the 339 pools were there signs warning against diving.

TABLE 2—Owners of the pools where injuries occurred.

Pool owner	Number
Residential	185
Motel/Hotel	62
Apt/Condo	53
City	16
School	14
Commercial	5
Private Club	2
Voluntary Agency	1
Military	1

10. Were There Rules for Use of Pool Posted?

Less than half (48%) of the pools had any kind of rules posted around the pool.

11. What Were the Various Shapes of the Pool Involved?

Most of the inground pools were rectangular while most of the above-ground pools were circular.

12. What Was the Profile of the Bottom of the Pools Involving Springboard/Jumpboard Diving?

Of the 72 springboard diving cases 37 occurred in spoon shaped pools, 34 in hopper bottoms, and one in a constant depth bottom.

13. Were the Victims Guests or Trespassers?

All but 12 of the injured were guests, or had paid a fee to get into the pool. The 12 were members of the household where the pool was located.

14. How Many Visits Had the Victim Made to the Pool?

232 of the 339 victims were visiting the pool for the first time.

15. How Many Dives Had Victim Made on the Day of the Accident Prior to Injury?

In 206 of the accidents the injured party was making his first dive or slide. For 96 victims it was their 2nd or third, and 37 had made more than 3 dives before being injured.

16. How Many of the Victims Had Used Drugs the Day of the Accident?

According to witnesses only 12 of the victims had used drugs. The specific quantity was unobtainable.

17. How Much Beer Was Consumed by the Victims the Day of the Accident?

Forty-five percent (155 victims) consumed some form of alcoholic beverage mostly beer the day of the accident.

18. How and Who Made the Rescue of the Victim?

Of the 339 victims 281 were rescued and removed from the pool by friends or other swimmers in the area. Only 46 were rescued and removed by lifeguards. Three of the victims were able to make it out of the pool by themselves. Rescue Squads (EMS) were responsible for removing seven victims, while in two cases a security guard for the motel removed the injured diver.

19. To What Extent Were Spineboards Used?

In only 22 of the 339 cases was a spineboard used to remove the victim from the water.

Question: Is the Sport of Diving Safe?

Not Safe—According to the University of Alabama in Birmingham database of spinal cord injuries, 14.2 percent of spinal cord injuries were sports-related accidents. Sixty-six percent of these sports-related spinal cord injuries were attributed to diving [*1*].

Safe—In 88 years of competitive diving in the United States, there has been no record of a fatality or a catastrophic injury connected with a supervised training session or diving competition [*2*].

The Purpose

These two seemingly contradictory facts are both true statements. Which one, safe or unsafe, is the informed answer to the question? Facts and figures need interpretation. This document has been published for U.S. Diving (USD) members, administrators, health officials and insurance underwriters to:

1. Set the record straight by exposing the "sport of diving is unsafe" myth, and
2. Focus the reader on aspects of user behavior in the aquatic environment that need to be addressed in order to elevate safety awareness and reduce the risk of injury.

Sponsors, diving administrators, parents, coaches and athletes involved in USD's programs are aware of the sport's commendable safety record and its benefits to the youth of our country (see Appendix, Dick Wilson testimonial). For those who are not personally involved, justification for the continuation of USD programs and for support of new programs is provided in this position paper. This publication includes information from the Lancaster Springboard Diving Booster Club (LSDBC) in California and two high school groups, the Illinois Swimming Association (ISA) and the New York State High School Athletic Association (NYSHSAA), that have been successful in thwarting attempts to remove diving boards.

The Definitions

Diving—the water entry activity that involves plunging head-first into any body of water.

Sport of diving—the supervised sport that provides instruction and/or coaching in dives with head- and feet-first entries from 1 and 3 meter competitive springboards or 5, 7.5, and 10 meter platforms into the deep diving area of a pool.

Spinal Cord Injury (SCI)—"Diving" SCI usually are the result of flexion or flexion-rotation injuries generally associated with compression fractures/dislocations that cause direct injury to the spinal cord at that site. The magnitude of motor and sensory impairment that results is based on the location of injury in the spinal cord. If a diving accident results in injury at the C4 level of the cervical spine, all of the functions at or below that level could be affected [*3*].

Catastrophic Diving SCI—a spinal cord injury sustained by entering the water head-first resulting in a fatality or a non-fatal permanent severe functional disability.

An Overview of Issues

Issue

A misconception exists that the sport of diving is unsafe.

USD Position—The 'sport of diving is unsafe' myth is inaccurate because it is based on incomplete information. Worse yet, it is a dangerous belief because it focuses the problem on the wrong aspect of user behavior. There is a risk of catastrophic SCI on *all* diving water entries into shallow (5 feet or less), mid-range or deep water (9 feet or over). Appropriately supervised competitive and recreational diving is a safe sport. Careless diving water entries into shallow water (5 feet deep or less) is an extremely dangerous activity.

Safety Record of Instructional Diving Programs

U.S. Diving, NCAA and NFSHSA, competitive diving organizations have no record of a catastrophic diving SCI. A study of diving cases within the Lexis System (electronic retrieval system which identifies reported decisions of various courts of law) indicates no catastrophic diving SCI cases in a teaching or school environment involving a 1 or 3 meter board (Clements, 1989) [4]. The competitive swimming and diving organizations, USS, NCAA, FINA* and the NFSHSA have had great influence on public pool design, both for swimming and diving. This influence is seen in the favorable safety record of the well-supervised programs in these locations [5]. Just as drowning victims were not actually swimming (competitive connotation) when they drowned, the so-called 'diving' victims were not involved in competitive diving at the time the SCI was sustained.

Statistical Limitations

Spinal Cord Injury: The Facts and Figures [6]—Presents data from 1973—August 16, 1985 based on almost 10,000 spinal cord injured persons, some of whom have been followed for more than 10 years. The University of Alabama at Birmingham Spinal Cord Injury Data Management Service (UAB-SCI-DMS) collects objective information on 108 critical variables. The distribution by SCI etiology is listed by percentage as follows:

Motor vehicle accidents	47.7
Falls	20.8
Acts of Violence	14.6
Sports	14.2
Other	2.7

In the report, a distribution of sports-related SCI are listed by percentage as follows:

Diving	66.0
Football	—
Snow skiing	—
Surfing	—
Trampoline	—
Other Winter Sports	—
Wrestling	—
Gymnastics	2.2
Horseback Riding	2.0

---

*FINA (Federation Internationale de Natation Amateur) is the international governing body for competitive diving. USD recommends FINA dimensions for newly constructed competitive diving facilities or any facility that will install a board at least 1 meter in height.

Other   9.6

As these statistics provided by the database relate to diving safety issues, the information is more remarkable for what variable is does *not* include. There is no information in this national database concerning depth of the water in which diving injuries occurred [7]. For clarification, we must then look elsewhere for additional information. The 1988 White Paper on Diving Accidents (Appendix) from the National Spa and Pool Institute executive summary of the Arthur D. Little studies diagrams the annual number of spinal cord injuries. Seventy-five percent (75%) of the 'diving' SCI occurred in the natural environment. Competitive divers use swimming pools, not oceans, lakes and rivers. Only twenty-five percent (25%) of the 'diving' SCI resulting in quadriplegia occurred in swimming pools. Approximately ninety-five percent (95%) of the 'diving' SCI resulting in quadriplegia in pools occurred in the shallow rather than in the deep diving area of the pool. Careless diving into shallow and mid-range water depths is the aspect of user behavior that needs to be addressed.

"Whenever two or more things are compared with respect to one characteristic, it is taken for granted that 1) the characteristic in question is the same for each, and 2) other relevant factors are close enough to the same that they won't invalidate the comparison. But comparisons are often invalid because one or the other part of this implicit assumption is not met" [8].

Comparing the water entry activity of 'diving' into any body of water with other competitive sports like football, wrestling, gymnastics etc. is an apples and oranges comparison that falsely implicates the sport of competitive diving. It is inaccurate to conclude that the sport of diving is unsafe based on the statistics that 'diving' accounts for sixty-six percent (66%) of sports SCI. Misconceptions are perpetuated when this statistic finds its way into newspapers, magazines etc. without the limitations of the information thoughtfully pointed out to the reader [9]. The myth that the sport of diving is unsafe is compounded by magazines reporting statistics that reflect the water entry activity of 'diving' juxtaposed with a photographic illustration of a competitive diver [10]. The epitome of this misconception is like building an all-shallow pool as a deterrent to 'diving' SCI [11].

Focus on Problem

Clearly there is a problem if sixty-six percent (66%) of sports-related SCI are represented by one activity. "Over 100 million... Americans... have taken up swimming, making it the number one participatory sport in the United States... There are roughly 2.5 million in-ground pools plus over 1 million spas and hot tubs in use in this country today (1985)" [12]. There are a very large number of tragedies involving these products—many of which do not necessarily involve product design or maintenance problems but instead, aspects of user behavior that may be addresssable [13]. What makes the drownings, near-drownings, quadriplegia, and eviscerations so irrevocably tragic is that they are preventable through consumer awareness, training and supervision [14]. Public education about water hazards has occurred for years via television in countries such as Australia and New Zealand which have been much more aggressive about addressing these problems than we have been in our country [15]. Appropriate solutions to the problems will not be forthcoming until the problems are clearly identified. Safety awareness can only be achieved when individuals with different responsibilities—be they facility users, parents, instructors, coaches, lifeguards, pool managers, administrators, insurance underwriters or lawyers come together in a concerted effort to reduce the risk of injury.

Issue

Catastrophic 'diving' SCI can effectively be prevented by removing all diving boards.

USD Position—The shotgun approach to removing diving boards is not the cure-all to reduce the real risk of 'diving' SCI injury. There is no justification to remove competitive diving boards in sites with excellent safety records that provide appropriate supervision (lifeguard and/or diving coach, instructor present) and sufficient room to maneuver.

Participants in the sport of diving need a water envelope that provides sufficient room to maneuver. The American Red Cross recommends a 9 feet minimum depth for a 1 meter springboard. U.S. Diving sanctions 1 meter competitions with a minimum depth of 11 feet. There is no record of a catastrophic diving SCI from impact with the bottom in a diving area that meets the competitive diving organization's facility dimensions recommendations. Yet, Richard Stone of Arthur D. Little calculated that depths of 20–22 feet deep under a 1 meter springboard would be needed to eliminate the risk of injury from potential head impact with the pool bottom. Such an over-built diving area design is considered impractical. Competitive facility dimensions followed for the Olympic Games do not even recommend that much depth under the 10 meter platform.

If all diving boards were removed or diving areas built 22 feet deep, the real reduction in catastrophic 'diving' SCI would amount to only 1.25% (5% occurring in the deep end times 25% occurring in pools). Ninety-nine percent of the 'diving' SCI victims would still have sustained catastrophic injury since these injuries occurred in the nondiving area of the pool and in the natural aquatic environment [16].

Removing competitive diving boards in supervised sites with excellent safety records is unwarranted. Although there is a risk of injury in any practically built diving area, the real risk statistically comes from diving into shallow water five feet deep or less. There is a more subtle aspect of user behavior that needs to be addressed to reduce the risk of shallow water diving injuries. Although learning to dive in shallow water may be safe for youngsters 4–8 years old, the risk of injury from head impact with the bottom increases as the child matures into an adult-sized body with increased height and weight. Facility users need to appreciate this increased risk and adjust their behavior accordingly.

Given the facts, removing shallow water, not diving boards, is the obvious solution. However eliminating shallow water, like eliminating diving boards, is a 'Catch 22' situation. Overall, 'diving' accounts for only eight percent (8%) of the risk for spas, pools and associated equipment. Drowning accounts for seventy-five percent (75%) of risk [17]. The shallow water cannot be removed to prevent 'diving' SCI without increasing the risk of drowning. Likewise, removing diving boards used by instructional, competitive and recreational programs eliminates programs with excellent safety records that teach safe water entry skills.

Appropriate supervision is a key factor in reducing the risk of injury. Providing appropriate supervision enables continual monitoring of user behavior. A classic 'diving' injury profile based on over 200 'diving' SCI that occurred in pools, presented by Milton Gabrielsen, Ph.D., at the 1984 National Pool and Spa Safety Conference, points to the lack of supervision as a prominent predisposing factor [18]:

- In 89% of the time the location of a spinal cord injury was a residential, motel, hotel or apartment pool.
- In 85% of the accident sites, no qualified lifeguard, instructor or coach was present.
- In 57% of the cases there was evidence the victim had consumed some form of alcoholic beverage, mostly beer.

These statistics identify diving in an unsupervised pool as one critical factor in the 'diving' SCI profile. One variable motel, hotel and apartment pools have in common with oceans, lakes, rivers, and quarries and aquatic sites where alcohol is not prohibited is that they are all likely to be unsupervised sites.

Although the annual number of catastrophic 'diving' SCI in swimming pools is relatively small given the U.S. population of about 238 million [19] (annual estimates for catastrophic diving SCI vary in range from 500 (63 quadriplegics year in pools—see White Paper on Diving Accident in the Appendix) to 713 [20] to 1,000 [21]), the devastation to quality of the victim's life, the rehabilitation and care costs are staggering. The total rehabilitation cost per case for the more severely injured 'diving' patient was a high average of $88,000 [22]. The costs of taking care of the quadriplegics from 'diving' accidents run somewhere in the area of six to eight hundred million dollars per year [23]. Despite the removal of diving boards throughout the country, these tragic 'diving' SCI persists. There is a need to accurately identify the problems as they relate to SCI in order to formulate appropriate solutions.

(Note: the 713 estimate for 'diving' spinal cord injuries was derived from the UAB-SCI-DMS national capture rate of 32 cases/million population incidence of SCI for all accident modes (238 × 32 = 7616; 7616 × 14.2% sports-related = 1082; 1082 × 66% 'diving' = 713)

Impact on Competitive Programs

Throughout the country, divers are having the diving boards taken out from under them. The big community pool, country club or resort pool with diving boards seems to be a thing of the past. Only 15.2% of nonresidential pools have diving boards of any kind [24]. Diving programs have been canceled in Parks and Recreation, YMCA, high school, club and local pools in Wisconsin, California, Connecticut, Rhode Island, Massachusetts, Ohio, Texas, and Washington. One mother of two prospective young divers wrote to express her concern. The local YMCA permanently removed the diving boards because the insurance company would no longer cover them. This concerned parent sent in a copy of an advertisement acknowledging Phillips Petroleum's sponsorship of U.S. Diving since 1979. The Phillips' ad declares, "We'll support them in the future, as well" [25]. Without the opportunity to be introduced to the sport on the local level, this mother inquired, "who will 'they' be and how many of them?" [26] Olympic gold medalist, Greg Louganis, agrees, "the sport of diving has the potential of becoming extinct" [27].

The removal of diving boards throughout this country comes at a crucial time for USD's future Olympic efforts. While the numbers of young Americans with access to diving boards is diminishing, the Chinese have developed a large base of young age group athletes from which to field their future Olympic teams. Up until now, the U.S.has dominated the sport of diving internationally. In fact, based on a recent study of medals available versus medals won in all sports, the U.S. has enjoyed its greatest Olympic success in competitive diving. The U.S. has won 45 of 70 gold medals and 121 of 210 total medals [28]. Yet, this increasing disparity in the talent pool will effect our ability to maintain our dominance in the international arena in the very near future.

The Liability Crisis

The problem is not simply limited to the issue of 'diving' safety, but is part of a greater liability crisis this country is now experiencing. "Over the years, courts have increasingly based liability 'more on the theory that the defendant has deep pockets or the insurance coverage to pay and not because they have really done anything wrong,' said Richard K. Willard, U.S. assistant attorney general and chairman of the Justic Department's Tort Policy Working Group" [29].

In response to diving coach Wayne Oras' letter to President Reagan regarding the liability problem facing diving programs, the office of the General Counsel of the U.S. Department of Commerce offered the following concluding remarks: "This Administration is committed to tort reform. We are actively working with all segments of our society and the Congress to bring about a solution to the liability problems" [30]

The economics (medical, actuarial, business) and judicial complexities of the liability issue will eventually be resolved at some future point in time by the U.S. Congress. Reform bills, which are hotly opposed by consumer advocate groups, are currently being considered. Ultimately, the cost of liability is absorbed by the consumer or organization participant [31].

References

[1] *Spinal Cord Injury: Facts and Figures,* 1986, Available from the National Spinal Cord Injury Statistical Center, SRC, Room 522, University Station, Birmingham, AL 35294, pp. 9 and 15.

[2] Ron O'Brien, Head Coach U.S. Olympic Diving Team 1972, '76, '80, '84, '88, '92 personal correspondence, (November 5, 1984).

[3] Martha Scotzin, New York Regional Spinal Cord Injury System, Rusk Institute of Rehabilitative Medicine, in proceedings of the *National Pool and Spa Safety Conference* (NPSSC), co-sponsored by the U.S. Consumer Product Safety Commission (CPSC) and the National Spa and Pool Institute (NSPI), Arlington, Virginia (May 14, 1985), p. 36.

[4] Annie Clement, "Current trends in aquatic litigation", Council for National Cooperation in Aquatics National Conference, Indianapolis, November 8–12, 1989.

[5] Milton Gabrielsen, Ph.D., Nova University, in the proceedings of the *National Pool and Spa Safety Conference,* p. 29.

[6] *Spinal Cord Injury: Facts and Figures,* pp. 9 & 15.

[7] Janet L. Gabriel, personal correspondence from J. Scott Richards, Ph.D., Professor, Director of Research, Rehabilitation Medicine, The University of Alabama at Birmingham, April 12, 1991.

[8] Stephen K. Campbell, *Flaws and Fallacies in Statistical Thinking,* Prentice-Hall, Inc., Englewood Cliffs, New Jersey, 1974, p. 99.

[9] Robert McG. Thomas, Jr. "Lineman for Lions is Paralyzed Below Chest", New York Times (November 20, 1991).

[10] Joseph S. Torg, M.D. and Joseph J. Vegso, M.S., A.T.C., "Head-smart for safety", *SportCare & Fitness* (September/October 1988), p. 38.

[11] Barbara E. Sorid, "The Demise of the Diving Board", The Philadelphia Inquirer (Neighbors section), July 19, 1989.

[12] Terrance Scanlon, Chairman Consumer Product Safety Commission, in the proceedings of the *National Pool and Spa Safety Conference,* p. 1.

[13] Stuart Statler, Commissioner of the U.S. Consumer Product Safety Commission, in the proceedings of the *National Pool and Spa Safety Conference,* p. 1.

[14] Con Ducy, Curtis Plastics, in the proceedings of the *National Pool and Spa Safety Conference,* p. 14.

[15] Dr. Steven Cavalier, Department of Pediatrics and Neonatology, Kaiser Permanente Foundation Hospital, in the proceedings of the *National Pool and Spa Safety Conference,* p. 12.

[16] Leif Zars, Executive Summary of the Arthur D. Little Diving Studies (May 3, 1982, provided courtesy of Lester Kowalsky, p. 3. (The ADL Studies are available as NSPF's "Detailed Diving Studies by Richard S. Stone of Arthur D. Little, Inc.", as a set of 10 studies, from NSPF, 10803 Gulfdale, Suite 300, San Antonio, TX 78216 (512) 525-1227)

[17] Gail E. McCarthy, Ph.D., P.E. and J. Neil Robinson, Ph.D., "Spa and Pool Safety: A Quantitative Risk Analysis", prepared for the National Spa and Pool Institute by Failure Analysis Associates (FaAA) (September 3, 1984), p. 1.

[18] Gabrielsen, pp. 28–29.

[19] *World Almanac,* Newspaper Enterprise Association, Inc., 1989.

[20] *Spinal Cord Injury: Facts and Figures,* p. 8.

[21] Martha Scotzin Shaver, "Data Collection Subcommittee Report for the National Swimming Pool Safety Committee, December, 1987.

[22] Scotzin, p. 36.

[23] John S. Young, Peter E. Burns, A. M. Bowen and Roberta McCutchen, "Spinal Cord Injury Statistics", Good Samaritan Medical Center.

[24] Bob Greene, "Diving Boards are Leaping to Oblivion", Chicago Tribune (April 18, 1989).

[25] Phillips Petroleum Advertisement, National Geographic (July, 1987).

[26] Carol L. Trippel, concerned parent, personal correspondence (November 15, 1987).

[27] Linda G. Green, "Blunting the Competitive Edge?" Pool & Spa News (February 8, 1988), pp. 74–76.

[28] United States Olympic Committee, correspondence to USD, 1991.

[29] Carolyn Lochhead, "All are Liable in Product Liability", Insight (February 15, 1988), p. 46.

[30] Douglas A. Riggs, Office of the General Counsel of the United States Department of Commerce, personal correspondence (April 10, 1986).

[31] Lochhead, p. 47.

Risk Factors

J. W. Thomas Byrd[1]

RISK FACTORS OF HEAD AND NECK INJURIES IN EQUESTRIAN ACTIVITIES

REFERENCE: Byrd, J. W. T., "Risk Factors of Head and Neck Injuries in Equestrian Activities," Head and Neck Injuries in Sports, ASTM STP 1229, Earl F. Hoerner, Ed., American Society for Testing and Materials, Philadelphia, 1994.

ABSTRACT: Equestrian activities represent a very heterogenous population. The risk of injury varies greatly among the various disciplines. Most injuries do not occur in organized competition but occur in the leisure, recreational or working environment.

Factors associated with mounted injuries include lack of adequate protective headgear and a significant incidence of ETOH intoxication. Unmounted cranial injuries usually occur from being kicked, reflecting the significance of exercising precaution at all times, even in unmounted situations.

Helmets that meet the ASTM standards have been found to significantly reduce head injuries. Protective vests, although popular, are unproven. A properly constructed vest may give some added protection from a direct blow but they will offer no protection from major spinal injuries.

KEY WORDS: Head, Neck, Injury, Equestrian, Horse

INTRODUCTION

There is very little scientific data to define precisely factors and parameters associated with head and neck injuries in the equestrian world. Other organized sports such as football have developed excellent registries for cataloging significant injuries and influencing factors. Unfortunately, these resources are much more fragmented in horseback riding.

Even at the advanced competitive levels, equestrian sports still represent a very heterogenous group. The demands upon the participants and the associated levels of risk vary greatly and each group has its own governing body. The likelihood of potential exposure to injury (falling) ranges from rare in Dressage to more likely in Steeplechasing and anticipated in Rodeo.

---

[1]Orthopaedic Surgeon, Southern Sports Medicine & Orthopaedic Center, 2021 Church Street, Nashville, TN   37203; Assistant Clinical Professor, Department of Orthopaedics and Rehabilitation, Vanderbilt University School of Medicine, Nashville, TN   37203

The individual governing bodies each take significant steps towards emphasizing rider safety. They are now expanding this to share information among the organizations in an effort to learn from each other. Much of this is occurring through the medium of the American Medical Equestrian Association whose sole purpose is emphasizing safe riding through injury prevention, education, rule changes and ongoing studies of protective equipment. As this networking evolves, greater appreciation of injury patterns and risks will be gained.

The impact of this cooperative effort among the governing bodies will still be somewhat limited due to the large numbers of participants who do not belong to any organization. These leisure or recreational participants make up the largest population of horseback riders. It is in this population that most of the injuries occur and, in fact, the risk of injury per exposure is probably higher than in the competitive arena.

For this large population of recreational equestrians, the greatest impact on injury prevention will probably occur through education. It is unlikely that regulation alone will significantly affect such a poorly defined group.

RISK FACTORS

The single most unique aspect that separates equestrian sports from other groups is that these are team sports comprised of individuals of different species. They are intimately dependent upon one another, both for success as well as safety. Both are also capable of making their own decisions, but the horse is usually the less predictable of the two. The horse also outweighs the human by between one and two thousand pounds.

Depending on the sport, these animals may achieve speeds of 35 to 40 miles an hour with the rider's head being carried approximately nine feet off the ground.

There is no such thing as a safe horse. Even a quiet animal may be spooked. In fact, placing undue confidence in a seemingly quiet horse may increase the risk of injury if one misinterprets this to mean that routine safety precautions are not necessary.

The risk of injury just from handling horses in an unmounted fashion is significant. In one physician's [1] experience of 83 central nervous system injuries (cranial and spinal), 22 (26.5%) occurred unmounted (all cranial).

In this series of 83 patients, there were 72 cranial injuries and 11 spinal cord injuries. Of these, seven were fatal. Of the 61 injuries that occurred mounted, only 22 (36.0%) were wearing helmets. All spinal cord injuries occurred from a fall. Of the 83, 23 (27.7%) were legally intoxicated with an ETOH level greater than 0.1. Also of the 83, only 20 (24.1%) occurred during some form of organized competition.

With regards to risk factors, this emphasizes a significant number of injuries (approximately one-quarter) occur unmounted. Of the individuals who were mounted, most were not wearing helmets. Alcohol was a significant factor in over one-quarter of the injuries, and less than one-quarter occurred during some form of organized competition.

BIOMECHANICS OF INJURY

Unmounted cranial injuries occur from a direct blow such as being kicked. Mounted cranial and spinal injuries result from the forces generated during a fall. These forces represent the summation of the speed of the animal and the height from which the fall occurs, both of which may be considerable. Added to this is the potential component of being trampled, dragged or kicked after falling.

In racing, the rider leans forward over the shoulders of the horse and his head becomes the leading part of his body. As the rider falls, he tends to duck his head, curl up and roll. This helps dissipate the energy of the impact and also makes the rider a smaller target for the hoofs of other horses.

As a consequence, axial loading of the cervical spine is rarely a mechanism of injury. Most are pure flexion injuries and are more likely to be associated with significant neurological deficit. Extension injuries are less common, and when they occur, tend to be more stable.

Also relatively unique to equestrian sports is the flexion injury to the thoracolumbar spine. The incidence of neurological deficit is significant and the injury usually occurs from landing in the seated position.

PROTECTIVE EQUIPMENT

Helmets

The ASTM [2] has established excellent standards for the manufacture of equestrian helmets. Much thought went into the design features of these helmets.

Equestrian helmets need to be lightweight and comfortable. They must protect against penetrating injury and be round in shape to turn direct blows into glancing blows. The contour needs to be such that it protects the vulnerable areas of the skull without hindering mobility or obstructing vision. In addition to cushioning the brain, the helmet must have a harness assembly adequate enough to prevent the helmet from being dislodged during a fall.

Helmets meeting the current ASTM standards far exceed the quality of any helmet on the market prior to initiation of these standards in 1987. Although initial acceptance of these new designs was slow, it has gradually increased as their efficacy has been proven. The final hurtle to be surmounted is to assure proper fit and comfort for various shaped heads.

Protective Vests

Much attention has been given to protective vests and, in fact, their acceptance rate has been high. Despite their popularity, little scientific information is available to support their effectiveness.

Currently, there are no American standards for protective vests. The British Equestrian Trade Association (BETA) does have a standard that tests the impact protection of vest materials but does not address the issue of vest design.

It seems apparent that a properly constructed vest will give some added protection to lessen the severity of injury from a direct blow to the thorax such as would be expected from a contusion or possibly even a cracked rib.

However, it seems equally apparent that protective vests will offer no protection from major spinal injuries. In fact, a poorly constructed, overly rigid vest could potentially heighten the likelihood of a major spinal injury.

CONCLUSIONS

The equestrian world is a very heterogenous bunch. With few exceptions, there is very little hard scientific data to define accurately the risks of head and neck injuries.

However, several glaring factors do stand out. One of these is the importance of approved, fitted and secured protective head gear in all mounted situations and the need for caution even in unmounted encounters with horses. Another is the role of alcohol in a significant number of severe equestrian injuries.

Most injuries do not occur in the competitive arena, but occur in the leisure, recreational or "working" environment. This area is especially difficult to regulate and again emphasizes the importance of education as a part of injury prevention.

The sparsity of data emphasizes our need to generate data collection and structure scientific studies to provide better education and awareness in the equestrian community.

REFERENCES

[1]   Brooks, William H., M.D., Neurosurgical Associates, 1401 Harrodsburg Road, Suite B485, Lexington, KY   40504.

[2]   American Society for Testing and Materials, 1916 Race Street, Philadelphia, PA   19103 - Designation F1163-88.

onald R. Gilbert[1]

UNIFORM MINIMUM SAFE DIVING DEPTH FOR SWIMMING FACILITIES

EFERENCE: Gilbert, Ronald R., **"A Uniform Minimum Safe Diving
epth for Swimming Facilities,"** Head and Neck Injuries in Sports,
STM STP 1229, Dr. Earl Hoerner, Ed., American Society for
esting and Materials, Philadelphia, 1994.

BSTRACT: Sports medicine physicians have estimated as many as
800 spinal cord injuries from "shallow water" diving annually
n our country. These injuries are devastating (usually high
ervical injuries) resulting in quadriplegia. This high number
f injuries is unacceptable and preventable. It is preventable
y establishing a minimum safe diving depth in all bodies of
ater of 5 feet. The minimum depth of 5 feet has been recognized
y a number of state public health codes and has been
tatistically documented by research and studies done by Dr.
ilton Gabrielsen through Nova University. The establishment of
 minimum safe diving depth is a "passive" safety system which
romises to greatly reduce and eliminate the tragedy, economic
oss, litigation resulting from the spinal cord injuries, and
lso result in millions of dollars of savings of medical care and
osts for these tragic quadriplegic victims. In addition to a
umber of state public health codes, the American Red Cross and
he Aquatic Injury Safety Group have advocated a minimum diving
epth of 5 feet for many years. The establishment of a minimum
afe diving depth of 5 feet does not eliminate diving, but rather
romotes **safe diving**.

YWORDS: diving, 5 feet, starting blocks, minimum depth, neck
         injury, quadriplegic, spinal cord injury, shallow
         water

"The greatest danger in diving is hitting the
bottom with the head. It is the self-taught
diver who is most prone to this sort of
accident. *** He is in danger because he is
unaware of danger."[1]

"More quadriplegics result each year from the
head first entry into water than all other

[1]Chairman, Foundation for Spinal Cord Injury Prevention,
46 Penobscot Building, Detroit, Michigan 48226

sports combined. That grim reality requires
action which combines education, communication
and regulation to all who use water."[2]

The above quotes highlight the purpose of this article which
is to advocate a uniform and accepted minimum safe diving depth
for the one hundred million recreational swimmers in our country
Physicians in the Sports Medicine area have estimated that
as high as 1 800 spinal cord injuries (nearly all cervical) occur
annually as a result of diving injuries.[3]   This statistic is
not only unacceptable, but also unnecessary.
In the course of the paper, I will explain the reasons for
accepting a uniform minimum depth.   I also will review the
literature which supports this view. At the present time, there
are only two groups that have advocated and endorsed a minimum
safe diving depth. For the first time in 1985 the American Red
Cross came out in their publications advocating diving in no less
than 5 feet of water.[4]   In the same year, the Aquatic Injury
Safety Group began advocating the same with its publications.
Unfortunately since that time, there's been nothing but confusion
as to what the minimum safe diving depth is for the hundred
million recreational swimmers in our country. By establishing a
uniform, minimum safe diving depth for the average recreational
swimmer, we can:
1.   Decrease the human tragedy associated with head and
neck injuries;
2.   Increase the saving of lives;
3.   Decrease litigation.
These are the ultimate goals and purposes of this article.
The 5 foot minimum diving depth which has been adopted and
recommended by the American Red Cross and the Aquatic Injury
Safety Group has a foundation based both on statistical evidence
as well as common experience. For example, Dr. Milton
Gabrielsen's statistics demonstrate that 89% of shallow water
dives resulting in spinal cord injury occurred in water of 5 feet
or less.[5]   This is a significant figure which could eliminate
most diving quadriplegics each year.
In 1984, a somewhat publicized meeting of a number of
aquatic safety experts from the swimming pool industry met and
endorsed the 5 foot depth. However, it was never publicly or
officially adopted or accepted.
On the other hand, a number of public health departments
throughout the United States have already adopted and
incorporated into state law, the minimum safe diving depth of 5
feet.[6]
In addition, the 5 foot depth is reasonable at this point in
time and accommodates safe diving in most multi-use pools in the
country without the need for reconstruction of pools. There are
very few pools in the United States which do not have areas which
are 5 feet in depth. However, all types of diving must be
prohibited in any pool that has a depth of less than 5 feet.
Safe pools must be promoted with safe diving areas
supervised by knowledgeable lifeguards who enforce these safe
diving areas.

One of the aquatic myths in our country is that young
people, ages 4 to 8, are taught to dive into shallow water less
than 5 feet deep. Statistics by NEISS and Gabrielsen demonstrate
shallow water diving (5 feet or less) is safe at ages 4-8. The
youngest reported shallow water diving quadriplegic is age 9.[7]
The myth is that these young people can continue diving into that
depth because they have done so safely in the past. As they
become older, 13, 14, etc., they are not aware of the fact a
rather serious and dangerous risk faces them each time they dive.
They become familiar and comfortable with the idea that they
themselves have dove hundreds and perhaps thousands of times into
3 or 4 feet of water safely. In fact, they often are oblivious
to the idea that they could possibly hurt themselves by diving
into less than 5 feet of water.
Tragic and unfortunate evidence of approximately 30 diving
quadriplegics occurring from diving off starting blocks into 3 to
4 feet of water proves that even the most experienced diver and
swimmer can end up being quadriplegic by diving into less than 5
feet of water.[8] The 30 diving quadriplegics were certainly
experienced swimmers and divers. If it can happen to them, it
can happen to anyone, especially less skilled individuals,
recreational swimmers. The way to avoid injury is to avoid
diving into less than 5 feet of water. The U.S. Swim Association
has acknowledged this fact by advocating the moving of starting
blocks into deeper water, 4 1/2 feet.[9] This author does not
feel that 4 1/2 feet is deep enough. At least it's better to
move the starting blocks into 4 1/2 feet of water than not to
move them at all!
Further evidence of the problem of people diving to a "false
sense of security" is the well known speech given by Robert
Weiner, a noted aquatic person, at the 1984 Worldwater Park
Association meeting.[10] Mr. Weiner indicated at that time that
even if there were a no diving sign, people would go ahead and
dive into 3 feet of water because of the fact that they had dove
before themselves, and also because they've seen others dive into
3 feet of water and not be injured. We all know that this is not
safe practice and "diving by example" must be stopped. The
only way to stop it is to have a minimum uniform depth, 5 feet to
stop all diving by all persons of any age into less than 5 feet
of water. Coaches and instructors and other aquatic safety
personnel must be trained to educate and train all the young
people from the very first day they start to swim and dive that
it is not safe to ever dive into less than 5 feet of water.
Furthermore, they must train and educate these young people the
reason why it is not safe to dive into 5 feet of water or less.
They must train these persons to carry the message to others.
With many of the prevention programs that I have worked with, it
would be recommended to have a quadriplegic sitting in a
wheelchair come out and participate in some of these training and
education sessions to emphasize the seriousness as well as the
reality of what can happen by diving into less than 5 feet of
water.
Another reason that a minimum safe diving depth needs to be
adopted immediately and endorsed by all the aquatic safety groups

is the tremendous confusion that has occurred since 1982 when the A.D. Little, Richard Stone, and the National Spa and Pool Institute and National Spa and Pool Foundation studies came out recommending "steering up". To this author, "steering up" is more of a myth than a fact and it is therefore difficult for me to define what "steering up" means. However, in the Swimming Pool Industry literature, they show an individual making what appears to be a shallow dive into deep water. Part of the myth is that this document showing this type of dive is circulated to people who purchase the several hundred thousand above ground pools sold each year, as well as inground pools. Apparently, "steering up" is meant to be some type of manoeuvre using the hands and back and other parts of the anatomy to avoid hitting the bottom. This author submits that the average recreational swimmer is unable to comprehend and understand and execute the "steering up" principle in a manner so as to avoid hitting the bottom and suffering injury. As indicated by Gabrielsen's research and interviews with over 300 quadriplegics from diving accidents, as well as interviews with over 100 quadriplegics from diving accidents by this author, every diver was totally unaware of the danger or believed that he could do a "shallow dive" which would not involve hitting the bottom. The fact that nearly 1 000 quadriplegics each year are created by diving, proves the fact that the average recreational diver is not able to control his dive nor "steer up".[11]

Further confusion and myth surrounds "steering up" when swimming pool industry people who created this "myth" are asked to define what a minimum safe depth of water is for "steering up". Dr. Stone who appears to be the author of "Steering Up" indicates 18 inches is safe for himself to dive into and furthermore that 2' 9" is safe for the average recreational swimmer. However, Dr. Stone further indicates that the average recreational swimmer can safely dive into 2' 9" of water with "steering up" or without "steering up".[12]

In deposition after deposition, industry people have consistently testified that the diagram of "steering up" shows diving into 1 1/2 feet of water. We go back to the diving by example propounded by Robert Weiner and if we show pictures of people diving safety into 1 1/2 feet of water, why should they not dive into shallow above ground pools and other shallow bodies of water? Furthermore, the "Sensible Way to Enjoy Your Pool", continuously uses the word "shallow water" but never once defines it. The industry recently admitted in response to several questions that were raised, that the industry itself does not know what the depth of "shallow water" is or should be. Specifically, this question was responded to by the NSPI representative at the CPSC meeting in Phoenix, Arizona on September 19, 1988. Certainly, if the industry and representatives of the industry do not know what shallow water is, how can the one hundred million recreational swimmers know? At that same meeting, a pool dealer, who sells pools in the Phoenix areas, was asked what shallow water meant to him. He indicated 2 feet. In other words, he felt that it was okay to dive into water 2' 1" deep.

Unfortunately, this is not an isolated incident. The director of beach safety at an east coast beach, who is a certified Red Cross lifeguard and director of beach safety for 8 years, recently testified under oath that he saw nothing wrong with diving into as shallow as **two inches** of water, at least for himself.[13] Whether that is correct or not, the problem is that we go back to the diving by example where other people see him doing this type of behavior and believe that they can do it too, only hey do not know that they cannot do it safely. Likewise, a judge who lives on the east coast, recently indicated that he had been body surfing and diving into the waves consisting of 3 feet of water or less all of his life and that he saw nothing wrong with it. Again, when confronted with questions, he admitted that he had not taken into account the fact that there might be people from the midwest come to his beaches and see him do it, not knowing that it cannot be done safely by all persons. In all of these examples, we have one common theme. The common theme is that there are many people who are experienced, who apparently, believe that they can safely dive into less than 5 feet of water and they go ahead and do it anyway and, in the meantime, lead others to do it. By adopting a minimum safe diving depth, all of these problems and temptations and examples will be eliminated.

Along these same lines, as far as training and supervision is concerned, there is deposition testimony after deposition testimony, all under oath, by lifeguards throughout the United States indicating they constantly see people diving into 3 or 4 feet of water and do nothing to warn these people to stop, nor to prohibit them from doing so by threatening to remove them from the pool.[14] While there are isolated instances where lifeguards do warn people, the all too common experience is that our lifeguards allow people to continue to dive into shallow water. If we have a uniform minimum safe diving depth, and our lifeguards are taught to enforce it, we will again remove this problem and this risk and substantially reduce the number of living quadriplegics each year in our country.

If the true immensity of this problem is not obvious to everyone, we should keep in mind the fact that there are over five million backyard residential pools in our country today. There also are between three and four hundred thousand new ones being sold and installed each year.[15] This does not even take into account the open bodies of water, as well as the commercial and public and semi-public pools. If this is not enough to indicate the immensity of the potential risk problem, certainly, we must take into account the findings of the Consumer Product Safety Commission and Regional Spinal Cord Reporting Centers in their recent reports and studies as to the cost of these tragic accidents.[16] According to recent reports by the National Spinal Cord Injury Association, as well as the Consumer Product Safety Commission, the cost of taking care of the quadriplegics from diving accidents run somewhere in the area of six to eight hundred million dollars per year.[17] Certainly, if we could contribute just one percent of that amount of money toward education and training of the above principles, the payback would be well worth the effort. Sober recognition must be given to the fact that we need an immediate solution to the problem. The most immediate and feasible solution is to adopt a minimum uniform safe diving depth.

Perhaps someone reading this article may question how do we know that it will work? Will it work? There is a firm proof of the fact that this system will work. The Feet First--First Time (now called THINK FIRST) program out of northern Florida, has resulted in a 40% reduction of spinal cord injury from diving accidents over 4 years it has been in existence.[18] Although this program does not specifically endorse a minimum safe diving depth, the principle is similar since people are taught to go into the water feet first, instead of head first, regardless of the depth of the water. It is my belief that, while feet first entry is a good principle, diving in our country should not be banned. I have never advocated, as an individual or aquatic safety advocate, banning of diving. Therefore, I believe the alternative and equally workable solution is to come up with a minimum safe diving depth.

CONCLUSION

The goal of this article is to stimulate those who are reading this article, as well as other groups to whom this article will be circulated, to adopt and endorse a uniform minimum safe diving depth. Furthermore, an additional goal is to see that every aquatic facility, swim club and all aquatic environment participants, are trained and educated not to dive in any water less than 5 feet deep under any circumstances. If this program is adopted by every aquatic facility in our country and enforced the way it ought to be, I am certain that, within the next 3 years, we will see a substantial reduction in the number of diving quadriplegics in our country, perhaps even greater than the 40% reduction through the Feet First--First Time (now called THINK FIRST) program.

REFERENCES

[1]   Rackman, G., "Diving Complete" (Faber and Faber, Ltd., 1975), 39.

[2]   Gabrielsen, M. Alexander, Ph.D., "Diving Injury Parameters and Prevention", presented at the National Safety Congress Seminar on Diving Injuries: Mechanics & Prevention, on October 16, 1983, Chicago, Illinois. Gabrielsen is the author of Swimming Pools: A Guide to their Planning, Design and Operation, a project of the Council for National Cooperation in Aquatics.

[3]   Torg, Joseph S., "Epidemiology, pathomechanics, and prevention of athletic injuries to the cervical spine", Medicine and Science in Sports and Exercise, Vol. 17, No. 3, 1985

[4]   American Red Cross, Swimming and Aquatics Safety, 5 foot
      diving depth, 1985.

[5]   Gabrielsen, M. Alexander, Ph.D., "Case studies of Spinal
      Cord Injury Victims Who Were Injured as a Result of Diving
      or Sliding Into Swimming Pools", May, 1985.

[6]   Illinois, Michigan, Ohio, Iowa, New Jersey, Minnesota,
      Pennsylvania. California (6 feet) and New York (8 feet
      effective 1992). (New York beginning October 7, 1992
      requires starting blocks to be placed in at least 6 feet of
      water)

[7]   Gabrielsen, M. Alexander, Ph.D., "Etiology of Diving
      Injuries". Conference sponsored by Consumer Product Safety
      Commission, May 19-20, 1988.

[8]   Gabrielsen, M. Alexander, Ph.D., and Shulman, Stanley M.,
      M.A., Spivey, Mary, RRA and Sprain, Michael, BBA, "Starting
      Blocks: The Etiology of 30 Spinal Cord Injuries As a Result
      of Dives Made from Starting Blocks with Recommendations",
      February, 1992.

[9]   Counsilman, James E., Counsilman, Brian E., Nomura, Takeo,
      and Endo, Motohiro, Starts and Turns, "Three Types of Grab
      Start for Competitive Swimming", 1987.

      Welch, John H., and Owens, Virginia L., Ph.D, "Water Depth
      Requirements of Competitive Racing Starts", J. Swimming
      Research, Vol. 2, No. 3 (1986).

[10] Weiner, Robert, "Safety and Informational Systems in
      Waterparks", 1984 World Water Park Symposium.

[11] Shaver-Scotzin, Martha, "Data Collection Subcommittee Report
      for the National Swimming Pool Safety Committee", 1987. (For
      the fact that there are nearly 1 000 quadriplegic diving
      injuries per year).

[12] Stone, Richard and Little Arthur D., "Diving Safety in
      Swimming Pools". A Report to the National Swimming Pool
      Foundation, May 15, 1980.

      Stone, Richard deposition testimony, Rodriguez v S.R. Smith,
      Inc., et al, Case No. 86-2-01447-0, Superior Court of the
      State of Washington, In and For the County of Yakima;
      January 3, 1989.

[13] Dean, Robert Edgar, Jr. deposition testimony, Whalen v Town
      of Bethany Beach, et al, U.S. District Court for the
      District of Delaware, C.A. No. 86-405-JLL.

[14] Egstrom, Glen deposition testimony, Gifford v Coleco
      Industries, Inc., In the Circuit Court for the Tenth

Judicial Circuit of Illinois, Peoria County, Case No. 84-L-568; August 5, 1988.

Egstrom, Glen deposition testimony, <u>Riech v Hoffinger Industries, Inc.</u>, In the Circuit Court of the Seventh Judicial Circuit Sangamon County, Illinois, Case No. 86-L-462, February 9, 1989.

[15] 1986 Swimming Pool and Spa Industry Survey Report by NSPI. From 1986 there were 2.69 million inground pools and 2.269 million above ground pools and combine sales for $387,000. Projecting this to January, 1989, there are well over 5 million swimming pools.

[16] Young, John S., Burns, Peter E., Bowen, A. M., and McCutchen, Roberta, "<u>Spinal Cord Injury Statistics</u>", Good Samaritan Medical Center, Phoenix, Arizona.

Stover, S. L., M.D., Fine, P. R., Ph.D, M.S.P.H., "<u>Spinal Cord Injury, The Facts & Figures</u>", The University of Alabama, Birmingham, Alabama.

[17] Young, John S., Burns, Peter E., Bowen, A. M., and McCutchen, Roberta, "<u>Spinal Cord Injury Statistics</u>", Good Samaritan Medical Center, Phoenix, Arizona.

Stover, S. L., M.D., Fine, P. R., Ph.D, M.S.P.H., "<u>Spinal Cord Injury, The Facts & Figures</u>", The University of Alabama, Birmingham, Alabama.

[18] Feet First--First Time, (now called THINK FIRST) Sponsored by the Congress of Neurological Surgeons (statistical data over a 3 year period indicate 40% drop in spinal cord injuries from diving in Northern Florida).

Felice M. Duffy[1]

PSYCHOLOGICAL CHARACTERISTICS OF THE CHRONICALLY INJURED ATHLETE

REFERENCE: Duffy, F. M., "Psychological Characteristics of the Chronically Injured Athlete," Head and Neck Injuries in Sports, ASTM STP 1229, Earl F. Hoerner, Ed., American Society for Testing and Materials, Philadelphia, 1994.

ABSTRACT: The helpseeking literature is used to provide a theoretical framework from which to study athletic injuries. The literature suggests that athletes possess specific characteristics (high self-esteem, high need to achieve, internal locus of control, masculine sex-role orientation, independence) which highlight the negative aspects of seeking and receiving aid and athletes performing at a higher competitive level have a higher degree of these characteristics. In addition, the literature supports that people with these characteristics perceive seeking and receiving help as very threatening. It is hypothesized that this threat is manifested by the following: a) delay in seeking help; b) less use of help; c) more self help; d) non-compliance; and e) a high rate of drop out in rehabilitation. It is also hypothesized that these behaviors create an injury-prone athlete.

KEYWORDS: sports psychology, helpseeking, athletic injury, self-esteem, locus of control, sex orientation, achievement motivation, social psychology, sports medicine

---

INTRODUCTION

There is an overwhelming number of athletic injuries occurring at all levels of competition [1, 2]. Despite advances in fitness and conditioning, rule changes and improved equipment design, the injury rate continues to increase [3, 4]. Physical characteristics have long been examined as etiological factors in athletic injury. Physical characteristics as risk factors in athletic injuries are not useful in predicting injuries [3, 4].

Only recently has the role psychology plays in the injury process been investigated to any extent. The role of psychology has been approached from three perspectives. The role of life stress and the frequency of injury has received the majority of attention [5, 6]. The study of personality and motivational factors and their role in the injury process has received some attention [7, 8]. The third area is devoted to the role of psychological factors and situational predictors of adherence to treatment and compliance with athletic rehabilitation [9, 10].

---

[1]Head Coach, Athletic Department, Yale University, New Haven, CT 06520

The empirical findings in these three areas on the role of psychological aspects as etiological factors in athletic injuries provide scattered and inconsistent results. A major reason for the inconsistencies appears to be the lack of a theoretical model to guide the studies or interpret the results. The majority of studies claim there is a significant void in the literature. The need for theoretically grounded empirical work on the different mechanisms operating specially with regard to athletic injuries is stressed [1, 5, 8, 9 , 11, 12].

Introduced in this paper is an empirically-based theoretical model which may help explain the rising athletic injury rate from a psychological perspective.

Gross and McMullen's helpseeking model [13] is applied to create a model of helpseeking for athletic injuries. Based on Fisher's Threat to Self-Esteem Theory [14], it is suggested that psychological characteristics of the athlete could be a significant etiological contributor to the ever increasing number of athletic injuries. These characteristics interfere in the helpseeking process at various stages and actually create a chronically injured athlete.

REVIEW OF LITERATURE

Physical Etiology

As early as 1905, athletic injuries were serious enough for President Roosevelt to consider banning football from the United States. A series of rule changes in 1906 dramatically improved the safety of the game [3]. Many rule changes in sports in the last twenty years have been implemented to help offset the injury rate. The mandatory use of face masks in junior ice hockey levels was accepted and adopted in 1976 [15]. Spearing and crackback blocking in football has recently been eliminated. The prohibition of high sticking in ice hockey and field hockey and tackling from behind in soccer, are examples of hundreds of rule changes which have been executed to improve the safety of the sport [3].

Rule changes have led to improvements in the safety of the sport and prevention of sports injuries. For example, the elimination of spearing in football directly reduced severe head and neck injuries and the elimination of crackback blocking directly reduced knee injuries [3].

Despite this strategy, the volume of sports injuries is increasing 8% a year [3]. It is suggested that rule changes of one sort promote infractions of another sort which lead to different injuries [4].

Many attempts have been made to connect various physical variables to athletic injuries. This is typically done by trying to predict injury using results from studies which describe the epidemiological basis of athletic injury. Although many injuries are attributed to physical reasons (i.e., physical characteristics of the athlete, equipment, playing surfaces, etc.), they have been useless in predicting injury. There is too much interpersonal and situational variability to produce consistent results [4]. For example, artificial turf has long been suggested to produce more injuries. However, the overall injury rate for football due to playing surface is not affected by the type of surface [16]. Artificial turf may affect the type and severity of injury, but it does not affect the overall injury rate [4].

Equipment has been suggested as an etiological factor. Once again, equipment is found to be a cause for injury but is not able to

predict injury [17]. While use of mouthpieces show a marked improvement
in lowering dental injuries and contusions [3, 4], they do not seemingly
affect the overall rate of injury in any one sport [1]. The transition
to soft flexible helmets in ice hockey shows a 50% reduction in the rate
of serious injury [18], but this has not improved the injury rate in ice
hockey [1]. Vinger and Hoerner [4] provide an editorial comment which
examines the "trade-offs" in protective equipment. They suggest that by
fulfilling one need for protection, another may be created. For
example, energy absorbing material is necessary to bring the energy of a
blow to a stop before reaching the head. This material is of value for
reducing the impact of a blow, but, unfortunately, it increases the
degree and incidence of cerebral concussion. Helmets obviously reduce
the injury rates in football, ice hockey and lacrosse and are being
mandated in youth hockey leagues [19]. However, the force that a ridge
or edge of a helmet can impose on the neck could be tremendous. Studies
show that contact in these helmet edges in football generally occur at
the seventh cervical vertebrae, while in hockey it occurs at the sixth.
A force in this area of a magnitude, which would be entirely possible
from a mechanical viewpoint, could result in a broken neck. Another
problem with the elevation of the back rims in football and ice hockey
helmets is that the occipital area and upper cervical regions are
exposed to energy absorption when struck and are now more vulnerable
areas for future injuries [4]. These are some examples of trade-offs
with equipment changes in an effort to reduce injuries that actually
create different injuries. This is one explanation of why the injury
rate continues to increase despite improvements in the design and the
safety of equipment.

Inappropriate physical conditioning has been considered as an
etiological factor in athletic injuries. There are no consistent
results which show improved physical conditioning decreasing the injury
rate [1, 3, 20]. One study on football shows a reduction in the
severity of knee injuries when the players are put through a rigorous
physical conditioning program [21]. Research on racquetball injuries
suggests a high level of fitness and a pre-warm-up as good preventive
measures, although there are no supportive statistics to show a
reduction in injuries or injury rate [1]. A study conducted on soccer
players finds a reduction in traumatic injuries with increased training,
but the overuse and minor injuries remain constant [22]. Vinger and
Hoerner's [4] explanation of compensatory injuries is applicable in
relation to physical conditioning program. They suggest that some
injuries may be eliminated due to higher levels of fitness. However,
this may be compensated for by overuse, overtraining, and may make the
body more susceptible to other types of injury.

Although there are a number of physical characteristics of the
athlete that are suggested as risk factors for injury (i.e., tight
hamstrings, overpronated feet, muscle strength imbalance) they are not
useful in predicting injuries [3, 4, 20, 23]. No correlation is found
between muscle tightness and past injuries in soccer players [24]. There
are no data or physical measures which can identify boxers at risk, or
predict injury despite the extensive research on boxing injuries [1].
No physical patterns of injuries in wrestlers are detected [1].
Although joint stability and muscle tightness account for about twenty
percent of the injuries in one study [24], these factors are not useful
for further prediction of athletic injury [22].

On the whole, research suggests that searching for etiological
factors and then employing ways of preventing injuries from a
physiological/technical perspective has not produced a decrease in the
overall injury rate in athletics.

Psychological Etiology

Since 1965, little attention has been paid to the psychological aspects of athletic injuries. Crossman and Jamieson [8] note that medical personnel observe a lack of correlation between an athlete's response to an injury and the seriousness of the injury. These authors suggest that underlying psychological factors account for this discrepancy and need to be studied. Weiss and Troxel [10] found that athletes apparently separate into those who heal appropriately and those who linger in a chronically injured state. The distinct grouping is attributed to psychological factors particularly when this grouping occurs with the same injuries and the same treatments across groups. Rotella [25] a sport psychologist, also notes that some athletes appear to be more "injury-prone" than others and suggests it may be due to physical and/or emotional problems.

These noted differences between athletes are provocative and are not easily explained. These findings suggest that psychology may play a role in athletic injuries.

The literature on the role of psychology as an etiological factor in athletic injuries is classified in three groups. The social-psychological factors related to life stress and injury frequency among athletes comprises the majority of the literature [5, 6, 11, 26-28]. This approach is derived from the demonstrated relationships from a number of studies between stressful life events and illness [29-31]. Relatively little research has been done in this area.

The second area of psychological research on athletic injuries involves the study of personality and motivational factors, as they may account for the high observed rate of athletic injury. Four studies differentiate between injured and non-injured athletes on the basis of personality and motivational characteristics [32-35].

This scattered approach to personality factors as etiological factors in athletic injury is not only lacking in studies, but is clearly lacking in a theoretical foundation to guide the research.

The third area of psychology and its relation to athletic injury examines the role of psychological factors and situational predictors of adherence to treatment or compliance, as well as coping with athletic injury rehabilitation. There has been very little research in this area, despite the fact that this may offer an etiological explanation for part of the high level of athletic injury. Rehabilitation is critical to returning an athlete back to competition [3, 4, 9]. Inappropriate or incomplete rehabilitation may extend the original injury or make one very susceptible to re-injury [3, 22]. In a variety of medical regimens, forty to sixty-five percent of the patients drop out [36] and indeed, athletic trainers do report a problem of non-adherence to treatment protocols [10, 37].

These studies on the psychological aspects as etiological factors in athletic injury provide scattered and inconsistent results. The wide variety of methods used, particularly with regard to the psychological measures, definition of injury, the levels of competition and the subjects, may have contributed to the diversified results. However, it appears that a major reason for inconsistency is the lack of theoretical model to guide the studies or explain the results. The majority of the studies claim a significant void in the literature and stress the need for theoretically based empirical research on the different psychological mechanisms operating specifically with regard to athletic injuries [1, 5, 8, 9, 11, 12].

One area that has not been investigated with regard to athletic injury is the social psychological area of helpseeking. There are some

very interesting parallels in the research on helpseeking and the
athlete's response. These parallels may present the theoretical
framework that may be useful in explaining part of the complex injury
process. Interestingly, one of the reasons suggested for the high
injury rate with athletes is the underutilization of the health
professional [2, 20].

Several studies examine athletes and helpseeking behavior [38-42].
These studies show that athletes seek less help, have a more negative
view of emotional disturbance and are derogated more for seeking
psychological help when compared to their non-athletic counterparts.
Although the helpseeking task used in these studies is of a
psychological nature, it does suggest that athletes have different
mechanisms operating with regard to helpseeking than non-athletes.

This difference may have a significant effect on the injury
process. Some general factors may be identified in the helpseeking
literature which may affect the entire injury process, including
response to injury, helpseeking, and rehabilitation. A comprehensive
theoretical model derived from the helpseeking literature can be found.
Not only does it provide a comprehensive framework through which to view
athletic injuries, of all levels of severity, but also explains many of
the results of the earlier studies.

Theory—Threat to Self-Esteem

The formalized Theory to Self-Esteem Theory was proposed by Fisher
and Nadler in 1983. It is the first theory designed specifically to
account for reactions to help (See Figure 1). This theory is the most
comprehensive theory to date and is capable of predicting reactions to
aid most accurately across diverse aid contexts (For complete discussion
see Fisher et al [43]). The scope of this theory subsumes and extends
beyond prediction of earlier theoretical formulations used in predicting
recipients reactions to aid (i.e., Reactance theory [44]; The Theory of
External Attribution [45]; Attribution Theory [46, 47]; Indebtedness
Theory [48, 49]; and Equity Theories [50-53].

This theoretical approach assumes that the self-related
consequences of aid are the most important factors in determining
recipients reactions to aid [43]. In situations where the self
consequences of receiving aid are non-salient or of minimal importance
other conceptual approaches may be more appropriate (for discussion, see
Fisher et al.[43]). But, in instances where the receipt of aid affects
the recipient's self-esteem, this approach is the most comprehensive.
It is broader and clearer than any other, simplest in its explanation
and it is empirically supported (for complete review and discussion, see
Fisher et al.[43]).

The formalized threat to self-esteem theory predicts when aid will
be self-threatening or self-supportive. It specifies the relationship
between the self-implications of help and other reactions to help
(Fisher et al., [43]). The theory is based on five hypothesis, as
presented by Fisher et al.[43]) (See Figure 1).

Hypothesis 1). Most aid situations are both supportive and
threatening. The self-relevant messages contained in the aid itself will
be factors. The aid will be self-supportive or self-threatening
depending upon the extent to which those messages are positive or
negative. Values instilled during socialization will have an impact on
the supportive or threatening aspect of the aid. To the extent that aid
is consistent with these internalized social values, it will be self-
supportive and to the extent that it conflicts with them, it will be

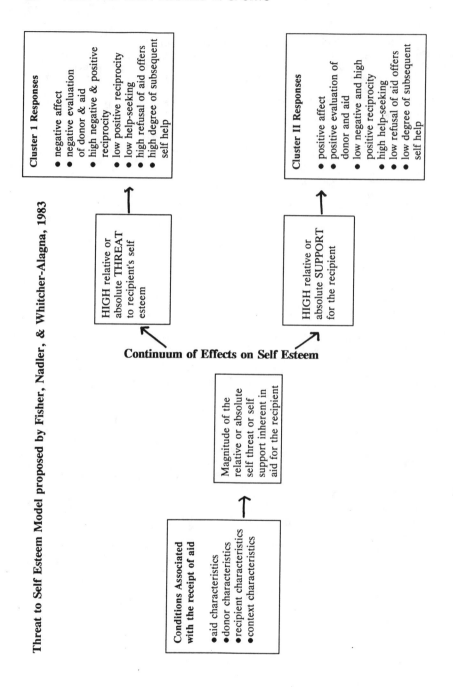

Threat to Self Esteem Model proposed by Fisher, Nadler, & Whitcher-Alagna, 1983

Cluster 1 Responses

- negative affect
- negative evaluation of donor & aid
- high negative & positive reciprocity
- low positive reciprocity
- low help-seeking
- high refusal of aid offers
- high degree of subsequent self help

Cluster II Responses

- positive affect
- positive evaluation of donor and aid
- low negative and high positive reciprocity
- high help-seeking
- low refusal of aid offers
- low degree of subsequent self help

HIGH relative or absolute THREAT to recipient's self esteem

HIGH relative or absolute SUPPORT for the recipient

Continuum of Effects on Self Esteem

Magnitude of the relative or absolute self threat or self support inherent in aid for the recipient

Conditions Associated with the receipt of aid

- aid characteristics
- donor characteristics
- recipient characteristics
- context characteristics

self-threatening. The inherent instrumental qualities of help will also determine the relative weights of self-threat and self-support.

Hypothesis 2). The situational conditions and the recipient's characteristics will determine the relative weights of self-support or self-threat. These variables determine whether the aid experience contains a favorable or unfavorable self-relevant message, the consistency or inconsistency with socialized values, and whether it meets one's needs or not. The relative weights of the self-relevant messages, socialized norms and the instrumental qualities will be determined by the recipient's characteristics and the situational conditions. Aid, therefore, will be threatening to the extent that the overall aid-related condition and recipient's characteristics highlight the aspects of aid that elicit self-threat relative to the aspects that elicit support and conversely with supportive aid.

Hypothesis 3). The self-supportive or self-threatening aspects of aid will determine the recipient's reactions to aid if all else is equal.

Hypothesis 4). The elements of self-threat and self-support are the intervening constructs which mediate the aid-related situational condition and recipient's characteristics and the recipient's reactions to aid.

Hypothesis 5). The self-supportive or self-threatening nature of the aid will determine the intensity of Cluster 1 (negative reactions) and Cluster 2 (positive reactions) responses. Self-threatening help elicits negative reactions which include unfavorable self-perceptions (i.e., affect and self-evaluation) and unfavorable external perceptions (i.e., increased self-help efforts and unwillingness to seek or receive future help). These are negative, defensive responses which, according to this theory, reaffirm the recipient's feelings of power and control. Aid that is predominantly supportive elicits positive reactions which include favorable self-perceptions, favorable external perceptions, and nondefensive behavior (i.e., fewer self-help efforts; greater willingness to seek and receive help).

Nadler and Fisher [54] add perceived control to the model in an effort to refine it. Perceived control incorporates the coping response and accounts for how the initiation of self-help occurs. Four additional hypotheses were added to the theory.

1). Perceived control mediates the self-threat and behavioral response, depending on whether or not the recipient expects to have control over subsequent outcomes.

2). If control over subsequent outcomes is associated with self-threatening aid, it will elicit short term psychological distress (negative personal and external perceptions) and instrumental behavioral responses (high self-help and low helpseeking).

3). If a lack of control over subsequent outcomes is associated with self-threat following the receipt of aid, a cluster of negative responses are elicited. Instrumental behavioral responses are not expected, and the recipient will continue to rely on external sources of help. This will persist over time.

4). Situational conditions and chronic beliefs about one's ability to end dependency through the investment of effort determines the degree of causal control.

The Formalized Threat to Self-Esteem Theory is the theoretical foundation for this study. Based on the following literature, this theory is comprehensive and encompasses many of the factors involved in the complex process dealing with athletic injury. This theory should be able to be used as an explanatory basis for determining which athletes are most threatened by the helpseeking process for athletic injuries, which includes the injury itself and rehabilitation.

THE HELPSEEKING MODEL

Helpseeking is a complex process with several stages and multiple decision making points [55]. It is not a simple, clear cut, linear path but, rather "an extended series of events, attributions and decisions which may or may not culminate in helpseeking" [55]. It is often a more tortuous route than a simple step by step process.

There have been many helpseeking models proposed and some cover very specific populations in special situations, such as teaching, medical helpseeking and mental health models. The medical helpseeking model focuses on disease and serious, traumatic illnesses [13] and does not incorporate different levels of severity found in athletic injuries, particularly minor ones. Therefore, the following model was chosen for its general stages incorporating common elements of other models and its' broad coverage of the many aspects of helpseeking.

Gross and McMullen [13] collapsed many models into three general stages (see Figure 2). The first stage is the perception, definition and labeling of the problem or symptoms as a problem [43]. Mere recognition of the problem is not enough, it must be perceived as problematic or harmful. The problem must also be perceived as amenable to help [13]. This perception varies from individual to individual [56]. It is apparent that some important factors other than just the mere presence of some objective disorder intervene in this labeling process [57-59].

Stage two is the decision to seek help. Self-help is usually attempted before other help. It is then determined if the problem can be solved alone with sufficient time and effort. The determination of whether help is necessary or convenient involves subjective judgments and individual variations in temperament and values [13]. These function in the cost-benefit appraisal. Choices are made that involve the assessment of costs. If the problem is amenable to self-help, then the costs are appraised in terms of time and effort. The decision to seek outside help is based on individual, personal and sociocultural values [13, 43, 60, 61]. If a problem necessitates outside help, some of the physical costs of not seeking help would be continuation and possible worsening of the problem. The psychological costs of seeking outside help is an assessment of personal costs related to self-esteem and self-concept (which operate at a level of less than full awareness) and social costs associated with interpersonal relationships and perceptions of others (which are consciously considered) [13]. In all cases the costs of not seeking help could be slight or significant [13]. A common theme in all medical models is the dimension of symptom meanings that are correlated with the readiness to seek help. They are disruptiveness or painfulness, novelty and embarassingness or social obtrusiveness [62].

Stage three involves the operationalization of strategies for seeking and receiving aid.

Each phase of the sequence is at least partially dependent on how the other steps are resolved. Steps can be revised, cycled several times or omitted [13]. This process is not orderly or logical. The individual acts on a belief that an option will produce certain consequences. This attitude equals the subjective probability of the outcomes occurrence times the evaluation of the consequences. This is not "reasoned" action [63] but semi-reasoned actions [64]. The

General Helpseeking Model
(proposed by McMullen & Gross, 1983)

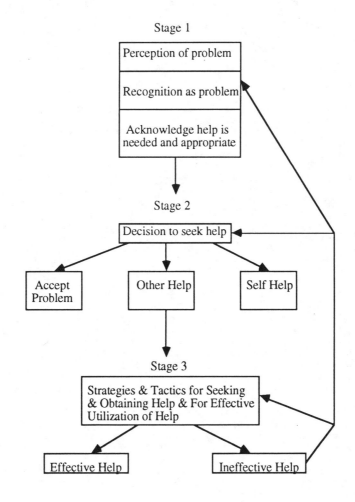

stressful conditions under which the victims operate cause them to make
less than objective rational decisions [64]. This helpseeking model
will be useful in illustrating the process of seeking help for
intercollegiate athletic injuries.

The following presentation will describe the problem
characteristics, situational conditions, and the recipient
characteristics for athletic injury. Application will be made to the
helpseeking literature. Risk factors will be discussed that may account
for differences between athletes in perception of the seriousness of an
injury, emotional response to an injury, compliance to rehabilitation
programs and may explain why some athletes appear more prone to injury.

PROBLEM CHARACTERISTICS

Minor/Chronic

This theory can be most useful in addressing minor, chronic
injuries. This focus addresses a significant portion of the injuries
occurring in sport and has been overlooked in past research.

Kraus and Conroy [1] find a direct correlation between the
severity of the injury and the associated amount of literature. In
general, minor injuries are not reported or studied and the majority of
studies use missed participation for one week as the minimum criterion
for definition of an injury. The two studies that include non-serious
injuries report an injury rate in an excess of 200% [65], and show that
two-thirds of bicycle related injuries are minor [66]. This oversight
in relation to minor injuries may account for the inability to detect
causes for athletic injury. In the relatively new studies not included
in this review, where minor injuries are reported, they account for a
significant proportion of the total [67]. One study which includes
injuries defined as precluding participation from one to seven days,
shows minor injuries accounting for 72.5 percent of the total [2].
Vinger and Hoerner [4], leading authorities on sport injury, claim that
90% of all sport related injuries are contusions and minor muscle pulls,
and that one half of an estimated fifty million reported sports injuries
require only brief medical attention with no restriction on the person's
usual activity. Tutko [68] states that an even more common source of
injury than traumatic contact injuries are those self-inflicted caused
by overtraining which begin as minor.

There is a problem with neglecting to study minor injuries and
their role in the total injury process. In an early address on the
concerns of sports medicine by a forerunner in the field [69], the
necessity of addressing chronic, minor injuries which do not improve is
emphasized. Small injuries, if left undiagnosed and untreated, can
hamper or end participation [3]. Minor injuries often precede major
back injuries [17]. Charles Moss, the trainer of the Boston Red Sox,
recognizes the importance of treating minor injuries. "Minor injuries
are a particular problem. It is tough to set a small injury to rest.
Minor injuries grow into major problems [3]." One of the leading sports
orthopedics in the United States, Southmayd [3] points out that even
small athletic injuries are serious. He notes that their role, in not
only precipitating major injuries, but is causing compensatory injuries.
Southmayd uses the analogy of the body being only as strong as the
weakest link in the chain, and uses the case of the Hall of Fame
pitcher, Dizzy Dean, to illustrate his point. When playing baseball for
the St. Louis Cardinals, Dizzy injured his big toe. Compensating for
the pain in his toe, Dizzy changed his pitching motion. This resulted

in damage to his throwing arm and the injury which ended his career. The lack of research on minor injuries may represent an oversight of a significant etiological factor in athletic injuries.

This theoretical approach does not account for traumatic, debilitating major or severe injuries which are results of exclusively external factors (i.e., collision, fall, faulty equipment, etc.). However, major or severe injuries that are a result of minor injuries or those that decrease in seriousness to a minor level are handled nicely by this approach. Also, minor and major injuries which continue to recur and become chronic are dealt with in this proposal.

It has been extensively demonstrated in the helpseeking literature that minor problems as opposed to major ones increase the self-threat to self-esteem in helpseeking. DePaulo [70] found a general disinclination to seek help for minor difficulties. Across helpseeking situations for a number of personal problems, psychological problems, worries [71], household emergencies [72], medical problems [73], it is found that people seek help from professionals only when the problem is severe (for review, see Wilcox and Birkel,[74]).

Chronicity, or the perception of chronicity promotes threat to self-esteem [43, 75], decreased helpseeking [76, 77] and less expectation of future helpseeking [78-80].

Centrality/Ego Relevance

The importance of an injury to an athlete can be assessed by determining how important participating in sports is to the athlete. A number of studies empirically support that the athletes' concept of physical ability, and the body and its ability to function is significantly more important to them than non-athletes [81-83].

It is consistently documented that individuals, especially those with high self-esteem, are more resistant to seeking help on ego-involving than non-ego-involving tasks [84-89]. A characteristic that makes receiving aid especially aversive to high achievers is when the task on which the aid is offered is especially meaningful [85].

RECIPIENT CHARACTERISTICS

There are particular recipient characteristics that athletes possess. These characteristics have been demonstrated to become stronger in the athletes as the level of competition and seriousness of the competition rises. Of interest is the empirical support for the fact that the injury rate increases as the level of competition increases [90-93].

Self-Esteem

Athletes have significantly higher self-esteem when compared to non-athletes [94-97].

It is consistently documented in social psychological research that aid recipients with high self-esteem are more threatened by help and display all defensive Cluster I behaviors [85, 98-100].

Need to Achieve

Both male and female athletes have been shown to be higher in the need to achieve than male and female non-athletes [101-103]. It is empirically supported that as the levels of competition increase, higher levels of achievement motivation are found [104-106].

Tessler and Schwartz [85] show, in one of the original and most widely cited studies on achievement motivation and helpseeking, that high achievers prefer not to seek help and are more threatened by aid than low achievers. DePaulo [70] and Morris and Rosen [107] provide additional support.

Internal Locus of Control

Athletes consistently show an internal locus of control for both success and failure [108-112] as a group and when compared to non-athletes.

The social psychology literature supports that internal perceptions of the cause affect (lowers) self-esteem and causes less helpseeking [13, 85, 113, 114].

Independence

Athletes have been shown to be more autonomous and independent than non-athletes by a number of researchers [102, 106, 115-120].

The lack of control and the dependence found in patient role studies suggest that a patient's desire for control (indicated by autonomy and independence) in medical aid settings may affect recipients reactions to aid. Negative reactions are expected only if the loss of control is significantly more than the patient desires [121, 122].

Studies in helpseeking which enhance perceived or actual control support this contention [123-127].

Studies on Type A individuals show that helpseeking negatively affects self-esteem in independent subjects [128-130].

Sex Role Orientation

It is consistently found that male and female athletes are more masculine-oriented than male and female non-athletes [83, 94, 131-133].

There is a widely supported and consistently found gender difference in helpseeking. Males are more likely to be threatened by helpseeking than females ([134]; for review see Gross and McMullen, [13]). Sociocultural values are reasons for these differences [13, 135]. Helpseeking for masculine sex-typed people is much more damaging to their self-esteem [43, 136, 137].

SITUATIONAL CONDITIONS

Request vs. Offer

Requesting help is more threatening than is receiving help that is offered [138-141].

Public vs. Private

It is well supported that public helpseeking causes self-threat [142-144].

Norm of Reciprocity

It is demonstrated that when one is unable to reciprocate, one will experience self-threat [43, 145].

An explanation of how these recipient, problem, and aid characteristics affect all stages of the helpseeking model will be presented using Fishers Threat to Self-Esteem Model. This summary is based on high levels of these particular recipient's characteristics and responses which would be supported by the previous research findings.

HELPSEEKING CYCLE FOR ATHLETIC INJURIES

Stage One

Stage one of McMullen and Gross' Helpseeking Model includes the perception of the problem, recognition of the incident or symptom as a problem and the acknowledgment that help is necessary and appropriate. The specific characteristics of the athlete and the problem affect each of these steps. The very nature of the minor athletic injury and the nature of the athlete's predisposition delays the perception of the problem. Distinguishing between "normal post-workout" muscle soreness and the onset of a minor injury is very difficult. Because of the personal characteristics of the athlete and due to the fact that the very definition of being an athlete is at odds with being injured [25], an athlete's natural bias would be to interpret these symptoms in the least threatening manner to their self-esteem [81]. Since athletics is based on physical prowess and depends largely on the strength of the body and its ability to function, the least threatening interpretation of pain to the athlete would be as a positive sign of muscle soreness and fatigue from a good workout in which they pushed themselves. This pain could even serve to positively reinforce an athlete's self-esteem if interpreted as if they were strong enough and capable of pushing themselves to their physical limit. Therefore, the perception of the symptoms as something beyond the expected results of hard work would be delayed for these athletes.

The perception or recognition of these symptoms, not merely as something beyond the ordinary but as an actual problem, would also be delayed for these athletes. Because of the athlete's high need to achieve being the predominant motivating force in playing sports [146], the symptoms would not even be perceived as a problem until it directly interfered with the actual performance. As long as the athlete was capable of functioning at a relatively high level, the symptoms would not actually constitute a problem for the athlete and would either be dismissed or ignored. Only until an injury became severe or prevented the athlete from achieving would the symptoms be recognized as a problem. This would be a significant delay at this step for appropriate helpseeking when compared to helpseeking in a population with different recipient characteristics.

Once the problem is recognized by the athlete, there would be a third delay in acknowledging that help is necessary. This is because seeking help for an athletic injury, particularly a minor injury, would signify a physical weakness and imply failure in the athlete's area of expertise [43]. Acknowledging that help is necessary would also negatively affect the athlete's self-esteem due to a conflict with needing help and their self-concept as an athlete of ability, of individual independence and self-reliance, and toughmindedness. Acknowledging that help is necessary would also conflict with their

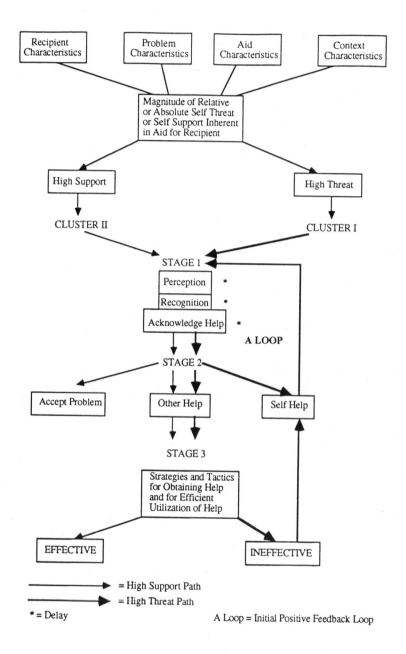

Chronic Injury Model

ability to be personally responsible for success and failure and the related desire to be in control. Therefore, acknowledging that help is necessary would be a very aversive psychological state for the athlete due to the self-threatening message inherent in needing help for minor athletic injuries. This delays the entire process and creates further problems for the athlete.

This delay causes a worsening of the physical problem and unnecessarily increases the magnitude of the injury, and this affects the second stage in a number of ways.

Stage Two

At this stage, the athlete has come to the decision that help is necessary. According to the Helpseeking Model, he/she has three choices. The athlete can accept the problem, can obtain self-help or can seek help from others. Since the athlete has not arrived at this point until the injury actually interferes with athletic functioning, an athlete at this level would not accept the problem. Accepting the problem would mean not performing or performing at a lesser level which would also severely affect the athlete's self-esteem. If the athlete could continue to perform at reasonable level, with the injury, the athlete would not have acknowledged help is necessary. As achieving is the primary concern of the athlete with these specific characteristics, accepting the problem and its accompanying inability to perform is not an option. Severity mediates this point in the model. The problem must be severe enough to interfere with the achievement of the athlete and override the costs to the athlete's self-esteem when acknowledging he/she requires help.

Of the other two alternatives, self-help or other help, the athlete will prefer self-help, regardless of the medical appropriateness of this choice.

The perceived control portion of the Fisher et al. [43] model incorporates the coping response and accounts for the motivation of self-help at this point in the model. As the hypothesis states, the degree of causal control is determined by an individual's chronic belief about his/her ability to end dependency through the investment of effort. As Weiner [147] and others have shown, the belief of one's ability to achieve mastery through effort is a characteristic of high achievers. An internal locus of control also points to the belief in causality being due to effort and ability. Therefore, an athlete at this stage would have a high initial perception of control.

This perceived control mediates the self-threatening aspects of aid and the behavioral response. The second hypothesis predicts a specific response when one expects to have control over subsequent outcomes when associated with self-threatening aid. The response is short-term psychological distress (negative personal and external perceptions) and an instrumental behavioral response (high self-help and low helpseeking).

So, self-help is predicted and empirically supported when one expects to have control. At this point in the model, an athlete would expect to have control and would thereby be directed toward self-help before other help.

At this point, other's perceptions play a significant role in the athlete's decision-making. Not only does acknowledging that one needs to help threaten the athletes personal self-perceptions, but seeking other's help would only serve to magnify this threat, by publicly exposing their inadequacy [43]. The public nature of seeking help, along with the necessity of requesting the aid and the inability to

reciprocate, greatly intensifies the already significant threatening
aspects of needing, seeking, and receiving aid. As the theory predicts,
when a helping situation is threatening, cluster one responses are
elicited. These clearly point to increased self-help over other's help.
The athlete's predisposition to take responsibility for failure and
believe that this injury is due to a personal shortcoming and therefore
is his/her fault, also steers him/her from other help and admitting
his/her perceived blame. Along with this, due to the delay in Step one,
the athlete actually is somewhat responsible for his/her condition as
earlier help would have been more appropriate. As research also shows,
when one suffers self-blame or is blamed by others, helpseeking is not
promoted [13, 140].

Due to the threatening nature of seeking other's help being
dependent on the personal and situational factors, the athlete will
choose self-help to avoid being placed in a public and, therefore, more
aversive situation. The athlete's independence and internal locus of
control, (not only desiring to be in control, but believing that he/she
is personally responsible for outcomes) also guides him/her to choose
self-help first.

Self-help will either work temporarily or fail. Generally, self-
help may get the athlete back to a functional level temporarily.
However, the athlete's achievement motivation continually pushes the
athlete to return to playing earlier and at a higher level than
appropriate when injured. This will only continue and most likely
worsen the injury. The athlete may also become more accustomed to
playing with the problem and may redefine his/her threshold for
perceiving and recognizing a problem and acknowledging the necessity of
help. Their idea of what is 'normal' may now include the injury or
symptoms associated with it. This is depicted in the model by the
positive feedback loop A (see figure 3). The athlete re-enters the
beginning of stage two after self-help and causes further delays in the
helpseeking process due to a higher threshold of perceiving a problem
exists. The problem will continue to worsen until the athlete has no
choice but to seek others help.

If the self-help fails immediately in Stage two, the athlete will
choose to seek other help. The decision to seek other help requires the
problem at this point to be serious enough to outweigh all of the
previously mentioned costs to the athlete's self-esteem. An athlete
will only seek other help when the only other alternative is to fail.
Failing for these athletes would be defined as the inability to perform.

Although an athlete's general disposition naturally allows him/her
to attribute success and failure to internal factors, the athlete is, in
a sense, again genuinely responsible for the magnitude of the injury.
This is due to the delay in the previous stage and in the decision to
attempt self-help first. This self-blame, coupled with the belief that
others blame them and the loss of control and dependency inherent in
seeking help for medical problems, gives rise to additional self-threat
when seeking other help. Also, the loss of self-esteem because the body
has failed along, with the accompanying implication that the athlete is
not physically or psychologically strong enough to "tough it out",
particularly for a minor problem, is heightened when made public. Also,
the lack of reciprocity, the public nature of seeking help and the act
of requesting help all foster an internal attribution of the cause of
the need of help by others. This reinforces the athletes pre-existing
perception of self-blame. The athlete's belief that the problem is due
to internal reasons, and the belief that others believe them
responsible, decreases the athlete's self-esteem. The athlete's self-
esteem has already suffered due to his/her inability to achieve and

exhibit physical prowess through performing. The recipient, problem and aid characteristics all function to make the act of seeking other's help very aversive. The stigma of being injured, as propagated by the coach and teammates, is felt by the athlete and also magnifies the threat involved in seeking other's help.

Stage Three

     This stage employs the operationalization of strategies for seeking and receiving help. Due to the magnitude of the threat to the athlete's self-esteem, help for athletic injuries is ineffective.
     Each time the athlete enters the helping situation, usually on a daily basis, he/she goes through this tortuous process where his/her self-esteem is threatened. Different situational conditions exacerbate the threat (discontinuity of treatment, different helpers, etc.) Because of the magnitude of the threat involved for the injured athlete in seeking help, the athlete will leave this threatening situation as quickly as possible. Due to the athlete's belief in personal responsibility for the outcome and subsequent desire for control and with the strong need to achieve being the primary force guiding the athlete's behavior the injured athlete will drop out of the helping interaction immediately upon reaching a performance criterion. This is generally before sufficient time has been allowed to properly heal the injury. This sets the athlete back into another positive feedback loop, elevating the thresholds of pain tolerance and problem perception and inevitably the injury resurfaces generally in worse condition. Severity again mediates the process. As severity decreases, the athlete leaves the helping situation. However, as this is too early for proper healing, ultimately the injury will become severe enough to temporarily outweigh the costs to self-esteem and the athlete will re-enter the helping situation.
     If forced to remain in the rehabilitation process, as the injury becomes less severe, the athlete will attempt to regain control and independence, either by doing too much or by not following their specific rehabilitation protocol. This illustrates the athlete displaying cluster one responses in response to the threat. This would be evidence of the preferred patient role of this population (characterized by independence, internal locus of control, and masculine sex role) reasserting itself as severity decreases [130]. Also, in an attempt to maintain his/her private and/or public self-image of mental and physical strength and ability, athletes can interfere with the diagnoses and treatment thereby causing further delay with the helping process. The athlete can do more than is appropriate in treatment to reaffirm his/her self-concept of strength and effort and may not publicly admit pain. This interferes with progress as appropriate responses are critical in making diagnoses and establishing treatment programs. This athlete is viewed as non-compliant by the therapist and creates more blame for the problem and places it on the athlete. This, again, makes the interaction more threatening by lowering the athlete's self-esteem. There is also potential for the therapist to take the athlete's non-compliant behaviors as a personal affront and create as additional unpleasant and blameful environment. The threat experienced at all stages may compound the injury directly. As pointed out by Weiss and Troxell [10], anxiety and worry about the injury can manifest itself physiologically in the weakened/injured area. This would serve to directly affect the injury negatively.
     For the athlete who has left the helping interaction earlier than is warranted, the injury will resurface and the cycle starts over.

Fisher's model would support the prediction of the establishment of chronicity at this point. Over time as the problem resurfaces or does not improve permanently, regardless of the athlete's behavior, illustrated by the feedback loops, the athlete perceives a lack of control over the outcomes. As Fisher's model shows when a lack of control is expected, the recipient will continue to rely on external sources of help and this persists over time [148]. This illustrates how the loss of control over the injury that the athlete experiences in this model, not only creates chronicity, but maintains it over time.

For the athlete who maintains an ineffective rehabilitation schedule, the problem also becomes chronic. However, the ensuing stages in this positive feedback loop are delayed even more. As the athlete then deals with the same problem, it becomes familiar, and familiarity of symptoms has been shown to decrease perceived severity [149]. As severity mediates the helpseeking process, it will take longer for the athlete to seek help if the problem is perceived as less severe.

Once the injury becomes chronic, the threat associated with seeking and receiving help for athletic injuries is compounded. Chronicity in, and of itself, fosters an internal attribution by oneself and others [75] and magnifies the associated self-threat. Chronicity increases self-threat by affecting the ability to reciprocate. The only possible way in this circumstance, of justifying help and indirectly reciprocating and maintaining equity, is by improving. Chronicity makes that impossible and increases the distress associated with inequity. Chronicity also directly negatively affects the patient-therapist interaction. It has been demonstrated that is some cases, the therapist's self-esteem is lowered when patients do not improve [150]. This is threatening to the therapist's self-esteem and results in the therapist avoiding the patient or displaying other defensive behaviors. This avoidance would magnify the threat already felt by the athlete. Also, as the therapist deals with a chronic injury, due to a realistic perspective of knowing they would continue to see the patient and in a subconscious attempt to maintain self-esteem and not feel exploited, the therapist would be more likely to give out smaller amounts of help. It has been shown that small amounts of help lead to increased threat [151]. This would be felt by the athlete. There is also evidence of a self-fulfilling prophesy. If therapists believe athletes will be non-compliant, they will be less motivated to correct those behaviors. Less information will be given to the athlete. This reduces the athlete's sense of control [152]. The therapist will not monitor the athlete and will not request the athlete's participation in treatment. This negatively affects the athlete's self-esteem.

The patient role has been shown to reassert itself with chronic problems [130] and an athlete who is independent, autonomous, high achieving, and masculine-oriented is more at odds with the inherent nature of the helping situation. The original factors that make helpseeking threatening to the athlete remain intact. But as the injury becomes chronic, due to the characteristics of the recipient, problem and aid, this chronicity only exacerbates the threatening aspects of the situation. This forces the athlete to delay entering or to leave the helpseeking situation as soon as possible, and maintains the chronicity as long as the athlete remains competitive, since help is necessary to remain functional.

When aid is threatening, cluster one negative responses are exhibited throughout the helpseeking process. There is negative affect, a negative evaluation of the donor and the aid, low future helpseeking and a high degree of subsequent self-help [43]. This compounds the negative aspects of future help and begins to create a cycle through which the athlete avoids future helping situations, due to the experienced threat in the initial interaction.

This creates a negative attitude which generalizes to other injuries. This particular athlete, in order to maintain self-esteem, is predisposed to avoid the helpseeking situation at all costs, there by setting up another delay with subsequent injuries. These characteristics of the recipient along with the specific problem, aid and situational characteristics, affects the athletes attitude and creates a chronically injured athlete.

This threat to self-esteem theory is useful in explaining and predicting helpseeking and receiving behavior for athletic injury across a wide array of situations. It encompasses all of the previous research findings and offers a comprehensive rationale for addressing needing, seeking, and receiving help and various aspects of the helping process. This synergy of the research in athletics and helpseeking and recipient's reactions to aid provides a theoretical rationale, which does not only consistently explains past research findings, but should be useful in guiding future research.

PRACTICAL APPLICATION OF THEORY

If valid, this theory would be extremely useful in predicting potential injury-prone athletes. The earlier this athlete could be identified, the earlier the interventions in this cycle could be accomplished. This would help stop the cycle of chronicity and the athlete would benefit both psychologically and physically.

This theory is useful for identifying and understanding the specific psychological mechanisms and their function. Understanding of the complex interaction of athlete's personality characteristics and the injury process is the first step in breaking the chain of chronicity. Once known, specific interventions can be used to make the injury process as positive as possible. The interventions should deal with the specific personality characteristics of the chronically injured athlete and how they would function at specific times of the process and under particular situations. This could certainly alleviate many of the negative factors which contribute to the threatening aspect of helpseeking for athletic injuries.

CONCLUSION

The literature clearly depicts a rising health problem from the increasingly high number of athletic injuries. The past routes that have been undertaken to discover the etiology of these injuries have not lead to the discovery of factors useful in predicting or preventing future injuries. The role that psychology plays in the injury process has only recently begun to be researched with any depth.

The study of the social psychological area of helpseeking has put forth a useful theoretical model. This has been borrowed and applied to athletic injuries. The model illustrates how current injuries may become worse and future injuries may occur due to the psychological nature of athletes and their response to helpseeking. It points out that this process may well be a significant etiological factor in athletic injuries for a particular group of athletes.

This theory does explain the majority of results presented in earlier papers on different responses to athletic injury,

rehabilitation, and compliance between abilities. It also provides a
rationale for the differences found between athletes and non-athletes.
     Despite no empirical support at the present time, the utility of
this theoretical model should not be overlooked. It provides a
comprehensive theoretical framework in an area that has been
atheoretical to date. It covers the entire injury process and explains
the past varied and, seemingly, inconsistent findings. The theoretical
model offers an explanation for the increasing number of athletic
injuries and it offers the predictive power. Interventions and
applications have been discussed to put this model to use in effectively
managing the problem of the high number of chronic athletic injuries.
     Future research is a necessity to examine the many different
aspects of this model. The general outline and hypothetical speculation
as to how this model operates in this study offers a solid foundation
from which other research should be generated. The application of the
social psychological area of helpseeking to the study of athletic
injuries offers a macrotheoretical conceptualization of how the injury
process operates. This is an important contribution to the study of the
role of psychology in athletic injury. Future research should be guided
by this paradigm.

REFERENCES

[1]   Kraus, J. and Convoy, C., "Mortality and morbidity from injuries
      in sports and recreation." Annual Review of Public Health, Vol. 5,
      1984, pp 163-92.

[2]   Lawrence, G., Connecticut Sports Medicine. Connecticut State
      Medical Society, 1990.

[3]   Southmayd, W. and Hoffman, M., Sports Health. New York: Quick Tex,
      1981.

[4]   Vinger, P. and Hoerner, E. Sports injuries: The unthwarted
      epidemic. London: John Wright Pub., 1982.

[5]   Passer, M. and Seese, M., "Life stress and athletic injury:
      Examination of positive vs. negative events and three moderator
      variables." Journal of Human Stress, 1983, pp 11-16.

[6]   Coddington, R. and Troxell, J., "The effect of emotional factors
      on injury rates: A pilot study." Journal Human Stress, Vol. 6,
      1980, pp 3-5.

[7]   MacDougall, J., Wenger, H., and Green, H., Physiological Testing
      of the Elite Athlete. Canada: Mutual Press, 1982.

[8]   Crossman, J. and Jamleson, K., "Differences in perceptions of
      seriousness and disrupting effects of athletic injury as viewed by
      athletes and their trainers." Perceptual and Motor Skills, Vol.
      61, 1985, pp 1131-34.

[9]   Duda, J., Smart, A., and Tappe, M., "Predictors of adherence in
      the rehabilitation of athletic injuries: An application of
      personal investment theory." Journal Sport and Exercise
      Psychology, Vol. 11, 1989, pp 367-81.

[10] Weiss, M. and Troxel, R., "Psychology of the injured athlete."
      Athletic Training, Vol. 21, 1986, pp 104-10.

[11] Bramwell, S., Minoru, M., Wagner, N., and Holmes, T.,
      "Psychosocial factors in athletic injuries." Journal Human Stress,
      June, 1975, pp 6-20.

[12] Wiese, D. and Weiss, M., "Psychological rehabilitation and
      physical injury: Implications for the sportsmedicine team." The
      Sport Psychologist, Vol. 1, 1987, pp B1.

[13] Gross, A. and McMullen, P., "Models of the helpseeking process."
      In New Directions in Helping, ed. B. M. DePaulo, A. Nadler, and J.
      Fisher. 47-72. Vol. 2. New York: Academic Press, 1983.

[14] Fischer, E., Winer, D., and Abramowitz, S., "Seeking professional
      help for psychological problems." In New Directions in Helping,
      ed. A Nadler, J Fisher, and BM DePaulo. 163-88. Vol. 3. New York:
      Academic Press, 1983.

[15] Trumble, H., "Rules Change: an example from ice hockey." In Sports
      Injuries: the unthwarted epidemic, ed. P. Vinger and E. hoerner.
      Boston: John Wright, 1982.

[16] Keene, J., Narenchania, R., Sachtjen, G., and Clancy, W., "Tartan
      turf on trial." American Journal of Sports Medicine, Vol. 8, 1980,
      pp 43-47.

[17] Ekstrand, J., Gillquist, J., and Liljedahl, S., "Prevention of
      Soccer Injuries." The American Journal of Sports Medicine, Vol.
      11, No. 3, 1983, pp 116-20.

[18] Kraus, J., Anderson, B., and Mueller, C., "The effectiveness of a
      special ice hockey helmetto reduce headf injuries in college
      intramural hockey." Medical Science in Sports, Vol. 2, 1970, pp
      162-64.

[19] Hulse, W., "Sport Equipment Standards." In Sports Injuries: the
      unthwarted epidemic, ed. P. Vinger and E. Hoerner. Boston: John
      Wright, 1982.

[20] Roy, S. and Irwin, R., Sports medicine: Prevention, evaluation,
      management and rehabilitation. Englewood Cliffs, NJ: Prentice
      Hall, 1983.

[21] Cahill, B. and Griffith, E., "Effect of preseason conditioning on
      the incidence and severity of high school football knee injuries."
      American Journal of Sports Medicine, Vol. 6, 1978, pp 180-84.

[22] Ekstrand, J., Gillquist, J., and Liljedahl, S., "Incidence of
      soccer injuries and their relation to training and team success."
      The American Journal of Sports Medicine, Vol. 11, No. 2, 1983, pp
      63-67.

[23] Kulund, D., _The Injured Athlete_. Philadelphia, PA: JB Lippincott & Co., 1988.

[24] Ekstrand, J. and Gillquist, J., "The Frequency of Muscle Tightness in Soccer Players." _American Journal of Sports Medicine_, Vol. 10, No. 2, 1982, pp 75-78.

[25] Rotella, R., "Psychological care of the injured athlete." In _The Injured Athlete_, ed. D. Kulund. 151-65. Philadelphia, PA: JB Lippincott C., 1988.

[26] Williams, T., Tonymon, B., and Wadsworth, C., "Stress and Injury." _Journal of Human Stress_, Spring, 1986, pp 38-43.

[27] Andersen, M. and Williams, J., "A model of stress and athletic injury." _Journal of Sports and Exercise Psychology_, Vol. 10, 1988, pp 294-304.

[28] Cryan, A. and Alles, W., "The relationship between stress and college football injuries." _Jouranl of Sports Medicine_, Vol. 23, 1983, pp

[29] Dohrenwend, B. and Dohrenwend, B., _Stressful life events: Their nature and effects_. New York: John Wiley and Sons, 1974.

[30] Rahe, R. and Arthur, R., "Life changes and illness studies: past history and future directions." _Journal of Human Stress_, Vol. 4, No. 1, 1978, pp 3-15.

[31] Johnson, J. and Saranson, I., "Recent Developments in Research on Life." In _Human Stress and Cognition_, ed. D. Hamilton and W. Warburton. pp. 205-233. Chichester England: John Wiley and Sons, 1979.

[32] Braun, R. and MacDougall, M., "Psychosomatic fitness." _Clinical Sports Medicine Journal_, Vol. 8, 1982, pp 11-13.

[33] Young, M. and Cohen, D., "Self-concept among female college tournament basketball players." _Journal of American Corrective Therapy_, Vol. 33, 1979, pp 139-142.

[34] Dahlhauser, M. and Thomas, M., "Visual disembedding and locus of control as variables associated with high school football injuries." _Perceptual & Motor Skills_, Vol. 49, 1979, pp 254.

[35] Diekhoff, G., "Running a mile; injuries in compulsive runners." _Journal of Sport Behavior_, Vol. 7, 1983, pp 120-29.

[36] Ice, R., "Long term compliance." _Physical Therapy_, Vol. 65, 1983, pp 1832-1839.

[37] Fisher, A., "Adherence to sports injury rehabilitation programmes." _Sports Medicine_, Vol. 9, No. 3, 1990, pp 151-158.

[38] Pinkerton, R., Hinz, L., and Barrow, J., "Utilization of professional service by athletes." Journal of American College Health, Vol. 37, No. 5, 1989, pp 218-26.

[39] Carmen, L., Zerman, J., and Blaine, G., "The use of Harvard psychiatric service by athletes and non-athletes." Mental Hygiene, Vol. 52, 1968.

[40] Smith, A., Scott, S., and Young, M., "The emotional response of athletes to injury." Canadian Assocaiation of Sport Sciences, 84p-85p, Spring, 1988.

[41] Pierce, R., "Athletes in psychotherapy: how many? how come?" Journal of the American College Health Association, Vol. 17, 1969, pp 247-9.

[42] Linder, D., Pillow, D., and Reno, R., "Shrinking jocks:derogation of athletes who consult a sports psychologist." Sport and Exercise Psychology, Vol. 11, No. 3, 1989, pp 270-280.

[43] Fisher, J., Nadler, A., and Whitcher-Alagna, S., "Four theoretical approaches for conceptualizing reactions to aid." In New Directions in Helping, ed. J. Fisher, A. Nadler, and B. M. DePaulo. 52-85. Vol 1. New York: Academic Press, 1983.

[44] Brehm, J., A Theory of Psychological Reactance. New York: Academic Press, 1966.

[45] Kelley, H., "Attribution theory and social psychology." In Nebraska Symposium on Motivation, ed. D. Levine. Lincoln, NE: University of Nebraska Press, 1967.

[46] Jones, E. and Davis, K., "From acts to dispositions: The attribution process and person perception." In Advances in Experimental Social Psychology, ed. L. Berkowitz. New York: Academic Press, 1965.

[47] Jones, E. and Harris, V., "The attribution of attitudes." Journal of Experimental Social Psychology, Vol. 3, 1967, pp 1-24.

[48] Greenberg, M., "A theory of indebtedness." In Social Exchange: Advances in Theory and Research, ed. K. Gergen, M. S. Greenberg, and R. Will. New York: Plenum, 1980.

[49] Gouldner, A., "The norm of reciprocity: A preliminary statement." American Sociologic Review, Vol. 25, 1960, pp 161-78.

[50] Adams, J., "Toward an understanding of inequity." Journal of Abnormal Social Psychology, Vol. 67, 1963, pp 422-36.

[51] Blau, P., Exchange and Power in Social Life. New York: Wiley, 1964.

[52] Walster, E., Berscheid, E., and Walster, G. "New directions in equity theory." Journal of Personality and Social Psychology, Vol. 25, 1973, pp 151-76.

[53] Walster, E., Walster, B., and Berscheid, E. Equity: Theory and research. Boston, MA: Allyn & Bacon, 1978.

[54] Nadler, A. and Fisher, J. "The role of threat to self-esteem and perceived control in recipient reaction to help: Theory development and empirical validation." Advances in Experimental Social Psychology, 1986.

[55] Wills, T. "Social comparison in coping and helpseeking." In New Directions in Helping, ed. B. M. DePaulo, A. Nadler, and J. Fisher. 109-42. Vol 3. New York: Academic Press, 1983.

[56] Mechanic, D. Medical Sociology. London: Collier-MacMillan, 1968.

[57] Hollingshead, A. and Redlich, F. Social class and mental illness. New York: Wiley, 1958.

[58] Koos, E., Health of Regionville. New York: Columbia University Press, 1954.

[59] Schenthal, J., "Multiphasic screening of the well-patient." Journal of the American Medical Association, Vol. 172, 1960, pp 51-64.

[60] Allen, G., "Reactions to help in peer tutoring; roles and social identities." In New Directions in Helping, ed. A. Nadler, J. Fisher, and B. M.DePaulo. 214-232. Vol. 3. New York: Academic Press, 1983.

[61] Pettigrew, T., "Seeking public assitance: A stigma analysis." In New Directions in Helping, ed. A. Nadler, J. Fisher, and B. M. DePaulo. 273-93. Vol. 3. New York: Academic Press, 1983.

[62] Jones, R., Wiese, H., Moore, R., and Haley, J., "On the perceived meaning of symptoms." Medical Care, Vol. 19, 1981, pp 710-714.

[63] Fishbein, M. and Ajzen, I., Belief, attitude, intentions and behavior: An introduction to theory and research. Boston: Addison Wesley, 1975.

[64] Greenberg, M., Ruback, B., and Westcott, D., "Seeking help from the police: the victims perspective." In New Directions in Helping, ed. A, Nadler, J. Fisher, and B. M. DePaulo. 71-103. 3. New York: Academic Press, 1983.

[65] McMaster, W. and Walter, M., "Injuries in soccer." American Journal of Sports Medicine, Vol. 6, 1978, pp 354-57.

[66] Waller, J. "Bicycle ownership and injury patterns among elementary school children." Pediatrics, Vol. 6, 1971, pp 1042-50.

[67] Duffy, F., Epidemiological study on intercollegiate soccer injuries. University of Connecticut, 1986. Unpublished Manuscript

[68] Tutko, T., "The Psychology of sports." In Sports Injuries: The Unthwarted Epidemic, ed. P. Vinger and E. F. Hoerner. 335-45. 2nd ed. Boston: John Wright, 1982.

[69] Ryde, D., "The role of the physician in soprts injury prevention." Journal of Sports Medicine & Physical Fitness, Vol. 5, 1965, pp 152-55.

[70] DePaulo, B., "Social psychological processes in informal helpseeking." In Basic Processes in Helping Relationships, ed. T. A. Wills. New York: Academic Press, 1982.

[71] Gurin, G., Veroff, J., and Feld, S., American's View Their Mental Health. New York: Basic Books, 1960.

[72] Litwak, E. and Selenyi, I., "Primary group structure and their functions:kin, neighbors and friends." American Psychological Review, Vol. 34, 1969, pp 465-481.

[73] Croog, S., Lipson, A., and Levine, S., "Help patterns in severe illness: the roles of kin network, non family measures and institutions." Journal of marriage and the Family, Vol. 34, 1972, pp 32-41.

[74] Wilcox, B. and Birkel, R., "Social networks and the help-seeking process: A structural perspective." In New Directions in Helping, ed. A. Nadler, J. Fisher, and B. M. DePaulo. 235-54. Vol. 3. New York: Academic Press, 1983.

[75] Brickman, P., Kidder, L., Coates, D., Rabinowitz, E., and Karuza, J., "The dilemmas of helping: Making aid fair and effective." In New Directions in Helping, ed. J. Fisher, A. Nadler, and B. M. DePaulo. 18-51. Vol. 1. New York:Academic Press, 1983.

[76] Brown, B. and Garland, H., "The effects of incompetency, audience acquaintanceship and anticipated evaluative feedback on face saving behavior." Journal of Experimental Social Psychology, Vol. 7, 1971, pp 490-502.

[77] Nadler, A., "Good looks do help: Effects of helpers physical attractiveness and expectations for future interaction on helpseeking behavior." Personality and Social Psychology Bulletin, Vol. 6, 1980, pp 378-84.

[78] Rosenthal, R. and Jacobson, L., Pygmalian in the Classroom. New York: Holt, 1968.

[79] Seaver, W., "Effects of naturally induced teacher expectations." Journal of Personality & Social Pscyhology, Vol. 38, 1973, pp 333-42.

[80] Beez, W., "Influence of bias psychological reports on teacher behavior and pupil performance." In 76th Annual Convention of the American Psychological Association, 1968.

[81] Loy, J., "The nature of sport: A definitional effort." Quest, Vol. Spring, 1968, pp 7-13.

[82] Coleman, J., "The adolescent society: The social life of the teenager and its impact on education." Free Press, 1961.

[83] Marsh, H. and Jackson, S., "Multidimensional self-concept masculinity and femininity as a function of women's involvement in athletics." Sex Roles, Vol. 15, No. 7/8, 1986, pp 391-99.

[84] DePaulo, B. and Fisher, J., "The cost of asking for help." Basic & Applied Social Psychology, Vol. 41, 1980, pp 478-87.

[85] Tessler, R. and Schwartz, S., "Helpseeking, self-esteem and achievement motivation: An attributional analysis." Journal of Personality and Social Psychology, Vol. 21, 1972, pp 318-26.

[86] Wallston, B., "The effects of sex-role ideology, self-esteem and expected future interactions with an audience on male help-seeking." Sex Roles, Vol. 2, 1976, pp 353-56.

[87] Morse, S., "Help, likeability and social influence." Journal of Applied Social Psychology, Vol. 2, 1972, pp 34-46.

[88] Nadler, A., "Personal characteristics and help-seeking." In New Directions in Helping, ed. B. M. DePaulo, A. Nadler, and J. Fisher. 303-40.Vol. 2. New York:Academic Press, 1983.

[89] Shapiro, E., "Is seeking help from a friend like seeking help from a stranger?" Social Psychology Quarterly, Vol. 43, 1980, pp 259-263.

[90] Garrick, J. and Requa, R., "Girls sports injuries in high school athletics." Journal of American medical Association, Vol. 239, 1978, pp 2245-48.

[91] Clarke, K. and Buckley, W., "Womens injuries in collegiate sports." American Journal of sports medicine, Vol. 8, 1980, pp 187-91.

[92] Lowry, C. and Leveau, B., "A retrospective study of gymnastics injuries to competitors and noncompetitors in private clubs." American Journal of Sports Medicine, Vol. 10, 1982, pp 237-9.

[93] Jeffrey, C., An epidemiological studyof injuries in American female gymnasts. Rainbow Sports Medical Center, Cleveland Ohio, 1975.

[94] Slusher, H., "Personality and intelligence characteristics of selected high school athletes and non-athletes." Research Quarterly, Vol. 35, 1964, pp 539-45.

[95] Valliant, P., Bezzubyk, I., Daley, L., and Asu, M., "Psychological impact of sport on disabled athletes." Psychological Reports, Vol. 56, 1985, pp 923-29.

[96] Hyland and Orlick., In Sports Psychology, ed. A. Carron. New York: Movement Publications, 1975, pp 228.

[97] Purdon, J., "Athletic participation and self-esteem." Masters Thesis, University of Western Ontario, 1978.

[98] Nadler, A., Fisher, J., and Streufert, S., "When helping hurts: The effects of donor-recipient similarity and recipient self esteem on reactions to aid." Journal of Personality, Vol. 44, 1976, pp 392-409.

[99] Fisher, J., DePaulo, B., and Nadler, A., "Extending altruism beyond the altruistic act: The mixed effects of aid on the help recipient." In Altruism and Helping Behavior, ed. J. Rushton and R. Sorrentino. New Jersey: Earl Baum Associates, 1981.

[100] Nadler, A., Aultman, A., and Fisher, J., "Helping is not enough: Recipients reactions to aid as a function of positive and negative self reguard." Journal of Personality, Vol. 47, 1979, pp 615-28.

[101] Ryan, E. and Lakie, W., "Competetive and non-competitive performance in relation to achievement motivation and manifest anxiety." Journal of Personality & Social Psychology, Vol. 1, 1965, pp 344-45.

[102] Neal, P., "Personality of Traits of US Women Athletes Who Participated in 1959 Pan-American Games as Measured by EPPS." Masters Thesis, Univerisity of Utah, 1963.

[103] Harris, D., "Psychological considerations of the female athlete." Journal Health and Physical Education Research, Vol. 46, 1975, pp 32-6.

[104] Johnsguard, K., "The competitive racing driver." Journal of Sports Medicine, Vol. 8, 1967, pp 87-95.

[105] Olgilvie, B. and Tutko, T., "What is an "athlete"." In American Association of Health, Physical Educaiton and Recreation Nation Conference in Las Vegas, 1967.

[106] Williams, J., "Personality characteristics of the successful female." In Sport Psychology: An Analysis of Athlete Behavior, ed. W.F.Strait. Ithaca, NY, 1978.

[107] Morris, S. and Rosen, S., "Effects of felt adequacy and opportunity to reciprocate on help-seeking." Journal of Experimental Social Psychology, Vol. 9, 1973, pp 265-76.

[108] Gilmore, T. and Minton, H., "Internal vs. external attribution of tastk performance as a function of locus of control, initial confidence and success-failure outcome." Journal of Personality, Vol. 42, 1974, pp 159-74.

[109] Lefevbre, L., "Achievement motivation and causal attribution in male and female athletes." International Journal of Sport Psychology, Vol. 10, 1979, pp 31-41.

[110] Duquin, M., "Attributions made by children in coeducational sports settings." In Psychology of Motor Behavior and Sport, ed. D.M. Landers and R.W. Christina. Human Kinetics Pub., 1977.

[111] Lynn, R., Phelan, J., and Kiker, V., "Beliefs in Internal-External control of reinforcement and participation in group and individual sports." Perceptual and Motor Skills. Vol. 29, 1969, pp 551-53.

[112] Kleiber, D. and Hemmer, J., "Sex Differences in the relationship of locus of control and recreational sport participation." Sex Roles. Vol. 7, No. 1, 1981, pp 801-810.

[113] Alkire, A., Collum, M., Kaswam, J., and Love, L., "Information exchange and accuracy of verbal communication under social power conditions." Journal of Personality and Social Psychology, Vol. 9, 1968, pp 301-8.

[114] Gerber, I., "Bereavement and the acceptance of professional service." Community Mental Health Journal. Vol. 5, 1969, pp 487-95.

[115] Greenwald, A., "Ego task analysis." In Cognitive social psychology, ed. A Hastorf and A Isen. New York: Elsevier, 1982.

[116] Hardman, K., "An investigation into the possible relationships between athletes ability and certain personality traits in third year secondary modern schoolboyes." University of Manchester, 1962.

[117] Rushall, B., "Personality profiles and a theory of behavior modification for swimmers." Swim Technique. Vol. 4, 33, 1967, pp 66-71.

[118] Schurr, K., Ashley, M., and Joy, K., "A multivariate analysis of male athlete characteristics: Sport Type and Success." Multivariate Experimental Clinical Research, Vol. 3, 1977, pp 53-68.

[119] Harris, A., Tessler, R., and Potter, J., "The induction of self-reliance: An experimental study of independence in the face of failure." Journal of Applied Social Psychology, Vol. 7, 1977, pp 313-31.

[120] Peterson, S., Ukler, J., and Tousdale, W., "Personality traits of women in team versus women in individual sports." Research Quarterly. Vol. 38, 1967, pp 686-90.

[121] Janis, I. and Rodin, J., "Attribution, control and decision making: Social psychology and health care." In Health Psychology: A Handbook, ed. G. C. Stone, F. Cohen, and N. E. Adler. San Francisco, CA: Jossey Bass, 1979.

[122] Taylor, S., "Hospital patient behavior: Reactance, helplessness or control?" Journal of Social Issues, Vol. 35, 1979, pp 156-84.

[123] Klein, R., Kliner, V., Zipes, D., Troyer, W., and Wallace, A., "Transfer from a coronary care unit." Archives of Internal Medicine, Vol. 22, 1968, pp 104-8.

[124] Langer, E. and Rodin, J., "The effects of choice and enhanced personal responsibility for the aged: A field experiment in a institutional setting." Journal of Personality and Social Psychology, Vol. 34, 1976, pp 191-8.

[125] Bowers, K., "Pain, anxiety and perceived control." Journal of Consulting & Clinical Psychology, Vol. 32, 1968, pp 596-602.

[126] Pranulis, M., Dabbs, J., and Johnson, J., "General anesthesia and the patient's attempt at control." Social Behavior and Personality, Vol. 3, 1975, pp 49-54.

[127] Staub, E., Tursky, B., and Schwartz, G., "Self-control and predictability: Their effects on reaction to aversion stimulation." Journal of Personality and Social Psychology, Vol. 18, 1971, pp 157-62.

[128] Friedman, M. and Rosenman, R., Type A Behavior and Your Heart. Greenwich, CT: Fawcett Co., 1974.

[129] Jenkins, C., "Psychological and social precursors of coronary disease." New England Journal of Medicine, Vol. 284, 1971, pp 244-55.

[130] Whitcher-Alagna, S., "Receiving medical help: A psychosocial perspective on patient reactions." In New Directions in Helping, ed. A. Nadler, J. Fisher, and B. M. DePaulo. 131-62. 3. New York: Academic Press, 1983.

[131] Kingsley, J., Foster, L., and Siebert, M., "Social acceptance of female college athletes by college women." Research Quarterly, Vol. 48, 1977, pp 727-33.

[132] Helmreich, K. and Spence, J., "Sex roles and achievement." In Psychology of Motor Behavior and Sport, ed. R. W. Christina and D. M. Landu. II. Human Kinetics Pub, 1977.

[133] Black, J., "MMPJ Results of female college students." In Basic Readings in the MMPJ, ed. G. Lambertini. Minneapolis, MN: 1961.

[134] DePaulo, B., Nadler, A., and Fisher, J., New Diections in Helping. New York: Academic Press, 1983.

[135] Gove, W. and Hughes, M., "Possible causes of the apparent sex differences in physical health: An empirical investigation." American Sociological Review, Vol. 44, 1979, pp 126-44.

[136] Margolis, R., "The effects of sex, sex-type and causal attribution on the helpseeking process." Doctoral Dissertation, Pennsylvania State, 1982.

[137] Voit, R., "Effects of student sex role identity and personality type on the likelihood of seeking counseling and preference for counselor sex." Doctoral Dissertation, University of Virginia, 1982.

[138] Piliavin, I. and Gross, A., "The effects of separation of services an income maintenance on AFDC recipient's perceptions and use of social services." Social Service Review, Vol. 9, 1977, pp 389-406.

[139] Broll, L., Gross, A., and Piliavin, I., "Effects of offered and requested help on helpseeking and reactions to being helped." Journal of Applied Social Psychology, Vol. 4, 1974, pp 244-58.

[140] Gross, A., Wallston, B., and Piliavin, I., "Reactants, attribution, equity and the help recipient." Journal of Applied Social Psychology, Vol. 9, 1979, pp 297-313.

[141] LaMorto-Corse, A. and Carver, C., "Recipients reactions to aid: Effects of locus of initiation, attributions and individual differences." Bulletin of Psychonomics Society, Vol. 16, 1980, pp 265-68.

[142] Clark, M., Gotay, C., and Mills, J., "Acceptance of help as a function of similarity of the potential helper and opportunity to repay." Journal of Applied Social Psychology, Vol. 4, 1974, pp 224-29.

[143] DePaulo, B., Brown, P., and Greenberg, J., "The effects of help on task performance in achievement context." In New Directions in Helping, ed. J. Fisher, A. Nadler, and B. M. DePaulo. 224-52. 1. New York: Academic Press, 1983.

[144] Stokes, S. and Bickman, L., "The effects of the physical attractiveness and role of the helper on helpseeking." Journal of Applied Social Pyschology, Vol. 4, 1974, pp 286-93.

[145] Gross, A. and Latane, J., "Receiving help, giving help and interpersonal attraction." Journal of Applied Social Psychology, Vol. 4, 1974, pp 210-223.

[146] Roberts, J. and Sutton-Smith, B., "Child training and game-involvement." Ethnology, Vol. 1, 1962, pp 165-85.

[147] Weiner, B., "Theories of motivation." In Mechanism to Cognition, Rand McNally, 1972.

[148] Fisher, J. and Nadler, A., "The effect of similarity between donor and recipient on reactions to aid." Journal of Applied Social Psychology, Vol. 4, 1974, pp 230-43.

[149] Ostrove, N. and Baum, A., "Factors influencing medical helpseeking." In New Directions in Helping, ed. A. Nadler, J. Fisher, and B. M. DePaulo. 107-30. 3. New York: Academic Press, 1983.

[150] Maslach, C., "The burn-out syndrome and patient care." In Psychological care of the dying patient, ed. C. Garfield. New York: MaGraw-Hill, 1979.

[151] Freeman, H., "Reward versus reciprocity as related to attraction." Journal of Applied Social Psychology, Vol. 1, 1977, pp 57-66.

[152] Forsyth, N. and Forsyth, D., "Internality, controllability and the effectiveness of attributional interpretation in counseling." Journal of Counseling Psychology, Vol. 29, No. 2, 1982, pp 140-150.

Eric D. Zemper[1] and Willy Pieter[2]

CEREBRAL CONCUSSIONS IN TAEKWONDO ATHLETES

REFERENCE: Zemper, E.D., and Pieter, W., **"Cerebral Concussion Rates in Taekwondo Athletes,"** Head and Neck Injuries in Sports, ASTM STP 1229, Earl F. Hoerner, Ed., American Society for Testing and Materials, Philadelphia, 1994.

ABSTRACT: Injury and exposure data were collected at eight major U.S. taekwondo tournaments between 1988 and 1990, involving 5 682 competitors and a total of 5 566 bouts. There were 802 recorded injuries, 292 (36%) severe enough to cause time-loss of one day or more from further participation. Injuries were equally divided between the head and lower extremities, each accounting for about 40% of the injuries, with the remainder to upper extremities and the body. Cerebral concussions were among the most serious injuries observed, with 58 recorded or approximately 1 for every 100 participants. The total cerebral concussion rate was 5.2/1 000 athlete-exposures or 1.1/1 000 minutes of exposure. These rates of concussions for taekwondo are 3.1 times higher than seen in college football games based on number of exposures, and 7.9 times as high based on time of exposure.

KEYWORDS: cerebral concussion, taekwondo, martial arts, injury rates, epidemiology

---

The Korean martial art form of taekwondo was a demonstration sport in the 1988 and 1992 Olympic Games, and it is a candidate to become a medal sport in the future. Despite the increasing popularity and increasing numbers of participants worldwide, little sport science research on taekwondo is currently available. The present study is derived from the injury surveillance phase of an ongoing

---

[1]President and Director of Research, Exercise Research Associates of Oregon, P.O. Box 10123, Eugene, OR 97440.

[2]Research Associate, Exercise Research Associates of Oregon, P.O. Box 10123, Eugene, OR 97440.

multi-disciplinary research project on taekwondo athletes initiated by one of the authors (Dr. Willy Pieter), and supported by the U.S. Olympic Committee and the U.S Taekwondo Union. Data reported here were collected at eight major competitions held in the U.S., including the 1988 U.S. Olympic Team Trials, the 1989 and 1990 U.S. Senior National Championships, the 1989 and 1990 U.S. Senior Team Trials, the 1989 and 1990 U.S. Junior National Championships and the 1989 World Junior Championships. These eight tournaments involved a total of 5 682 competitors, including 4 318 males and 1 364 females. There were 4 139 Junior competitors aged 6-17 years old (3 274 males and 865 females) and 1 543 Senior competitors aged 18 years and older (1 044 males and 499 females).

This sport involves kicks and punches to the body and kicks to the head (punches to the head are not allowed). Competitors are categorized into eight weight divisions. Protective equipment includes a chest and rib protector; padding on the forearms, lower legs and dorsal side of the feet; and a light helmet constructed of foam rubber material approximately 1/2 in. thick. Points are scored by well-placed blows to the head and a designated area of the chest and rib protector.

Summaries of results for the general injury patterns found during this study have been reported elsewhere [1-3]. This paper will focus on the occurrence of cerebral concussions during taekwondo competition.

METHODS

Injury data were collected with simple check-off forms that describe the athlete and nature, site, circumstances and severity of the injury. These forms are a variation of forms used by the Athletic Injury Monitoring System, a national sports injury data collection system designed and operated by one of the authors (Dr. Eric Zemper). The forms were completed by the authors or by the medical staff covering the competition at the time of treatment for every injury for which treatment was sought by the competitors. All forms were screened on-site by the lead author to ensure completeness and consistency of the completed forms. The classification of cerebral concussion used in this study is that of Nelson et al. [4]. Exposures for calculating injury rates were gathered from records of bouts actually fought. Injury rates are reported as injuries per 1 000 athlete-exposures or per 1 000 minutes of exposure. In this instance, an athlete-exposure is one athlete taking part in one taekwondo bout where he or she is exposed to the possibility of being injured. Since each bout involves two competitors, there are two athlete-exposures per bout. The basic formula for calculating injury rates is: (# of recorded injuries divided by the total number of athlete-exposures) x 1 000 = # injuries per 1 000 athlete-exposures.

In the case of injury rates per 1 000 minutes, the total
number of athlete-exposures is replaced by the total number
of minutes of exposure as the denominator in the equation.

RESULTS

In the eight competitions covered during this study the
5 682 participants were involved in 5 566 bouts for a total
of 11 132 athlete-exposures (A-E). Accounting for instances
where bouts were terminated early because of injury, there
were a total of 52 575 min (876.25 h) of exposure. Table 1
summarizes the calculated injury rates for all reported
injuries, by gender and level of competition. Two types of

TABLE 1--<u>Total injury rates in taekwondo competition.</u>

	Rate/1 000 A-E			Rate/1 000 min		
	Male	Female	Total	Male	Female	Total
Juniors	58.2	56.6	57.8	16.1	14.8	15.8
Seniors	93.2	120.7	102.7	13.7	16.1	14.6
TOTALS	67.8	84.9	72.0	15.1	15.6	15.3

injury rates are shown in Table 1, rate per 1 000 athlete-
exposure and rate per 1 000 min of exposure. Injury rates
based on the number of exposures to the possibility of being
injured and on the amount of time exposed are much more
precise and provide a more accurate picture of injury
patterns than the rates per 100 participants most often seen
in the literature on sports injuries. There were a total of
802 injuries recorded. For those more familiar with rates
per 100 participants, for purposes of comparison, this is
equivalent to 14.1 injuries per 100 competitors (13.2/100
competitors for males, 17.1/100 competitors for females,
10.6/100 competitors for Juniors and 23.5/100 competitors
for Seniors). The majority of these injuries (64%) were not
serious enough to cause termination of participation in the
competition. Table 2 summarizes the injury rates for time-
loss injuries. Thirty-six percent (292) of the recorded
injuries were severe enough to cause time-loss of one day or
more from further participation. Twenty-five percent of the
injuries to Senior competitors were time-loss injuries,
while 45% of the injuries to Juniors involved time-loss. The
difference may be explained by physicians being more
conservative in recommending a period of non-participation
following an injury for children and adolescents than they

would be for adult competitors. The total time-loss injury rates of 26.2/1 000 athlete-exposures or 5.6/1 000 min of exposure are equivalent to one time-loss injury in every 10 bouts. These rates are essentially the same for males and females.

TABLE 2--Time-loss injury rates in taekwondo competition.

| | Rate/1 000 A-E | | | Rate/1 000 min | | |
	Male	Female	Total	Male	Female	Total
Juniors	25.7	29.2	26.4	7.1	7.6	7.2
Seniors	27.7	22.2	25.8	4.1	3.0	3.7
TOTALS	26.3	26.1	26.2	5.9	4.8	5.6

Table 3 shows the distribution of injuries by area of the body. As can be seen, injuries were fairly equally divided between the head and lower extremities, each accounting for about 40% of the injuries, with the remainder occurring in the upper extremities and the body. As might be expected given the nature of this sport, the predominant type of injury was contusions (45%), most of which were not severe enough to cause any time-loss.

TABLE 3--Distribution of taekwondo injuries by body area.

	# of Time-Loss Injuries	Percent
Head & Neck	106	36.3
Upper Extremities	35	12.0
Torso	37	12.7
Lower Extremities	114	39.0
TOTALS	292	100.0

The most common of the more serious injuries observed during the eight tournaments covered in this study were cerebral concussions (Table 4). With 58 such injuries recorded, there was approximately one concussion for every 100 participants. Table 4 presents the cerebral concussion

TABLE 4--Cerebral concussion rates in taekwondo competition.

	Rate/1 000 A-E			Rate/1 000 min		
	Male	Female	Total	Male	Female	Total
Juniors	5.4	4.6	5.3	1.5	1.2	1.4
Seniors	6.1	3.3	5.1	0.9	0.4	0.7
TOTALS	5.6	4.0	5.2	1.3	0.7	1.1

rates by level of competition and gender. They ranged in severity from very mild, involving post-bout headache following a direct blow to the head (Nelson Grade 0), to severe concussions (Nelson Grade 4) involving extended loss of consciousness, retrograde amnesia and, in one case, seizures. There were 11 Grade 0 cerebral concussions recorded, 36 mild concussions of Nelson Grade 1 or 2, 8 moderate or Nelson Grade 3, and 3 severe or Nelson Grade 4. All of the Grade 3 and Grade 4 concussions occurred in males. The total rates for cerebral concussions were 5.2 per 1 000 athlete-exposures or 1.1/1 000 min. of exposure. Males have a somewhat higher rate of concussion than females, while Juniors and Seniors have about the same rate based on athlete-exposures, but Juniors have a higher rate based on minutes of exposure.

It should be noted in these tables for total injuries, time-loss injuries and concussions that Juniors generally have approximately the same or lower injury rates when calculated based on numbers of athlete-exposures (bouts), but the Juniors have higher rates when based on the number of minutes of exposure. This is due to longer rounds and more rounds per bout for Seniors, resulting in four minutes per bout for Juniors and nine minutes per bout for Seniors. Although the risk of injury per bout is greater for Seniors, the risk of injury per minute of competitive exposure is actually greater for the Juniors.

DISCUSSION

A comparison of injury rates in competition for taekwondo and in various intercollegiate sports shows that taekwondo has among the highest time-loss injury rates, exceeded only by football and wrestling [5]. However, when looking specifically at cerebral concussion rates, the situation becomes of more concern. The total concussion rate for collegiate football games is 1.7/1 000 athlete-exposures or 0.14/1 000 min of exposure [6]. College football generally has been considered to have one of the highest concussion rates in American sports, yet the concussion rate for taekwondo competition is 3.1 times higher based on number of athlete-exposures, and 7.9 times that seen in college football games when based on minutes of exposure. This becomes of major concern when considering the cumulative effects of concussion.

It has been shown that memory function and information processing capacity are measurably reduced for up to 30 days after a closed head injury, even those that do not involve loss of consciousness [7,8]. The degree of reduction in function not only is greater in those who have had a previous concussion, but the measurable cognitive deficits also last longer before returning to normal. These closed head injuries (defined as no skull fracture, no intracranial hematoma, no localized neurological signs) have three distinct and measurable effects on memory. First, there is reduction in information processing ability, related to tasks requiring complex processing or tasks with time constraints. Second, there are problems storing material in long-term memory and, third, there is a deficit in retrieval ability once material is stored. This has obvious implications for the classroom performance of school age competitors who sustain even mild head injuries during participation in any sport.

It has been noted that Senior taekwondo athletes can generate velocities of 13-16 m/s during the roundhouse kick, a circular kick most frequently used in competition [9]. The Junior girls who participated in the First Junior Taekwondo World Championships recorded a mean velocity of 12 m/s (range: 9-14.5 m/s) for the roundhouse kick, and the boys 14.7 m/s (range: 12-19.6 m/s). It was estimated that a punch velocity of 8 m/s would result in a peak acceleration of the head of about 200 g, assuming there is no deflection during the punch [10]. Head accelerations of 80 g are hypothesized to cause concussion in adults [11]. It is readily apparent that the velocities generated by even the Junior taekwondo athletes during kicking are more than sufficient to result in cerebral concussion in adults.

Based on the results presented here plus other observations made during this multi-disciplinary study, project staff are working with the U.S. Taekwondo Union Sports Medicine Committee to develop a series of recommendations aimed at reducing risk of cerebral concussion in this sport. These include measures such as requiring the use of mouthguards (currently, use is only recommended, and additional data from this project show that the more severe the concussion the less likely the competitor was wearing a mouthguard); requiring the use in competition of mats to help reduce the possibility of concussion if the head hits the floor during a fall (which was observed on several occasions where competition took place on concrete floors covered only by a thin layer of carpet); and improvements in protective equipment (particularly the helmet). Additional potential rule modifications include adopting a mandatory suspension from participation for a specified period for individuals suffering a knock-out, similar to the rules used in amateur boxing; or disqualification of a competitor who causes a knock-out of an opponent, which would return the emphasis to skill and technique rather than "going for the kill," particularly when behind on points. The two primary areas where this sport may be able to utilize assistance from standard-setting bodies will be in the development of minimum standards for competition mats, and in establishing helmet standards in cooperation with manufacturers to encourage development of headgear with better protective capability.

ACKNOWLEDGEMENTS

This study was funded by the U.S. Olympic Committee and supported by the U.S. Taekwondo Union. Thanks also are extended to Samuel Pejo, M.D., Marianette Bailey, R.N., and Charles Bailey for their help in data collection, and to the several attending physicians at the various tournaments for their cooperation.

REFERENCES

[1]   Zemper, E.D., and Pieter, W., "Injury Rates in Junior and Senior National Taekwondo Competition," in: Proceedings of the First IOC World Congress on Sport Sciences, USOC, Colorado Springs, 1989, pp 219-220.

[2]   Zemper, E.D., and Pieter, W., "Injury Rates at the 1988 U.S. Olympic Team Trials for Taekwondo," British Journal of Sports Medicine, Vol. 23, No. 3, 1989, pp 161-164.

[3]   Pieter, W., and Zemper, E.D., "The Oregon Taekwondo Project - Part II: Preliminary Injury Research Results," Taekwondo USA, Fall 1990.

[4]   Nelson, W.E., Jane, J.A., and Gieck, J.H., " Minor Head Injury in Sports: A New System of Classification and Management," The Physician and Sportsmedicine, Vol. 12, No. 3, 1984, pp 103-107.

[5]   McKeag, D., Hough, D., and Zemper, E., Primary Care Sports Medicine, Brown and Benchmark, Dubuque IA, 1993, pp 68-69.

[6]   Zemper, E.D., Unpublished data.

[7] Gronwall, D., and Wrightson, P., "Cumulative Effect of Concussion," Lancet, Vol. II(7943), 1975, pp 995-997.

[8] Gronwall, D., and Wrightson, P., " Memory and Information Processing Capacity after Closed Head Injury," Journal of Neurological Surgery and Psychology, Vol. 44, No. 10, 1981, pp 889-895.

[9] Pieter, F., and Pieter, W., "Speed and Force of Selected Taekwondo Techniques," (In Press).

[10] Whiting, W.C., Gregor, K.J., and Finerman, G.A., "Kinematic Analysis of Human Upper Extremity Movements in Boxing," American Journal of Sports Medicine, Vol. 16, No. 2, 1986, pp 130-136.

[11] Smith, P.K., and Hamill, J., "The Effect of Punching Glove Type and Skill Level on Momentum Transfer," Journal of Human Movement Science, Vol. 12, No. 3, 1986, pp 153-161.

Biomechanics, Laboratory Simulation, and Modeling

Patrick J. Bishop[1]

IMPACT POSTURES AND NECK LOADING IN HEAD FIRST COLLISIONS:
A REVIEW

REFERENCE: Bishop, P.J. "Impact Postures and Neck Loading
in Head First Collisions: A Review" Head and Neck Injuries
in Sports, ASTM STP 1229, Earl F. Hoerner, Ed., American
Society For Testing and Materials, Philadelphia, 1994.

ABSTRACT: Axial compression of the cervical spine is a
significant source of spinal cord trauma and quadriplegia.
This paper summarizes a number of studies related to injury
mechanisms and potential strategies for reducing the risk of
trauma. Head first collisions at 1.8 m.s^{-1} were conducted
with a mechanical test dummy fitted with a force and moment
transducer in the neck. Films taken at 500 fps confirmed
that the head-neck-torso system was decelerated in stages
rather than uniformly, so that the neck became trapped
between the fixed head and moving torso. Compression forces
were about 4800N for the neutral neck and 3800N for the
flexed neck. Further analysis with a post-processing
computer model of the cervical spine revealed compressive
forces in excess of 5000N in the lower regions (C_5, C_6, C_7)
for both the flexed and neutral postures. Simulations with
the neck extended suggest that the anterior longitudinal
ligament, the neural arches and spinous processes would
likely be damaged. When the ATD was subjected to blows that
produced side bending of the head and neck the compressive
force output from the transducer was 50% lower when compared
to direct axial loading. This side bending posture appears
to offer some promise in reducing the compressive loads on
the spine due to head first collisions.

KEYWORDS: Axial Loading, Cervical Spine, Impact Postures,
Flexed/Extended Neck, Lateral Bending

Axial compression of the cervical spine, associated
with head first collisions in sport or recreation is a
significant source of spinal trauma and quadriplegia. The
primary cause of these injuries is a collision in which the

---

[1] Professor, Department of Kinesiology, University of
Waterloo, Waterloo, Ontario, Canada, N2L 3G1

crown of the injured player's head either strikes or is struck by a fixed or moving object. The head is often partially flexed so that the cervical lordosis is removed and the cervical vertebrae became aligned one on top of the other. The compressive force is then distributed along the cervical spine resulting in compressive deformation of the vertebral discs, continued compressive deformation of the vertebral bodies, angular deformation of the cervical column and finally buckling. Cervical failure is often apparent between C_4 and C_6 and is manifested clinically as a burst fracture, vertebral subluxation or both [1].

While the problem of axial compressive loading is a significant issue for North American football, our concern has been with ice hockey where players have suffered quadriplegia after being propelled head first to strike the boards surrounding the ice surface with the top or crown of the head. This paper summarizes a number of studies conducted in our laboratory related to the mechanics associated with these injuries and with strategies for potentially reducing the risk of such injuries.

MECHANICAL SIMULATIONS

Head first collisions were conducted by propelling a mechanical anthropometric test dummy (ATD), wearing an ice hockey helmet, in free flight to strike a rigid barrier (Figure 1). These simulations have been described previously [2,3].

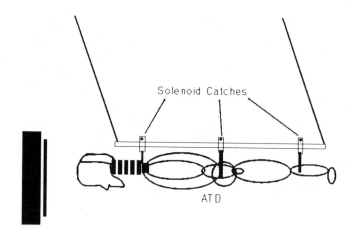

Fig. 1--ATD Impact Assembly Set-up (Schematic).

The ATD consisted of a Hybrid III head and neck fitted at the atlanto-occipital junction (a-o) with a transducer (Denton Electronics) that output three orthogonal forces and moments of force. The head and neck combination was affixed to a Hybrid II body which was modified so that it represented a standing rather than a seated ATD. The ATD was placed in the prone position and attached to a swing bar suspended from the ceiling. This enabled the entire assembly to be raised to the height required to produce a desired impact velocity. Upon release from the appropriate height, the ATD swing bar assembly travelled like a pendulum toward a rigid barricade. As it passed through a photoelectric light beam the solenoid catches on the swing bar, were released, permitting the ATD to travel horizontally in free flight to strike the rigid barrier. At impact, the force and moment signals from the transducer were amplified and digitally converted through a 12 bit A/D converter with a sampling rate of 2500 Hz per channel. The photoelectric beam system served to trigger the A/D converter. The A/D output was processed on an IBM-PC using specially written software to produce the force-time and moment-time curves. Collisions were filmed at 500 fps using a Locam movie camera.

It is well recognized that the Hybrid III neck is much stiffer than the human cervical spine [4, 5], and that it is limited both anatomically and physiologically. However, other models suitable for studying axial compressive loading, such as cadavers or animals, present substantial limitations as well. It is extremely difficult to obtain permission from ethics committees for the use of such models and, even if they were permitted, scientists are faced with issues of repeatability and reproducibility, items over which control is difficult when using animal or human specimens. It was decided on balance, therefore, that to overcome some of these limitations a durable mechanical surrogate, capable of repeated use, was suitable for investigating this injury producing mechanism. To partially account for the problem of stiffness, low impact velocities, which still produced large compressive forces, were used in the collision trials.

INJURY RISK REDUCTION

Since the majority of cervical spine injuries associated with axial loading are vertebral body fractures, injury risk reduction strategies should be directed toward lowering the large compressive forces acting on the cervical vertebral column.

One strategy often suggested is the use of protective padding. Certainly some padding materials placed on the floor can be helpful in reducing the risk of cervical trauma in a sport like gymnastics. However, the suggestion that placing additional padding material in the crown of a sport helmet would be helpful is indeed questionable. Previous studies have shown that the thickness of the padding material needed to keep the compressive force within tolerable limits is excessive and is not compatible for use in a sport environment

[3, 6]. Thus, in attempting to arrive at appropriate risk reduction strategies, our efforts have been directed toward active measures that players can potentially use to protect themselves when faced with an axial loading situation. These measures are related to the position of the head and neck at impact.

Conditions of axial loading occur in sport because the player's head and neck are placed in partial flexion, a vulnerable position that allows force to be directed along the straightened cervical spine. This can happen because of fear, for example, when a football player drops his head to make contact with an opponent. It can also happen to a hockey player who is struck from behind and is propelled forward to strike the boards, goalpost or another player. When struck from behind the natural tendency is for the head to move into extension due to indirect inertial loading. This is true if the player is upright. Often, however, hockey players are bent over at the waist and a check or push from behind will cause them to contact an immovable surface with a partially flexed neck. What then, can players do to avoid this vulnerable neck posture if they find themselves in such a predicament? Should the head be flexed further, extended or moved to the side? Given that players will not have a great deal of time to react, it may well be that they cannot do anything. If they can be prepared however, by placing the head and neck in an appropriate posture and actively contracting their muscles to stiffen the cervical spine, they may be able to reduce the risk of cervical quadriplegia. Various postures were investigated by using the ATD and placing the head and neck into flexion or extension or forcing it to lateral bending. The increased stiffness of the ATD, when compared to the human neck, helped to account for the condition of prepared, contracted musculature.

a) Neutral and Flexed Neck Postures

A series of experiments was conducted to investigate the loading on the cervical spine with both a neutral and a flexed neck in order to determine whether the flexed posture of the head and neck was protective (Figure 2). The ATD neck was held in flexion (30° below the horizontal) by means of a light breakable cord running from a hook inserted in the ATD mouth to another hook attached to the ATD chest. The neutral posture of the ATD was selected to represent pure axial loading. More complete details of these experiments were presented at the first ASTM Symposium in Safety in Ice Hockey and are published elsewhere [3].

Film observation of both the flexed and neutral collisions revealed that the head-neck-torso system was decelerated in stages rather than uniformly, so that the head stopped first, trapping the neck between it and the moving torso.

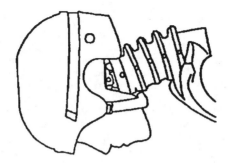

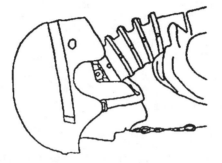

Fig. 2--ATD Neck Positions of Neutral (Top) and Flexed
        (Bottom).

When the compressive forces recorded from the transducer
were examined for both bareheaded and helmeted trials,
magnitudes of approximately 3800N (flexed) to 4800N (axial)
were obtained (Figure 3). Based on these results it appeared
that the flexed posture might indeed be protective.

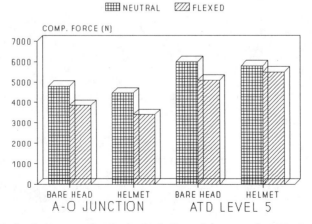

Fig. 3--Peak Compression at A-O Junction and ATD Level 5.

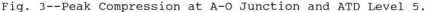

Since cervical injuries due to axial compressive loading usually occur lower in the cervical spine, and not at the atlanto-occipital region, an attempt was made to enhance the biofidelity of the ATD. This was done by combining the forces and moments of force obtained from the transducer with the neck position information obtained from the cine film for use as inputs to a previously described post-processing analytical computer model of the cervical spine [2]. Representative compressive forces at ATD neck level 5 (approximating C6), obtained when using the model for both the axial and flexed postures, are also shown in Figure 3.

The magnitude of the compressive forces in the lower cervical spine, for both the axial and flexed neck postures, was very large and the initially noted advantage of the flexed neck posture has disappeared. From these results it was concluded that a flexed neck posture at impact did not provide a reasonable measure of injury risk reduction in situations of axial loading. In fact, it is more reasonable to conclude that flexing the neck likely places players in positions which make them extremely vulnerable to cervical trauma.

b)   **Extended Neck Posture**

In discussing cervical spine injuries associated with diving, McElhaney [7] noted that catastrophic injuries related to axial loading were not generally observed when the head and neck were in extension at impact. This suggests that when the face or forehead makes contact (rather than the crown of the head) the cervical spine will be forced further into extension, possibly reducing the compression on the cervical vertebral bodies to tolerable levels. In such instances it is suspected that the spinous processes of the adjacent vertebrae would be forced together, allowing the compressive load to be shared by both the spinous processes in contact and by structures other than the vertebral bodies [8].

To investigate the loading distribution produced by a face first or forehead first collision, a number of trials with the Hybrid III ATD was again conducted. The head and neck were held in extension (20° above the horizontal) prior to impact by means of a light breakable cord as illustrated in Figure 4. To enhance the biofidelity of the ATD, the force, moment and positional outputs were post-processed using a quasi-static analytical sagittal plane model of the cervical spine in compression and extension. Essentially, this model partitioned the reaction forces and moments of force to several load bearing structures including the vertebral bodies, the anterior longitudinal ligament, the intervertebral discs, the anterior muscles of the neck, the neural arches and the cervical spinous processes. The anatomical link between real life, the ATD and the analytical model was provided by Magnetic Resonance Imaging (MRI) scans of the live human neck under forced extension. Complete details of the model and its

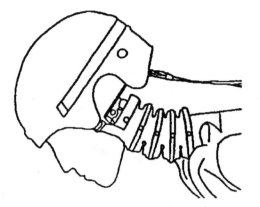

Fig. 4--Extended position of ATD Neck.

use in analyzing a face first collision are described elsewhere [9]. Since the most common sites of trauma in extension compression injuries include the anterior longitudinal ligament and the spinous processes [10, 11, 12, 13] the loading on these structures will be considered here.

i)   Anterior Longitudinal Ligament and Neck Musculature

One of the ways to examine the model's output is to consider the moments of force acting about the facets. These moments must be supported by the tissue structures involved in order to prevent spinal failure. Table I gives the transducer moment and the moments at each cervical segment modelled as well as the moments for the anterior longitudinal ligament (ALL) for bareheaded trials at 1.8 and 2.5 m.s^{-1}. Although the ALL is considered to be an important structure for resisting neck extension under normal circumstances [14, 15, 16] the model suggests that it accounts for only a small proportion (less than 2.5%) of the peak segmental load. Although not included in Table I, the longus colli and longus capitis muscles accounted for a maximum of 5% of the segmental moment and the intervertebral discs and the anterior neck muscles accounted for approximately 15% and 20% respectively.

Table II shows that below C_2/C_3 the modelled ALL forces for a 1.8 m.s^{-1} trial were within 50-60% of the failure loads provided by Yoganandan, et. al. [5] and were within 60-80% of failure for a 2.5 m.s^{-1} trial. Even though the ALL may not be critical for supporting the loads imposed by a face first impact, it does play on important role in resisting subluxation and thus contributes to spinal stability. Because the predicted loads borne on this ligament exceed 50% of failure tolerance, particularly in the lower cervical spine, it is likely that this structure would be close to its limits of extension under the forced neck extension expected from a face first impact, making it vulnerable to failure.

TABLE I-- Segmental and Anterior Longitudinal ligament moments obtained for two impact velocities

Spinal level	1.8 m.s^{-1}		2.5 m.s^{-1}	
	Seg. Mt, Nm[1]	Lig. Mt, Nm	Seg.Mt, Nm	Lig.Mt, Nm
A-O	-39.0	...	-74.2	...
C_1	-9.3	...	-10.9	...
C_2	11.9	4.6	22.3	0.6
C_3	34.0	7.0	62.1	0.7
C_4	59.9	9.3	95.7	1.2
C_5	68.0	13.1	97.9	1.6
C_6	71.8	11.4	106.4	2.2
C_7	80.7	10.9	108.4	1.9

TABLE II--Predicted Anterior Longitudinal ligament forces compared to failure forces at two impact velocities

Spinal level	Failure[2] Force, N (± SD)	Lig.Force, N 1.8 m.s^{-1}	Lig.Force,N 2.5 m.s^{-1}
C_1/C_2	281 ± 36	...	...
C_2/C_3	207 ± 98	18.0	27.0
C_3/C_4	47 ± 14	20.8	31.3
C_4/C_5	47 ± 14	40.2	49.2
C_5/C_6	89 ± 67	51.9	70.8
C_6/C_7	176 ± 67	82.9	102.9
C_7/T_1	97 ± 28	57.7	68.7

ii) Spinous Processes

The majority of the loading in these collisions would be borne by bony structures including the vertebral bodies, neural arches and spinous processes. The MRI scans of three

---

[1] A - sign indicates clockwise direction

[2] From Yoganandan, et al (1989)

volunteers verified that the spinous processes from adjacent vertebrae did indeed contact each other under forced neck extension. The extension angle at which contact was observed was 74.5° (SD 6.1°). This observation supported the assumption that spinous process contact was one mechanism for sharing or distributing the impact load. When the spinous processes were not in contact the loading would be supported, in part at least, by the neural arches.

Figure 5 illustrates the compressive loading on the vertebral spinous processes output from the model at C_4, C_5, C_6 and C_7 for impact velocities of 0.9, 1.8 and 2.5 m.s^{-1}. In Figure 5 the spinous process forces were normalized to a failure load determined indirectly from the cervical vertebral body failure tolerance of two age groups (20 to 39 years; 40 to 59 years) provided by Sonnoda [17], cross-sectional dimensions provided by Francis [18], cross-sectional area determined from the work of Nachemson and Morris [19], and spinous process contact area determined from graphical representations of the cervical vertebrae provided by Kazarian [11]. The failure loads for the cervical spinous processes were then obtained by scaling the tolerance of a given vertebral body according to the ratio of the contact area of the spinous processes to the cross-sectional area of the vertebral body [9]. Using this procedure the failure loads were estimated to range from 550N to 750N (age 20 to 39 years) and from 450N to 650N (age 40 to 59 years).

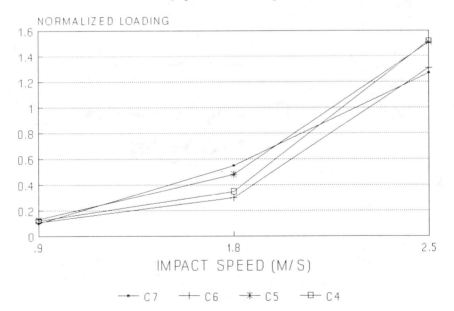

Fig. 5--Predicted Normalized Spinous Process Loading vs. Impact Speed.

Figure 5 suggests that 75% of failure would occur at an ATD impact velocity of 2.3 m.s^{-1} and that by 2.5 m.s^{-1} the failure load would be exceeded by as much as 50%. However, it is difficult to translate an ATD impact velocity to the velocity with which players strike the boards.

Based upon the results of this extension model it appears that the face-first or forehead-first impact mode may offer some protection against quadriplegia in head first collisions because of the ability to distribute the load across the entire cervical segment and to soft tissue structures of the cervical column. Other types of tissue disruption, in the form of ligamentatous and/or spinous process failure can be expected, however, likely at moderate impact velocities.

c)   Side Bending of the Head and Neck

An additional approach for reducing the magnitude of the compression on the neck that has been investigated is that of attempting to divert the axial force by means of a glancing blow that would produce lateral bending of the cervical spine.

A series of crash simulations was conducted as described previously but lateral bending of the ATD neck was produced by placing the impact barrier at different angles to the flight of the ATD as shown in Figure 6. The angle of incidence of the ATD was either 70° or 50° to the impact surface and the results were compared to those obtained from direct axial load collisions in which the angle of incidence was 90°.

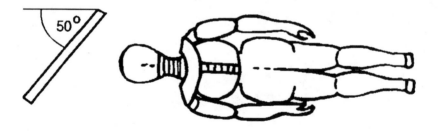

Fig. 6--ATD Lateral Bending (Top View).

Figure 7 summarizes the average peak compressive and lateral shear forces recorded at the transducer for three trials at each angle of incidence. When compared to the direct axial loading condition (i.e. 90°), the compressive force was not effectively reduced for the 70° impacts. However, at 50° the compressive force was reduced to about 2200N, a 50% and a 55% decrease compared to the 70° impact and 90° impacts respectively. The lateral shear forces increased from 50 Nm (90°) to 497 Nm (50°).

LATERAL SHEAR & COMPRESSION

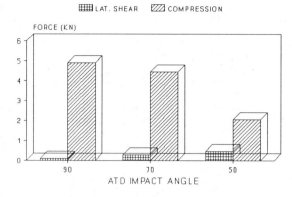

Fig. 7--Peak Lateral Shear and Compression vs. ATD Impact
      Angle.

        These results suggest that turning the head to the side
prior to impact may be effective in reducing the compressive
loading on the neck provided the glancing angle is large
enough.   High speed film of these collisions taken from above
the ATD showed that for the 90° and 70° conditions the ATD
head was restrained by the barrier during impact so that the
ATD neck became trapped between the fixed head and the moving
torso.   This produced large compressive forces on the ATD
neck.   For the 50° condition, the ATD head was not restrained
but was free to move (Figure 8).   Thus the ATD neck was not
trapped and the compressive load was substantially reduced.

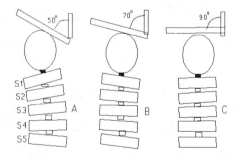

Fig. 8--ATD Neck Bending During 50° (A), 70° (B) and 90° (C)
      Impacts

These findings are similar to those of Meyers, et. al. (20)
who examined the influence of imposed end conditions on spinal

loading and found that full end constraint conditions produced large axial loads (and comparatively small flexion moments) but that unconstrained specimens developed both small axial loads and comparatively small flexion moments.

While this reduction in compression appears promising, it must be remembered that in real life the lateral shear forces and moments of force produced by forced lateral bending of the head would have to be borne by the vertebral bodies, the facets, the intervertebral discs, the ligaments and muscles of the cervical column [21]. Whether the loads measured in the ATD would produce failure in these tissues in live humans is uncertain. Lateral bending of the neck and associated nerve root injuries are common in football, yet this author is unaware of any football players who have suffered quadriplegia due to lateral neck bending. Based upon cadaveric observation, forced lateral bending of the neck may also lead to some torsion but the effect of this has not been investigated here.

From the results of these simulations it does appear that for conditions which produce enough lateral bending of the ATD head and neck, to prevent it from being trapped between the fixed head and moving torso, the amount of axial compression can be substantially reduced without producing large lateral shear forces. Further investigations to extrapolate these data to the human cervical spine are ongoing.

SUMMARY AND CONCLUSIONS

To effectively reduce the risk of cervical quadriplegia from head first collisions it is necessary to reduce the magnitude of the compressive force acting on the cervical spine. While rule changes and appropriate techniques may be helpful in keeping players from high risk predicaments, there are many instances where players are unwittingly placed in situations where a head-first collision is a distinct possibility. In these instances players need to be able to react appropriately in order to protect themselves.

Several impact postures were evaluated using a mechanical surrogate propelled to strike a rigid barrier. The results suggest that a flexed neck posture is not effective in reducing the magnitude of the compressive load on the neck. An extended neck posture, produced by a face-first or forehead-first collision may offer some protection but tissue disruption is likely even at moderate impact speeds. Lateral bending of the head and neck appears to be effective in reducing the magnitude of the compressive force on the neck, provided the head is bent far enough to the side. Further research is needed to examine the potential effects of such blows to other bony structures and soft tissues of the cervical spine.

ACKNOWLEDGEMENTS

Appreciation is extended to Sport Canada, the Canadian Amateur Hockey Association, The Defence and Civil Institute of Environmental Medicine and the Rick Hansen Man in Motion Legacy Fund for their support of this work.

REFERENCES

[1]   Torg, J.S., J.V. Vegso, M.J. O'Neill and B. Sennett. "The Epidemiologic, Pathologic, Biomechanical and Cinematographic Analysis of Football Induced Cervical Spine Trauma." American Journal of Sports Medicine, Vol. 18, No. 1, 1990, pp. 50-57.

[2]   Bishop, P.J. and R.P. Wells. "The Hybrid III Anthropometric Neck in the Evaluation of Head First Collisions", In Passenger Comfort, Convenience and Safety: Test Tools and Procedures, SAE Publication, p174, 1986, pp. 131-140.

[3]   Bishop, P.J. and Wells, R.P. "Cervical Spine Fractures: Mechanisms, Neck Loads and Methods of Prevention," in Castaldi, C.R. and Hoerner, E.F. (eds.) Safety in Ice Hockey, Philadelphia, Pa: ASTM STP 150, 1989, pp 71-83.

[4]   McElhaney, J., Doherty, B.J., Paver, J.G., Myers, B.S. and Gray, L. "Combined Bending and Axial Loading Responses of the Human Cervical Spine." Proceedings of the Thirty-Second Stapp Car Crash Conference, SAE, No. 88179, 1988.

[5]   Yoganandan, N., F. Pintar, J. Butler, J. Reinartz, A. Sances, Jr. and S.J. Larson. "Dynamic Response of Human Cervical Spine Ligaments." Spine, Vol. 14, No. 10, 1989, pp. 1102-1110.

[6]   Wells, R.P., Bishop, P.J. and Stephens, M. "Neck Loads During Head First Collisions in Ice Hockey: Experimental and Simulation Results," International Journal of Sport Biomechanics Vol. 3, No. 4, 1987, pp. 432-442.

[7]   McElhaney, J. "The Biomechanical Aspects of Spinal Trauma." Presented at the Second International Symposium on the Prevention of Catastrophic Sports and Recreational Injuries to the Spine and Head. The Canadian Sports Spine and Head Injuries Research Centre, Toronto Western Hospital, Toronto, January, 1989.

[8]   Prasad, P., A.I. King and C.L. Ewing. "The Role of Articular Facets During +Gz Acceleration." Journal Applied Mechanics, 1974, pp. 321-326.

[9] Li, Y., Bishop, P.J., Wells, R.P. and McGill, S.M. "A Quasi-Static Analytical Sagittal Plane Model of the Cervical Spine in Extension and Compression," Proceedings of the 35th Stapp Car Crash Conference, SAE, San Diego, Ca., Paper 912917, Nov. 1991.

[10] Bauze, J.R. and Ardran, M.A. "Experimental Production of Forward Dislocation in the Human Cervical Spine" Journal Bone and Joint Surgery Vol 60B, No. 2, 1978, pp. 239-245.

[11] Kazarian, L. "Injuries to the Human Spinal Column: Biomechanics and Injury Classification," Exercise and Sport Sciences Review Vol. 9, 1981, pp. 297-352.

[12] Maiman, D.J., A. Sances, Jr., J.B. Myklebust, S.J. Larson, C. Houterman, M. Chilbert and A.Z. El-Ghatit. "Compression Injuries of the Cervical Spine: A Biomechanical Analysis," Neurosurgery, Vol. 13, No. 3, 1983, pp. 254-260.

[13] Nusholtz, G., Huelke, D.E., Lux, P., Alem, N.M., and Montalvo, F. "Cervical Spine Injury Mechanisms," Proceedings of the Twenty Seventh Stapp Car Crash Conference, SAE: Philadelphia, 1989, pp. 191-214.

[14] Woodburne, R.T., Essentials of Human Anatomy, Sixth Edition, Oxford University Press, London, 1978.

[15] Sances, A. Jr., R.C. Weber and S.J. Larson. "Bioengineering Analysis of Head and Spine Injuries." CRC Critical Reviews in Bioengineering, Vol. 8, February 1981, pp. 79-122.

[16] Sances, A. Jr., J. Myklebust and D. Maiman. "Biomechanics of Spinal Injuries." CRC Critical Reviews in Biomedical Engineering, Vol. 11, 1984, pp. 1-76.

[17] Sonoda, T. "Studies on the Strength for Compression, Tension and Torsion of the Human Vertebral Column." Journal of Kyoto Prefectural Medical University, Vol. 71, 1962, pp. 659-702.

[18] Francis, C.C. "Dimensions of the Cervical Vertebrae." Anatomical Record, Vol. 122, 1955, pp. 603-609.

[19] Nachemson, A. and C.J.M. Morris. "In Vivo Measurements of Intradiscal Pressure." Journal of Bone and Joint Surgery, Vol 46, No. 5, 1964, pp. 1077-1092.

[20] Myers, B.S., McElhaney, J.H. Richardson, W.J., Nightingale, R.W. and Doherty, B.J. "The Influence of End Condition on Human Cervical Spine Injury Mechanisms," Proceedings of the Thirty Fifth Stapp Car Crash Conference, SAE: Philadelphia, Pa., 1991, pp. 391-399.

[21] Goel, V.K., Winterbottom, J.H., Weinstein, J.N., and Kim, Y.E. "Load Sharing Among Spinal Elements of a Motion Segment in Extension and Lateral Bending," <u>Journal of Biomechanical Engineering</u> Vol. 109, 1987, pp. 291-297.

Albert H. Burstein,[1] and James C. Otis[1]

THE RESPONSE OF THE CERVICAL SPINE TO AXIAL LOADING: FEASIBILITY FOR
INTERVENTION

REFERENCE: Burstein, A.H and Otis, J.C.,"The Response of the Cervical
Spine to Axial Loading: Feasibility for Intervention,"Head and Neck
Injuries in Sports, ASTM STP 1229, Earl F. Hoerner, Ed., American
Society for Testing and Materials, Philadelphia, 1994.

ABSTRACT: We present a two part study. The first part deals with the
mechanics of cervical spine injury and the injury mechanism. We have
established the parameters of a head first impact situation which gives
rise to catastrophic cervical spine injuries. We have examined the
parameters of head acceleration, time, neck and head force, and neck and
trunk displacement associated with such injuries. We will present data
on several types of football helmets, and show what alteration in the
mechanics of injury can be expected from a helmet.

The second part is the study of injury parameters which may be useful
in analyzing the efficacy of proposed protective devices. One such
device, a collar air bag, will be presented and its performance criteria
will be evaluated.

KEYWORDS: cervical spine, axial loading, football helmets, air bag,
computer simulation

Axial loading has been identified as the primary cause of catastrophic
cervical spine injury in athletes. These catastrophic injuries can
occur during head first tackles in football, head first impact with the
side board in hockey, head contact with the bottom of the pool during
diving, or head contact with a gym mat during an improperly executed
gymnastic maneuver. During each of these types of injuries, the
accident victim displayed the same posture and circumstance at the
moment of impact. First, the victim had his or her head flexed forward
slightly so that the cervical spine had been moved from its normal
lordotic position to one of axial alignment. Secondly, the victim was
moving in a direction coincident with the axis of the now straightened
cervical spine. Thirdly, impact occurred at or near the crown of the
head, allowing a resistance force to be directed through the head, and
co-linear with the axis of the straightened cervical spine.

Most accident configurations such as are found in diving and gymnastics
have the accident victim in motion with a velocity of approximately two
meters per second or more. Occasionally, as might be experienced in
football, the accident victim may not have been moving, but may instead
have been impacted by another moving player. In either circumstance,
there is considerable kinetic energy in the impact, and this energy
cannot be managed by the cervical spine, the skull, the protective
helmet or padding, or the combination of all three.

[1]Senior Scientist, Department of Biomechanics, Hospital for Special
Surgery, New York, NY 10021

The details of the mechanism of loading, as well as a model for its study, have previously been presented by the authors [1]. To summarize briefly, the model consists of the head, neck and torso of the accident victim, as well as the head and torso masses of the individual being struck. If it is a two person accident, the impacting masses are considered. If an immovable object is struck, a zero velocity boundary condition at the head or helmet is imposed. Associated with the head, and placed between it and the object being struck, is the load versus displacement description of the interface. This interface may represent either the helmet characteristics or the compliance characteristics of the head and scalp. The model also contains the load versus deflection characteristics of the cervical spine. The failure load of the cervical spine may be arbitrarily chosen to represent the appropriate failure mode. Thus, our recent interest in various buckling modes may be examined by the inclusion of appropriate critical loads [2], [3], [4]. As this current research indicates, the highest likely load at failure is approximately 4 500 N. We will continue to use this criteria as the limiting point of our analyses. Should it be desirable to investigate lower loads, these values may be read directly from the graphical presentations which will follow.

In this paper, we will review the mechanical performance of the neck in accidents which result in axial loading. We will look at the variables of energy, load, displacement and time. We will examine the parameters of impact velocity, equivalent torso mass, and load deflection characteristics of various helmets. Two cases will be examined, one in which the accident victim impacted a relatively immovable object, and the second in which the victim was impacted by an oncoming second person.

We first examined the kinetic energies in a typical impact situation in which an accident victim with a torso mass of thirty six kilograms impacted a relatively immovable stationary object at 4.6 meters per second velocity. We used, in this simulation, a helmet whose characteristics were modeled after a PAC 3 helmet, a variety which was popular for many years. In this simulation, we calculated the kinetic energy of the torso and of the head, and also calculated the strain energy stored in the helmet and the neck (Figure 1). For this set of parameters, the cervical spine would have fractured approximately eleven milliseconds after the onset of helmet contact, and we see that during this entire time, the torso retained approximately 95% of its kinetic energy. At the time of neck fracture, the head had lost virtually all its kinetic energy, save for a very small amount which it recaptured when it rebounded from the helmet. The helmet had stored approximately the same amount of kinetic energy which was possessed by the head, and this was just slightly more than the strain energy stored by the cervical spine before it failed. What is immediately apparent from examination of these factors is that there was a gross imbalance between the amount of kinetic energy which was available in the torso prior to impact, and the amount of energy which could be stored in both helmet and neck. The kinetic energy of the head appeared to be mostly transferred into strain energy in the helmet, and thus, there was virtually nothing but the cervical spine which was available to absorb the huge quantity of kinetic energy of the torso. Therefore, if the cervical spine is in the straightened position, and if axial loading occurs, failure of the spine is inevitable and no reasonable design of helmet or surface padding can prevent the catastrophic cervical spine injury which will ensue.

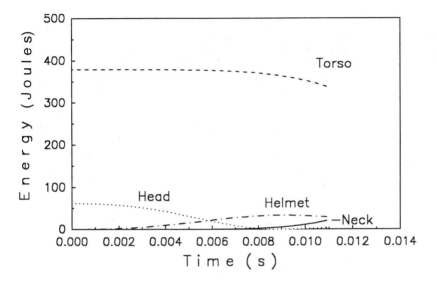

Figure 1   The relationship between the kinetic energies and the strain
energies   for a typical head first tackle while playing football.

We next ask the question: What is the sensitivity of this mechanism to
impact velocities? To answer the question, we repeated the impact with
the identical model presented, but at three velocities, 2.3 meters per
second, 4.6 meters per second, and 6.1 meters per second. This
represented a range of running velocities from modestly slow to
moderately fast. It is also representative of velocities obtained from
falls from rather modest heights. The results of the simulation showed
that for the highest velocities, the force on the cervical spine reached
critical buckling values in about seven milliseconds, whereas those same
forces were achieved at the low velocity at about eighteen milliseconds
after the initiation of contact (Figure 2). We observed, of course,
that the kinetic energy available at the higher impact speed, 6.1 meters
per second, presented an even more hopeless picture with regard to the
helmet's ability to protect the neck than was seen in the example
presented with a 4.6 meters/second velocity (Figure 1). Note, however,
that even at the low velocity (2.3 meters per second), the kinetic
energy of the torso was still about four times more than was needed to
cause cervical spine buckling.

We next examined the effect of the equivalent torso mass on the injury
mechanics. Varying the effect of torso mass is equivalent to examining
the effects of the line up between the cervical spine and the torso. In
those instances where the accident victim's body was well aligned, i.e.
head, cervical spine and torso are along a common axis, we have assigned
full torso mass to the model. If alignment was not perfect, it is
reasonable to assign a lesser fraction of torso mass to the analytical
model. In this analysis, in addition to the full thirty six kilograms
of torso mass, we examined the effect of half torso mass (eighteen
kilograms) and one quarter torso mass (nine kilograms)(Figure 3). In
all three instances, we see that the time to develop critical load in
the cervical spine was virtually identical. Since the kinetic energies
are proportional to the masses, we can imagine that we are dealing with

one half of the kinetic energy and one quarter of the kinetic energy
respectively, in the one half and one quarter mass simulations, but
these kinetic energies were more than sufficient to overcome the energy
absorbing capacity of the cervical spine.   Note that the time
relationships in developing the force in the cervical spine were not at
all sensitive to the equivalent mass of the torso.   Similar results, of
course, would be seen at different velocities.

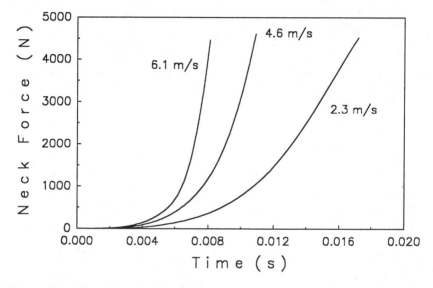

Figure 2   The effect of impact velocity on the load time history of the
cervical spine.

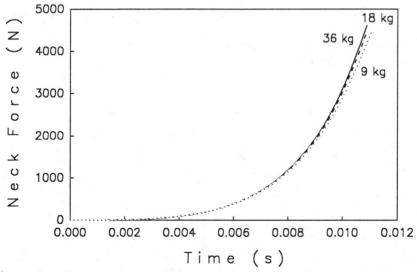

Figure 3   The neck force time history is shown for different equivalent
torso masses.

We next examined the effect of the load deflection characteristics of
various commercial sports helmets. Five varieties have been chosen,
some of which were used for historical comparison only. The neck force
is shown as a function of time for each simulated impact (Figure 4).
What we note is that the helmets produced different load time histories,
dependent upon the stiffness of the helmet padding in the initial
loading region. Those helmet pads which produced "softer" initial
loading responses required more time to stop the head. This response of
the head to the initial stiffness of the helmet pad resulted in a time
delay for compressing and loading the cervical spine. This initial
effect can be appreciated if we examine the time required for each of
the helmets to increase the neck force from one thousand N to forty five
hundred N. This time varied only from approximately two to three
milliseconds depending upon the helmet characteristics. In each of
these loading simulations, however, the strain energy absorbed by the
helmet represented little more than the kinetic energy lost by the head.

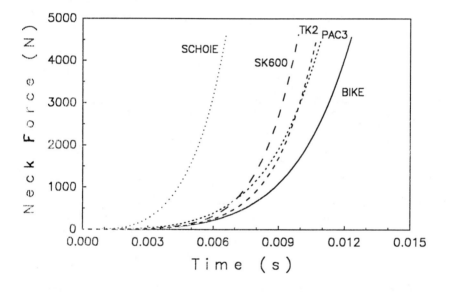

Figure 4   Neck forces are shown for different helmets.

We next examined the acceleration of the head in the simulated
catastrophic neck injury model. For this study, we chose to look at
five helmets whose load deflection characteristics vary most widely from
one another. These helmet manufacturers have apparently chosen somewhat
different load deflection characteristics as a way to achieve head
protection performance, and we examined the consequences of these
choices on head acceleration. We observed that associated with
different stiffnesses were different peak head accelerations (Figure 5).
The stiffest device (Schoie) produced higher initial head accelerations
and, after the peak acceleration, fairly large reductions in
acceleration. Note, however, that no matter what head acceleration time
history the helmet produced, peak acceleration occurred well before neck
failure. We note, also, that at modest velocities represented by the
4.6 meters per second case, head accelerations in catastrophic cervical

spine trauma peaked between less than 100 g's to slightly over 175 g's. These are fairly modest accelerations with regard to head trauma, and one could certainly expect g loadings of the head of equal or greater value in contact situations which do not result in catastrophic cervical spine injury.

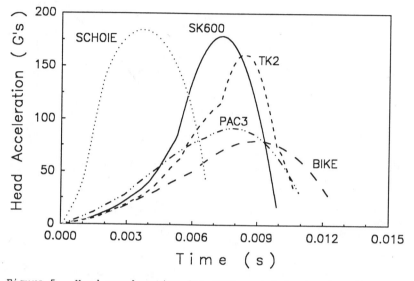

Figure 5   Head acceleration for different helmets show differing acceleration patterns during the simulated head first impacts.

Let us now integrate all of these findings in a review of the mechanics of cervical spine trauma for both the moving victim (4.6 meters/sec) and the stationary victim. We examined the forces in the neck and in the PAC 3 helmet suspension system, as well as the relative displacement between the torso (36 kg mass) and the fixed coordinate system, and the head (5.9 kg mass) and the fixed coordinate system. For the parameters chosen, which are typical of modest velocity impact, the head was brought to a stop after a displacement of about three centimeters (Figure 6). This occurred at about the eight millisecond time mark, and for the last three milliseconds of loading, the head displacement was actually reversed as it rebounded slightly from the compressed helmet energy absorbing system. The displacement of the torso, however, continued throughout the impact at almost constant velocity. The relative displacement between head and torso represented the compression of the cervical spine. Little shortening occurred before three milliseconds, after which the spine became progressively shorter, until at about eleven milliseconds, when there was approximately two centimeters of axial shortening induced in the cervical spine. This corresponds to a compressive force in the cervical spine which before three milliseconds was negligible, but quickly increased between four milliseconds and eleven milliseconds to the catastrophic level of approximately 4 500 N. During this time period, the force on the head had peaked at over 6 000 N, and then corresponding to the head rebound, dropped off just before cervical spine failure.

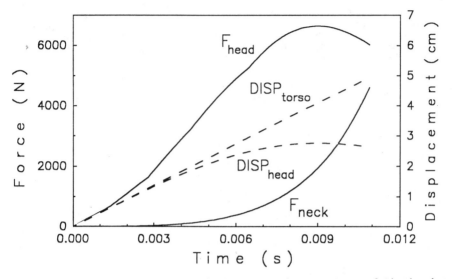

Figure 6   The force time and displacement time response of the head,
torso and neck are illustrated for the 4.6 meter per second impact
velocity, 36 kilogram torso mass, and 5.9 kilogram head mass.

We also examined the case of a stationary helmeted victim with identical
physical characteristics to those in the above case, being impacted by a
thirty six kilogram mass (Figure 7). We observed a set of functional
relations which imposed exactly the same condition on the cervical
spine. In this case, the displacement of the torso of the accident
victim remained essentially zero, while the displacement of the head
showed a progression towards the torso terminating in a displacement of
slightly over two millimeters at the time of cervical spine failure.
The force on the head showed an identical peaking at approximately eight
plus milliseconds, with a drop off by the time cervical failure
occurred. This result is, of course, no surprise, as the symmetry of
the laws of mechanics simply require that irrespective of which end of
the chain the energy is inputted, the response of the cervical spine
will be identical.

Recently the popular press has reported on a new device in progress, the
RushAir SpineSaver football helmet.[5] [6] The device, which is a
product of Rush Sportmedical Inc. consists of a collar shaped air bag
mounted on a helmet with a triggering device which responds to the axial
load between the head and the helmet, i.e. the head force. As currently
constituted, the collar air bag initiates its activation cycle when 2
250 N of axial load is applied to the head. In its current
configuration, the time delay between the onset of the 2 250 N head load
and the deployment of the bag is fifteen milliseconds. [7]

The bag functions by providing a force transmission mechanism between
the player's helmet and shoulders. When the bag is deployed, a large
force can be provided between the helmet and shoulders. The design
objective of the collar air bag is to provide a sufficiently large force
to allow the energy of the trunk to be absorbed by the bag, This would
protect the cervical spine.

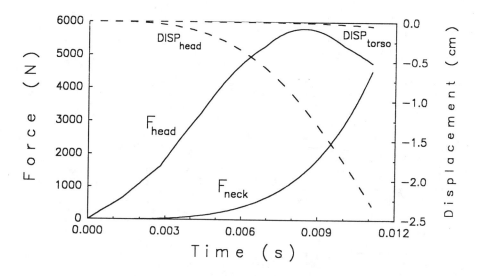

Figure 7   The impact situation illustrated in Figure 6 is altered in that the injured player is stationary and is impacted by a player traveling at 4.6 meters per second.

As the second aim of this paper, we examine the design parameters necessary for the appropriate function of a collar air bag. Let us first examine the feasibility of using this device with a fifteen millisecond time delay. We note from Figure 6 that if the air bag would trigger when the head force reaches 2 250 N, a fifteen millisecond time delay puts the deployment of the bag well after the time that the neck has reached a critical buckling load. We see that in order for the air bag to deploy before the neck has approached its critical load, the deployment delay time must be of the order of milliseconds, and not tens of milliseconds. We therefore examined deployment delay times of six and four milliseconds to see if these would present sufficient time to allow the air bag collar to act as an efficient protective device.

The second issue we will examine concerns the axial force generating capacity of the collar air bag. As we previously noted, the kinetic energy of the torso during typical impact situations was approximately 400 joules. In order for a collar air bag to be able to absorb that energy, its generated compression force would have to be quite high. The stiffness characteristics of an inflating air bag are rather complex. As the bag inflates, it has the capability of exerting progressively larger loads on the shoulders and helmet. During this inflation phase, the bag may do work against the shoulders thereby decreasing the velocity and hence kinetic energy of the torso. At some point, the bag reaches maximum pressure, but will, as it deflates still sustain a load between the helmet and the shoulders. Again, the air bag can continue to decelerate the torso, reducing its kinetic energy. While the actual force time history of the collar air bag are bell shaped, for purposes of the analysis, we make the assumption that the force time history is a constant, time independent value. Thus, we model the collar air bag as a device capable of providing constant resistance between the helmet and shoulders. Our justification for this assumption is two fold. First, we do not know the actual

characteristics of a collar air bag. Secondly, the assumption of a
constant relationship will give the designer an accurate estimate of the
average force which must be provided between the helmet and shoulders
over the time duration of bag deployment and shoulder contact. We will,
therefore, examine collar air bag forces of 22 500 N and 45 000 N.

For each of the following studies, we used the same parameters as were
used in our previous example (Figure 6). In that study, the compression
force between the head and helmet reached a triggering value of 2 250 N
at just over three milliseconds. We used this as the time to initiate
the triggering mechanism in all our subsequent studies. For our first
study, we assumed an air bag deployment delay time of six milliseconds
(approximately ten milliseconds faster than what is currently
achievable), and an average force between helmet and shoulders of 22 500
N. With this delay time, the force becomes effective at slightly over
nine milliseconds after initiation of helmet contact (Figure 8).
Results, perhaps somewhat surprisingly, are virtually identical to those
shown in Figure 6. The neck still fractures at eleven milliseconds, but
the collar air bag, with the six millisecond deployment delay and 22 500
N load characteristics, absorbed an additional 32% of the energy over
and above that absorbed in the impact situation without a collar air
bag. Since the energy absorbed from the torso was 11% of its initial
energy without the collar air bag, the total energy absorbed with the
air bag was 43% of the initial torso kinetic energy. This still leaves
a significant amount of energy, and considering the modest impact speed
used in this example, it was decided that a simulation of successful
protection of the cervical spine would require a decrease in the delay
time of the air bag.

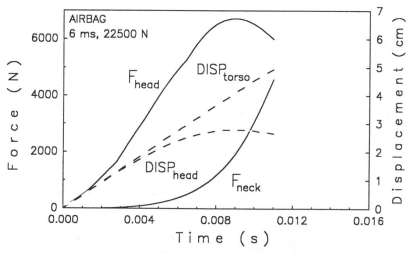

Figure 8   The simulation of Figure 6 is repeated, but with the addition
of an air bag interposed between the helmet and the shoulders of the
player. The air bag has a deployment lag time of six milliseconds from
the onset of firing, which occurs when the head force reaches 2 250 N.
The collared air bag is assumed to generate a constant force of
22 500 N.

We next examined the situation in which the air bag deployment delay
time was reduced to four milliseconds, while the air bag force was
maintained at 22 500 N (Figure 9). The air bag was thus deployed at

slightly over seven milliseconds after head first contact, but the
cervical spine still reached its critical failure load in approximately
twelve milliseconds. On the positive side, the collar air bag absorbed
an additional 80% of the kinetic energy of the torso over the non-air
bag simulation for a total energy absorption of 90% of torso kinetic
energy. While this was encouraging, the combination of a four
millisecond delay time and 22 500 N deployment force still would not
provide cervical spine protection.

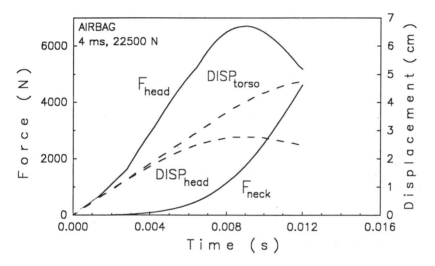

Figure 9   The simulation presented in Figure 8 is repeated, but with a
four millisecond inflation time lag.

We then examined the behavior of a stiffer air bag. We reverted to the
six millisecond time delay, and saw that the cervical spine was still
not afforded protection (Figure 10). Failure of the cervical spine
again occurred at slightly above eleven milliseconds, and this set of
air bag parameters absorbed only an additional 63% of the torso energy
for a total energy absorption of 74% of the kinetic energy of the torso.
Thus, maintaining a six millisecond deployment delay time , but doubling
the compressive force produced by the air bag did not show as much
promise as reducing the deployment delay time from six milliseconds to
four milliseconds in absorbing the kinetic energy of the trunk.

Therefore, for our final simulation, we chose to maintain the air bag
force at 45 000 N, but reduced the deployment delay time back to 4
milliseconds (Figure 11). With this combination of parameters, we
simulated a head first impact that did not result in force levels
sufficient to produce failure of the cervical spine. The air bag
initiated the application of shoulder force at slightly over seven
milliseconds, at which point the neck force was approximately 900 N.
The neck force peaked at approximately 12 1/2 milliseconds at slightly
over 2 800 N and thereafter decreased. At about eleven milliseconds,
the torso energy was completely absorbed, and thereafter the torso
rebounded.

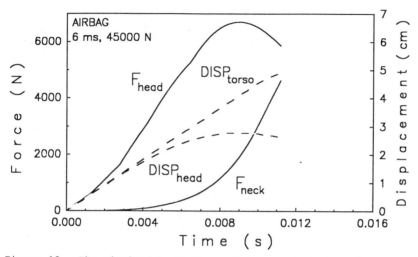

Figure 10   The simulation of Figure 9 is repeated, but the force generated by the collared air bag is assumed to have doubled to 45 000 N.

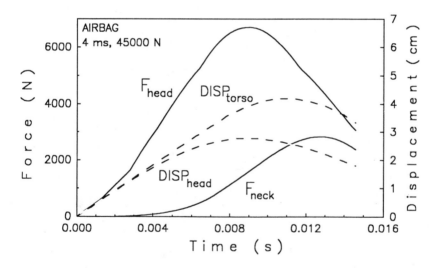

Figure 11   With the deployment delay time reduced to four milliseconds, and the collared air bag force maintained at 45 000 N, the simulation produces no fractured cervical spine.

The combination of a four millisecond deployment delay and 45 000 N of compression force capability represent exceedingly difficult performance characteristics to incorporate in a collar air bag cervical protection

device. Even in the presence of these design parameters, the modest
impact situation we examined showed an axial compression load on the
cervical spine which was two thirds of the assumed critical level of 4
500 N. It should be realized that some modes of failure of some
cervical spines may occur within this range of 3 000 N. Moreover, the
assumed impact velocity of 4.6 meters/sec was quite modest. Thus, while
a collar air bag of the stated characteristics was successful in the
chosen simulation, in the real world it might prove marginal.

It might be possible to provide collar air bags with even more favorable
characteristics than those investigated in this study. At the present
time, the parameters identified as being required for successful
deployment in the illustrated case are well beyond the technical means
available. However, future development may dramatically improve the
state of the art. Should such parameters become practical, then it
would be important that the designer of the collar air bag system
optimize the performance of the system by appropriately modifying the
helmet compression characteristics so as to make the entire system more
reliable.

As a final note, we have not examined the effect of a collar air bag on
the mental state of the wearer or the physical damage inflicted on a
player struck by the tackler wearing this device. The cervical spine
will always be vulnerable to injury in a contact sport, and to encourage
a perception to the contrary would be a disservice to the user of a neck
protection device. And, while the collar air bag may provide the wearer
with a degree of cervical spine protection, what injuries would be
inflicted upon the impacted player, who would receive considerably more
energy from the tackler?

REFERENCES

[1]   Otis, J.C., Burstein, A.H and Torg, J.S.:"Mechanisms and
Pathomechanics of Athletic Injuries." In Athletic Injuries to the Head,
Neck and Face (Second Edition). Mosby-Year Book, St. Louis, pp. 438-
456, 1991. Edited by J.S. Torg.

[2]   Pintar, F.A., Sances, A.Jr., Yoganandan, N., and Cusick,
J.:"Experimental Production of Head-Neck Injuries Under Dynamic Forces."
Head and Neck Injuries in Sports, ASTM STP 1229, Earl F. Hoerner, Ed.,
American Society for Testing and Materials, Philadelphia, 1994.

[3]   Voo, L.M. and Liu, Y.K.: "Buckling Analysis - A Model Method of
Predicting Cervical Spine Injuries Due to Crown Impact." Head and Neck
Injuries in Sports, ASTM STP 1229, Earl F. Hoerner, Ed., American
Society for Testing and Materials, Philadelphia, 1994.

[4]   Myers, B.S., McElhaney, J.H., Richardson, W.J., Best, T.M. and
Nightengale, R.W.: "The Effect of End Condition on Neck Injury
Potential." Head and Neck Injuries in Sports, ASTM STP 1229, Earl F.
Hoerner, Ed., American Society for Testing and Materials, Philadelphia,
1994.

[5]   U.S.A. Today. Feb.12,1993. "Doctor Develop Helmet Air Bags."

[6]   The Meridian Star. Dec.14,1992. p.1B. "Coaches Excited by
SpineSavers Potential."

[7]   Personal communication with developer Gus A. Rush, M.D.
May19,1993, Atlanta, Georgia.

C. Edward Dixon[1]

THE APPLICATION OF RODENT MODELS TO THE STUDY OF BRAIN INJURY
BIMECHANICS.

REFERENCE: Dixon, C.E., **"The Application of Rodent Models to the
Study of Brain Injury Biomechanics,** Head and Neck Injuries in Sports,
ASTM STP 1229, Earl F. Hoerner, ED., American Society for Testing and
Materials, Philadelphia, 1994.

ABSTRACT: The primary objective of this investigation was to
determine the relative contributions of contact velocity and
compression to acute neurological deficits and gross histologic
changes following either central or lateral cortical impact with
systematic, independent variations of contact velocity and depth of
deformation.   To investigate the response to midline and lateral
cortical impact, rats were injured, under anesthesia, at 1 of 18
different combinations of impact velocity and compression parameters.
Following injury, neurological response and the contusional state of
the brain was noted.   For both studies, acute neurologic responses
correlated better with velocity compression product (VC) than with
either velocity or compression alone.   At low contact velocity,
functional impairment is best predicted by maximal compression.
However, as velocity increases, injury severity becomes a function of
(VC), demonstrating the rate sensitivity of brain tissue.
The central and lateral impact data support the viscous response
(VmaxCmax) as a biomechanical predictor of rat brain injury.

KEYWORDS: brain injury, cortical contusion, bimechanics, rats

---

When mechanical impact occurs to the head, there is a rapid
displacement of the skull. If severe enough, this displacement can
cause differential motion between the brain and the skull.   The
severity of the brain displacement is related to the path of motion of
the head, the anatomical surfaces surrounding the brain and the
violence of the motion.   The displacement causes deformation of brain
tissues, which is felt to be a primary factor in brain damage [1,2].
Since biological tissues are viscoelastic, the amount and speed of
brain deformation are likely to be important and interactive factors
in tissue damage [3].   The biomechanical determinants of traumatic
brain injury related to deformation may be discussed in terms of
velocity and displacement of neural tissue [4-6].   These variables, in
turn, depend on the onset, duration, and magnitude of acceleration of
the head which produces the deformation, and on the material
properties of brain tissue.   Thus, a desirable model of brain injury
should make possible quantitative measurements of, and allow changes
in, the parameters influencing brain deformation.

Acceleration has a rich history as an engineering measure of
head injury risk from impact and the currently accepted criteria are
derived from acceleration.   The Head Injury Criterion (HIC) is based

---

[1]Assistant Professor, Department of Neurosurgery, University of
Texas - Houston Health Science Center, 6431 Fannin St., Suite 7.149,
Houston Texas   77030.

on the average level of head acceleration and its duration and recognizes that the tolerance to acceleration increases as the duration of the impact decreases. This approach to injury assessment treats the head as a rigid body and deals only with translational acceleration measured near the center of gravity of the head as the mechanical imput responsible for producing brain injury. While this criterion incorporates the best information on human tolerance from the 1960s and 1970s, considerable new biomedical data are now available on the mechanisms of brain injury. Differential motion within the brain is the principal cause of brain tissue deformation. Both amount and velocity of local tissue deformation may be critical to the severity of neural injury, and these deformations depend on both the translational and rotational components of head acceleration. The full three dimensional motion of the head is fundamental to the resulting local deformations of neural tissue [7,8].

Any biomechanical characterization of brain injury begins with a model that has precise, controllable loading conditions. Dynamic direct deformation of the brain, using a variety of methods, has been used successfully to reproduce some characteristics of human brain injury and avoids the necessity of more complex test situations involving head impact and the possibility of skull fracture [9]. Focal cortical deformation using weight drop devices and gas pressure jets can produce localized cortical contusions and distributed cerebral metabolic effects [10-13]. The restricted pattern of injury observed with these models may be due in part to mechanical properties of the dura and the viscoelastic properties of cortical tissue, which may damp the propagation of the input energy to the remainder of the brain and reduce the extent of global brain injury. The absence of biomechanical data in these injury models prevents any further conclusions. Focal brain deformation can be used as an alternative to whole head-impact [14-17] and non-impact head acceleration models [18-20] because it is comparatively easy to implement, and poses some potential advantages for biomechanical analysis of the injury event. However, these advantages remain a potential area of study since little or no analysis of the dynamics of the brain tissue deformation has been performed [9].

Recently, the controlled cortical impact technique has been developed in which the biomechanical events contributing to injury can be analyzed. This technique allows independent control of contact velocity, tissue deformation, and impact interface geometry and enables a quantifiable relationship between measurable biomechanical parameters and the magnitude of tissue damage and/or functional impairment to be made. The application of a constrained stroke pneumatic impactor allows accurate, reliable, and independent control of the compression parameters over a wide range of contact velocities, and has been demonstrated in spinal cord injury models to produce contusion and allow a reproducible gradation of injury outcome severity [21,22].

Experimental traumatic brain injury, employing a pneumatic impactor, has been well characterized in the laboratory ferret [23,24] and rat [25]. In general, the injury responses resembled aspects of severe closed head injury in humans. It has been difficult to measure impact dynamics using fluid percussion models of traumatic brain injury. However, the innovative use of physical models has provided insight into the biomechanics of fluid percussion injury [26]. In contrast to in vivo fluid percussion models of traumatic brain injury [27-30], a cortical impact model of experimental brain injury uses a known impact interface, and a measurable, controllable impact velocity and cortical compression. These controlled variables enable the amount of deformation and the change in deformation over time to be accurately determined.

The primary objective investigation of this study is to
determine the relative contributions of contact velocity and
compression to acute neurological deficits and gross histologic
changes to varying levels of controlled cortical impact in the rat at
two loci: (1) midline impact and (2) lateral impact.

MATERIALS AND METHODS

Injury device

Our injury device is modified from similar devices developed at
the Biomedical Science Department of the General Motors Research
Laboratories.   Built in the Bioengineering Department at the Medical
College of Virginia, the pneumatic impactor consists of a small (1.975
cm) bore, double acting, stroke-constrained, pneumatic cylinder with a
5.0 cm stroke (Figure 1).   The cylinder is rigidly mounted in a
vertical position on a crossbar, which can be precisely adjusted in
the vertical axis above the rigidly stabilized head.   The lower rod
end has an impactor tip attached (i.e., that part of the shaft that
comes into contact with the exposed dura mater).   The upper rod end is
attached to the transducer core of a linear variable differential
transformer (LVDT). The impact velocity can be adjusted between 1.0
and 7.0 meters/sec by controlled compressed nitrogen.   The impact
displacement/time history is directly measured by the LVDT (Shaevitz
Model 500 HR) which produces an analog signal that is recorded by a
PC-based data acquisition system (R.C. Electronics) for analysis of
time/displacement parameters of the impact.

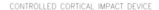

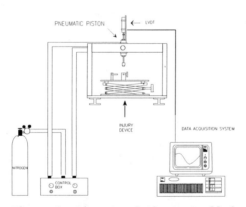

Figure 1 Diagram of the controlled
cortical impact model of traumatic
brain injury in the rat.

Surgical preparation

All animals were initially anesthetized with 4% isoflurane with a 2:1
N_2O/O_2 mixture in a vented anesthesia chamber. Following endotracheal
intubation, rats were mechanically ventilated with a 2% isoflurane

mixture. The rats were mounted in the injury device stereotaxic frame
in a prone position secured by ear bars and incisor bar. The head was
held in a horizontal plane with respect to the interaural line. In
rats receiving a midline impact, a midline incision was made, the soft
tissues reflected, and a 10 mm craniectomy was made centrally between
bregma and lambda (Figure 2). In rats receiving a lateral impact, a 6
mm craniectomy was made midway between bregma and lambda with the
medial edge of the craniotomy 1 mm lateral to midline (Figure 2)
Core body temperature was monitored continuously by a rectal
thermistor probe and maintained at 37-38°C by a thermeostatically
controlled warming pad. Immediately after injury the anesthetic gases
were discontinued in order to minimize the anesthetic effects on the
acute neurological assessments.   In uninjured rats, reflexes are
suppressed 2-4 min. after the anesthesia is discontinued.

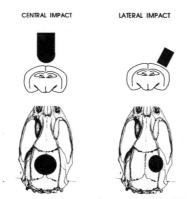

Figure 2 Orientation of the midline
and lateral impacts.

Test Matrixes

    Midline Impact: A total of 62 rats were injured at 1 of 18
different impact parameter combinations.

    Lateral Impact: A total of 52 rats were injured at 1 of 18
different impact parameter combinations.

Acute Neurological Assessments

    A battery of tests that have shown to be sensitive to varying
magnitudes of fluid percussion brain injury in the rat were employed
to assist in determining the relative contributions of impact velocity
and compression on acute neurological deficits and pathology.

I.   Simple Non-postural Somatosensory Functions

a)   The pinna reflex was assessed by touching the auditory meatus of
      the animal's ear to elicit a vigorous head shake.

b)   The corneal reflex was evaluated by lightly touching the cornea
      with a blunt instrument to elicit an eyeblink.

II.   Simple Postural Somatomotor Functions

a)   The assessment of the paw and tail flexion reflexes, consisted
of the gradual application of pressure on the hindpaw or tail
until paw or tail withdrawal was noted.

b)   The head-support response was assessed by noting the duration of
suppression of the animal's ability to support the weight of its
head. Inability of the animal to support its head is associated
with a generalized loss of muscle tone.

III.   Complex Postural Somatosensory Functions

a)   The righting response was defined as the animal's ability to
right itself three times consecutively after being placed on its
back.

b)   The escape response was assessed by briefly pinching the tail of
the animal to elicit locomotive activity away from the noxious
stimulus.

Data Analysis

Two hours after injury, the animals were transcardially perfused
with 10% buffered formalin while under deep surgical anesthesia.
After fixation, the brain and spinal cord tissue were removed and
macroscopically examined for the presence of hemorrhage, contusion,
and laceration. Either the presence or absence of such lesions were
recorded in a log and photographed.

Biomechanical Analysis

For each case the duration of suppression of each acute
neurological response was summed up to a single value. Also, for each
case the presence or absence of a brain contusion was noted. The
dependent variables for the biomechanical analysis were presence or
absence of: (1) a summed neurologic score $\geq$ 50 min., (2) a fatality
within the 2 hour post injury observation period, and (3) a brain
contusion.

All data was subjected to repeated logistic regression analysis
using the Statistical Analysis Package (SAS) and a procedure recently
developed by Ridella and Viano (1990). In brief, logistic regression
models a dependent binomial variable response against an independent
variable. The probability that the dependent variable equals 1 is
related to an exponential function of shape and intercept determined
parameters α and β. The LOGIST function related the probability of
injury occurrence P(x) to the magnitude of a response variable x based
on a statistical fit to a sigmoidal function $P(x) = [1 + \exp(\alpha - \beta x)]^{-1}$. The LOGIST procedure in SAS calculates test statistics for the
regression such as Chi-square (for goodness of fit) and correlation
coefficient, R. These two test statistics form the basis for the
conclusion presented in this section.

RESULTS

Midline Impact

The results of the LOGIST analysis for the midline impact are shown in Table 1. Summed acute neurologic responses < 50 min. correlated slightly better with the velocity-compression product than with compression alone. Figure 3 plots the function by which the probability of a high score increases as the VC increases. Fatality also correlated best with the velocity-compression product. However, compression alone was a major component. Figure 4 plots the function by which the probability of a fatality increases as the VC increases. The compression parameter was a better predictor of gross histologic responses than either velocity or the velocity-compression product. Figure 4 plots the function by which the probability of a contusion increases as compression increases. Thus, while the biomechanical determinants of acute neurological deficits may be different from the determinants of gross histologic change, a major contribution to all injury outcomes is level of tissue deformation.

Outcome	ED_{25}	ED_{50}			X^2	R
Behavioral Sum $\geq$ 50						
VC max(m/s)	0.97	1.27	4.73	3.73	24.52*	0.549
Cmax (%)	21.6	28.7	5.78	21.62	21.05*	0.505
Vmax (m/s)	-	-	2.48	0.33	3.43NS	0.138
Fatality						
VC max(m/s)	1.73	2.02	7.64	3.78	11.50**	0.566
Cmax (%)	32.3	37.2	8.45	22.74	6.83#	0.403
Vmax (m/s)	-	-	6.58	0.73	3.46NS	0.222
Contusion						
VC max(m/s)	0.59	1.17	2.19	1.87	4.79***	0.285
Cmax (%)	20.1(%)	26.6(%)	4.88	16.82	8.55**	0.437
Vmax (m/s)	-	-	.286	0.1	0.00	-

*=$p<0.0001$, **=$p<0.001$, ***=$p<0.05$, #=$p<0.01$, NS=Not Significant

ED_{25}, ED_{50} = 25% or 50% probility of designated outcome

Table 1: Logistic regression statistics for midline rate brain impacts.

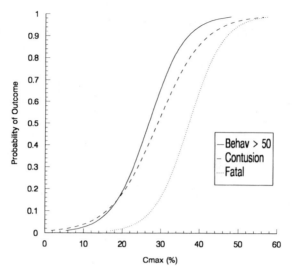

Figure 3: Midline LOGIST plot showing the functions by which the probability of a summed behavioral score > 50, a contusion, and fatality increase as compression increases.

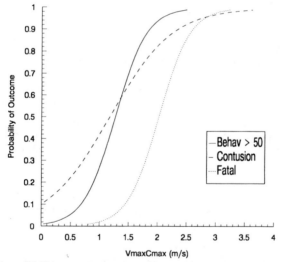

Figure 4: Midline LOGIST plot showing the functions by which the probability of a summed behavioral score > 50, a cortical contusion, and a fatality increase as VC increases.

Lateral Impact

The results of the LOGIST analysis for the lateral impact are shown in Table 2. For the neurologic score, compression, velocity and the viscous response showed significant correlation with the viscous response exhibiting the highest goodness of fit values. Contusion correlated with the viscous response and velocity of compression, but showed no dependene on compression. The highest correlation coefficients showed strong associations of the outcome with the input variable. Multifocal contusion correlated well with the viscous response and velocity, but showed no velocity dependence. for the multifocal contusion cases, compression exhibited the highest correlation with the viscous response exhibiting a slightly lower correlation. Figure 5 plots the function by which the probability of a behavioral sum > 50 increases as VC increases. Figure 6 plots the functions by which the probability of a cortical contusion increases as VC increases. Figures 7 and 8 compare the LOGIST plots between midline and lateral impacts on neurological and contusion variables. Figure 8 illustrates two distinctly different functions in regard to contusion. Lateral impacts appear to be more likely to produce cortical contusions when VC<1 than midline impacts.2

LOGISTIC REGRESSION STATISTICS FOR RAT BRAIN IMPACT DATA

OUTCOME	ED_{25}	ED_{50}	α	β	χ^2	R
Neurosum > 50						
$V_{max}C_{max}$ (m/s)	1.01	1.62	2.90	1.78	12.90[**]	0.414
V_{max} (m/s)	3.94	5.72	3.54	0.62	8.94[#]	0.331
C_{max} (%)	22.8	37.2	2.84	7.65	5.82[***]	0.245
Contusion						
$V_{max}C_{max}$ (m/s)	0.28	0.30	12.66	41.81	16.84[*]	0.813
V_{max} (m/s)	1.42	1.68	7.09	4.22	11.59[**]	0.654
C_{max} (%)	-	5.04	0.53	10.51	2.42[NS]	0.136
Multifocal Contusion						
$V_{max}C_{max}$ (m/s)	0.50	0.86	2.59	2.99	20.50[*]	0.529
V_{max} (m/s)	-	3.42	0.96	0.28	2.27[NS]	0.064
C_{max} (%)	17.7	23.7	4.39	18.56	25.70[*]	0.598

* = $p < 0.0001$, ** = $p < 0.001$, *** = $p < 0.05$, # = $p < 0.01$, NS = not significant

Table 2: Lateral Impact Statistics

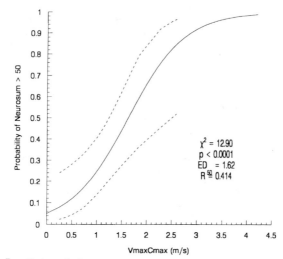

Figure 5: Lateral impact LOGIST plot showing the probability of a summed behavioral score > 50 increase as VC increases.

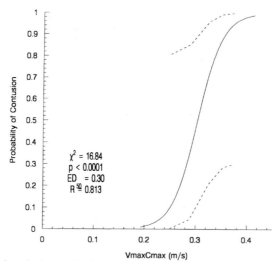

Figure 6: A lateral impact LOGIST plot showing the function by which the probability of a contusion increases as VC increases.

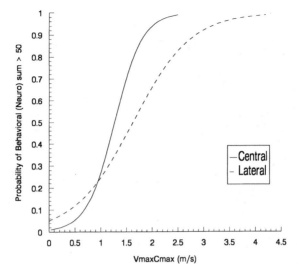

Figure 7: A comparision between midline and lateral impact.
LOGIST plots showing the function by which the probability of
a behavioral sum > 50 increases as VC increases.

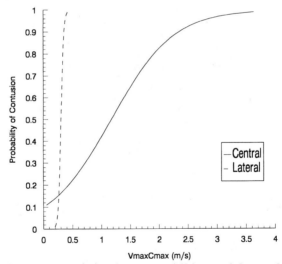

Figure 8: A comparision between midline and lateral impacts.
LOGIST plots showing the functions by which the probability of
a cortical contusion increases as VC increases.

DISCUSSION

The biomechanics of brain injury has become better understood over the past twenty years. Closed head injury is caused by impact resulting in rapid changes in the velocity of the head, which are secondary to a combination of translational and rotational acceleration. If the motion is violent enough the brain can deform and move within the skull. Motion between the brain and skull or relative motion of the brain hemispheres can deform local brain tissue and concentrate responses at different anatomical locations depending on the movement of the head. The differential motion can also result in shear which is suspected of causing the diffuse axonal injuries. While neural injury is caused by local tissue deformations, there are global parameters of biomechanical responses that strongly correlate with the severity of injury.

Much is known about the mechanism of direct deformation of soft biological tissues and organ systems [3,7]. While acceleration of the body has a rich history as an injury criterion, it is not a principal mechanism of injury. Rather, deformation of tissue is critical to injury. There are two mechanisms possible. One involves slow compression of the tissue and if sufficient in extent, causes injury by a crushing mechanism. The second mechanism may involve violent impact in which the speed and extent of tissue deformation are critical to the injury occurrence. Injury may be by a viscous mechanism which quantifies the tolerance of soft tissues to rate-dependent deformation [31]. This mechanism recognizes that the tolerance of tissue to compression decreases as the speed of the energy absorbed by the tissue and combines the velocity (V) and Compression (C) into a single mechanial parameter of injury.

The Viscous response is a critical parameter of injury to soft tissues including the heart, lung, liver and spinal cord [3]. There is extensive evidence that VC is a principal biomechanical parameter of impact injury. Many studies have found that injury risk is causally related to VC, that injury severity increases with increasing VC, and that the moment of greatest injury risk occurs when VC reaches maximum value much earlier in an impact than peak compression of the tissue--actually VC is zero at maximum compression because the velocity of deformation is zero. The viscous response may also be an important biomechanical parameter of brain injury. Experiments by Kearney et al., [22], Dixon [32] and Lighthall [23] with a controlled compression methodology have shown that VC is a parameter of neural injury related to spinal cord and brain injuries that are similar to clinical injury.

The results of this study suggests that the relative contributions of contact velocity and compression to neurological deficits and histopathology are similar to both midline and lateral cortical impacts. In the data set from midline impacts, the viscous response was a good predictor of fatality, contusion, and neurological score. Contusion was best predicted by compression and the behavioral score has a strong compression dependence. Velocity of impact was not correlated with any outcome. In the data set from lateral impacts, the viscous response is also a biomechanical predictor of rat brain injury. It best predicted the probability of an unfavioral neurosum score or contusion and was strongly associated with probability of contusions distant from the impact site. In contrast to midline impact, lateral impact was only weakly associated with the neurological response.

The controlled cortical impact rat model makes possible the study of many aspects of traumatic brain injury in a single model.

For example, this model offers a high level of mechanical control over the impact parameters and will be useful in relating measurable loading parameters with morphologic and functional outcome. This model also reproduces many features of severe human traumatic brain injury including neurological [25] and cognitive [33] deficits, cortical contusions and axonal injury. The present data will allow investigators to select loading parameters that produce specific clinical features of traumatic brain injury. The controlled cortical impact rat model should be an effective experimental tool to investigate the causes and treatment of traumatic brain injury.

ACKNOWNOWLEDGEMENTS

This research was supported by a CDC research grant number R49/CCR606659.

REFERENCES

1.   Goldsmith, W. (1972) In Fung, Y.G., Perrone, N. and Anlike, M. (Eds.): Biomechanics- Its Foundations and Objectives, Prentice-Hall, New Jersey, pp. 585-634, 1972.

2.   Lindgren, S., and Rinder, L. (1965) Experimental studies of head injury. I. Some factors influencing results of model experiments. Biophysik 2:320-329.

3.   Viano, D.C., King, A.I., Melvin, J.W., and Weber, K. (1989) Injury biomechanics research: An essential element in the prevention of trauma, Journal of Biomechanics, 22(5);403-417, 1989.

4.   Gierke, H.E. (1966) In. In Head Injury Conference, W.F. Caveness and A.E. Walker, eds, J.B. Lippincott Co., 383-396, 1966.

5.   Goldsmith, W. (1966) In Head Injury Conference, W.F. Caveness and A.E. Walker, eds, J.B. Lippincott Co., 350-382.

6.   Stalhammar, D. (1975) Acta Neurologica Scandinaica, 52:7-26.

7.   Viano, D.C., and Lau, I.V. (1988) A viscous tolerance criterion for soft tissue injury assessment, Journal of Biomechanics, 21(5);387-399.

8.   Ueno, K. and Melvin, J.W. (1990) Analysis of translational and rotational acceleration effects of head impact. 1st World Congress of Biomechanics, LaJolla CA, pp. 288.

9.   Lighthall, J.W., Dixon, C.E., and Anderson, T.E. (1989) Experimental Models of Brain Injury, J. Neurotrauma, 6(2):83-98.

10.   Dail, W.G., Feeney, D.M., Murray, H.M., Linn, R.T., and Boyeson, M.G. (1981) Responses to cortical injury: II. Widespread depression of the activity of an enzyme in cortex remote from a focal injury, Brain Research, 211:79-89.

11.   Feeney, D.M., Boyeson, M.G., Linn, R.T., Murray, H.M., and Dail, W.G. (1988) Responses to cortical injury. I: Methodology and local effects of contusions in the rat. Brain Research, 211:67-77, 1981.

12.   Gurdjian, E.S., Lissner, H.R., Webster, J.E., et al. (1954)
      Studies on experimental concussion. Relation of physiologic
      effect to time duration of intracranial pressure increase at
      impact, Neurology, 4:674-681.

13.   Ommaya, A.K., and Gennarelli, T.A. (1974) Cerebral concussion
      and traumatic unconsciousness. Correlation of experimental and
      clinical observations on blunt head injuries, Brain, 97:633-654.

14.   Denny-Brown, D. and Russel, W.R. (1941) Experimental cerebral
      concussion, Brain, 64:93-164.

15.   Hodgson, V.R., Thomas, L.M., Gurdjian, E.S., Fernando, O.U.,
      Greenber, S.W., and Chason, J.L. (1969) 13th Stapp Car Crash
      Conf. Proc., SAE, New York, NY, 13:18-37.

16.   McCullough, D., Nelson, K.M., Ommaya, A.K. 1971) J. Trauma,
      11:422-428.

17.   Tornhein, P.A., McLaurin,R.L., Thorpe, J.F. (1976) Surg
      Neurol.171-175.

18.   Adams, J.H., and Doyle, D. (1984) Diffuse brain damage in non-
      missle head injury, in:Recent Advances in Histopathology, 12th
      ed. p.p. Anthony and R.N.M. MacSween (eds), Churchhill
      Livingstone: Edinburgh, pp.241-257.

19.   Gennarelli, T. A., Segawa, H., Wald, U., Czernicki, Z., Marsh,
      K., and Thompson, C. (1982) Physiological Response to Angular
      Acceleration of the Head. In R.G. Grossman and P.L. Gildenberg
      (Eds.), Head Injury: Basic and Clinical Aspects, Raven Press,
      New York, 129-140.

20.   Unterharnscheidt, F.J. (1969) Acta Neuropath, 12:200-204.

21.   Anderson, T.E. (1982) A controlled pneumatic technique for
      experimental spinal cord contusion, J. Neurosci. Methods, 6:327-
      333.

22.   Kearney, P.A., Ridella, S.A., Viano, D.C., and Anderson, T.E.
      (1988) Interaction of contact velocitry and cort compression is
      determining the severity of spinal cort injury, J. Neurotrauma,
      5(3):187-208.

23.   Lighthall, J.W. (1988) Controlled cortical impact: A new
      experimental brain injury model, J. Neurotrauma, 5(1), 1-15.

24.   Lighthall, J.W., Goshgarian, H.G., and Pinderski, C.R. (1990)
      Characterization of axonal injury produced by controlled
      cortical impact, J. Neurotrauma, 7(2):65-76.

25.   Dixon, C.E., Clifton, G.L., Lighthall, L.W., Yaghmai, A.A., AND
      Hayes, R.L. (1991) A controlled cortical impact model of
      traumatic brain injury in the rat, J. Neurosci. Methods, 39,
      253-262.

26.   Thibault, L.E., Meaney, D.F., Anderson, B.J., and Marmarou, A.
      (1992) Biomechanical aspects of a fluid percussion model of
      brain injury, J. Neurotrauma, 9(4):311-321.

27.   Lindgren, S., and Rinder, L. (1966) Experimental studies in
      head injury. II. Pressure propagation in "percussive
      concussion," Biophysik, 3:174-180.

28.   Hayes, R.L., Stalhammar, D., Povlishock, J.T., Allen, A.M.,
       Galinat, B.J., Becker, D.P., and Stonnington, H.H. (1987) A new
       model of concussive brain injury in the cat produced by
       extradural fluid volume loading: I. Physiological and
       neuropathological observations, Brain Injury, 1(1):93-112.

29.   Dixon, C.E., Lyeth, B.G., Povlishock, J.T., Findling, R.L.,
       Hamm, R.J., Marmarou, A., Young, H.F., and Hayes, R.L. (1987) A
       fluid percussion model of experimental brain injury in the rat,
       J. Neurosurgery, 67:110-119.

30.   Dixon, C.E., Lighthall, J.W., and Anderson, T.E. (1988) A
       physiologic, histopathologic, and cineradiographic
       charaterization of a new fluid percussion model of experiment
       brain injury in the rat, J. Neurotrauma, 5(2): 91-104.

31.   Lau, I.V. and Viano, D.C. (1986) The viscous criterion: Bases
       and applications of an injury severity index for soft tissues,
       SAE Transactions, 95:189, 30th Stapp Car Crash Conference, SAE
       Technical Paper 861882, pp. 123-143, October, 1986.

32.   Dixon, C.E., Moore, G.L., Clifton, G.L., Viano, D.C., Lighthall,
       J.W., Ridella, S.A., Worrel, P.J., and Hayes R.L. (1990) A
       controlled cortical contusion model of traumatic brain injury in
       the rat: Biomechanical and neurological observations, Proc.
       Soc. Neurosci., 16:779.

33.   Hamm, R.J., Dixon, C.E., Gbadebo, D.M., Singha, A.K., Jenkins,
       L.W., Lyeth, B.G., AND Hayes, R.L. (1992) Cognitive deficits
       following traumatic brain injury produced by controlled cortical
       impact, J. Neurotrauma, 9(1), 11-20.

Liming M. Voo[1] , and Y. King Liu[2]

BUCKLING ANALYSIS -- A MODAL METHOD OF
ESTIMATING CERVICAL SPINE INJURY POTENTIAL

REFERENCE: Voo, L. M. and Liu, Y. K., "**Buckling Analysis -- A Modal Method of Estimating Cervical Spine Injury Potential,**" Head and Neck Injuries in Sports, ASTM STP 1229, Earl F. Hoerner, Ed., American Society for Testing and Materials, Philadelphia, 1994.

ABSTRACT: The whole straightened ligamentous cervical spinal column (C0/C1-T1) was represented by a three-dimensional segmented beam-column computer model, where vertebral bodies were treated as three-dimensional rigid body elements and intervertebral joints as three-dimensional joint elements having stiffness in axial compression-tension, antero-posterior and lateral shears, and flexural rotations (flexion-extension and lateral bending). Buckling modal analysis of this model estimated the potential responses of the cervical spine subjected to "axial" head impact. The calculated theoretical buckling loads are in agreement with the peak forces obtained in some of the in vitro cadaveric experiments of the cervical spine subjected to axial compressive loading.

KEYWORDS: biomechanics, cervical spine, spinal trauma, impact, mathematical modeling, buckling analysis

The human cervical spine connects, at the caudal end, to the thorax and supports the head at the other. It provides the head with motion while protecting the most fragile tissue of the body: the spinal cord. The cervical spine is, functionally, the most flexible part of the spinal structure and is particularly vulnerable to catastrophic injury. In events such as motor vehicle accident, tackle football, fall, diving, hockey, etc., the cervical spine is frequently exposed to traumatic loading which causes vertebral fracture and/or dislocation [1,2,3,4]. Consequences of severe neck injuries range from fatality to complete or incomplete quadriplegia. Injury mechanisms need to be understood before meaningful tolerance levels of the cervical spine can be established and reliable preventive measures developed.

The straightened cervical spinal column was postulated by Burstein et al. (1982) as potentially the most dangerous configuration of the

---

[1] The work was completed as a Graduate Research Assistant at the Department of Biomedical Engineering, The University of Iowa, Iowa City, Iowa 52242, USA. Currently a Research Scientist at the Department of Neurosurgery, Medical College of Wisconsin, Milwaukee, WI 53226

[2] Professor, Department of Biomedical Engineering, The University of Iowa, Iowa City, Iowa 52242, USA.
* Current Address: 101 S. San Antonio Rd., Petaloma, CA 94952, USA

cervical spine when subjected to "axial" head impact loading [1]. Liu
and Dai (1989) developed the concept of the stiffest and second stiffest
axes of the straightened cervical spine based on a continuous beam-
column model [5]. Analysis of the stiffness distribution of beam-column
with respect to the direction of loading also revealed that the beam-
column, when loaded along its stiffest and the second stiffest axes,
gives the least amount of "axial" displacement [6]. In other words, the
head and neck structure is a "loosely coupled" segmented beam-column
except in its first and second stiffest configurations. When the head
is prevented from moving laterally and rotationally upon impact, and the
neck is straightened, loading along the first or second stiffest axis of
the cervical spine may cause it to buckle. Other loading configurations
of the cervical spine bend in response to load [7]. The failure of the
cervical vertebral column, as a structure, can be due to local material
failure or structural buckling, depending on when and where the
tolerance limit is exceeded first [7]. The local material failure could
be the result of the post buckling behavior or beam deformation. Some
material and/or structural properties of spinal elements have already
been documented in the literature. However, the buckling behavior of a
straightened cervical spine is not yet known.

    In this study, buckling modal analysis of a segmented beam-column
model was performed to estimate response patterns and injury potential
of the cervical spine due to "axial" head impact.

MATERIALS AND METHODS

    The whole straightened ligamentous cervical spinal column (C0/C1-
T1) was represented by a three-dimensional segmented beam-column
computer model (Fig. 1). Cervical vertebral bodies were treated as
three-dimensional rigid bodies while intervertebral joints were
represented by three-dimensional joint elements having stiffness in
axial compression-tension, anterior-posterior and lateral shears, and
flexural rotations (flexion-extension and lateral bending) (Fig. 1).
The stiffness values of the joint elements were taken from the
literature [8,9,10,11]. The rigid element representing T1 vertebral
body was assumed fixed. The rigid element representing the head was
either free or prevented from moving laterally simulating the situations
where the head is either free to move or held by the contact surface
upon impact.

    The published average stiffness values of a cervical
intervertebral joint vary widely [8,9,10,11] as shown in Table 1. A
preliminary study was conducted to determine the influence of varying
individual stiffness values on the buckling behavior of the model. It
was found that the intervertebral joint stiffness in flexion-extension
was the primary determinant of the critical buckling load while the
stiffness values in axial compression, shears and axial torsion were
secondary [12]. Based on that initial finding, more attention was paid
to choosing and distributing the flexion-extension stiffness value,
which ranges from 2.9 N.m/rad to 19.1 N.m/rad depending on the spinal
level (Table 1), for each joint element of the model. In this study,
the flexion-extension stiffness data were taken from Liu et al. where 6
young male cadaveric specimens were used [9]. The magnitude at each
level varied as shown in Table 2. Other stiffness data were taken as an
average of the Liu [9] and Coffee [8] results. These values did not
vary with the spinal levels, as shown in Table 2. The model used to
represent the cervical spine in this study assumed an axial symmetry and
limited to the analysis of sagittal plane buckling behavior. The AP

shear stiffness was the same as the PA stiffness, as Table 2 implies.
Likewise, the flexion bending stiffness was the same as the extension
bending stiffness.   The stiffness in the lateral plane were not used in
this study.   Hence, the does not differentiate between the AP shear and
PA shear, nor between flexion and extension bending.

A general purpose structural analysis software ANSYS® was used for
the numerical solution of the model.   In this study, a linear eigenvalue
buckling analysis technique was employed.

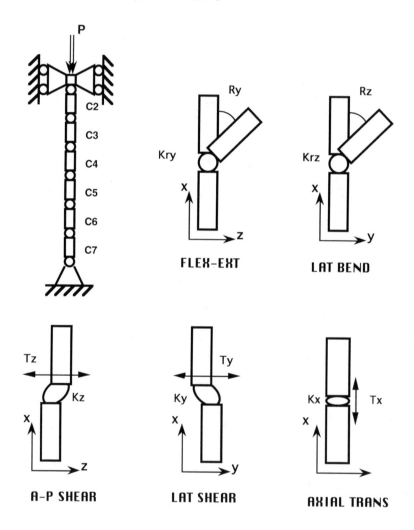

Fig. 1--Model configuration and specified stiffness

® ANSYS Revision 4.0, Swanson Analysis Systems, Inc., Houston, PA, USA.

TABLE 1--Stiffness data of the cervical motion segment

AUTHOR	REGION	(N/mm) COMPR	(N/mm) +SHEAR	(N/mm) -SHEAR	(N.m/rad) FLEX	EXTEND	LAT BEND
Liu [9]	Middle	3690	...	...	29	71	158
	Lower	4120	...	...	169	219	219
Coffee [8]	Middle	5180	580	220	86	...	...
	Lower	1360	104	130	166	191	...
Moroney [10]	All	1080	140	50	152	186	172
Panjabi[11]*	All	140	34	52	...	...	...

* Measured at 25-N force

TABLE 2--Intervertebral joint element stiffness values

	C0-C1-C2	C2-C3	C3-C4	C4-C5	C5-C6	C6-C7	C7-T1
Flex-Ext (N.m/rad)	29	29	57	85	113	141	169
Shear (N/mm)	200	200	200	200	200	200	200
Axial Compr (N/mm)	3500	3500	3500	3500	3500	3500	3500
Lat. Bend(N.m/rad)	180	180	180	180	180	180	180

TABLE 3--Critical buckling loads (N)

END CONSTRAINTS	FIRST MODE	SECOND MODE	THIRD MODE
Fixed-pinned	1498	3294	6106
Fixed-free	421	2269	5695

RESULTS

The buckling loads corresponding to the first three mode shapes
(Fig. 2) are summarized in Table 3. The model was first solved with
fixed-pinned end-constraints. The first (critical) buckling load was
1498 N with the corresponding mode shape depicting shear-dislocation at
the joints with simultaneous bending. The second buckling load was
3294 N with a single-curve buckling mode shape. The third buckling load
was 6106 N with a double-curve mode shape.
Releasing the pinned-end constraints, the critical buckling loads
and buckling mode shapes changed drastically. The first buckling load
decreased to 421 N while the corresponding mode shape suggests that the
load tend to deflect the loading end such that hyperflexion or
hyperextension may results. The second and third buckling modes were
similar to those of the pinned-end with non-zero free-end deflection and
reduced corresponding buckling loads.

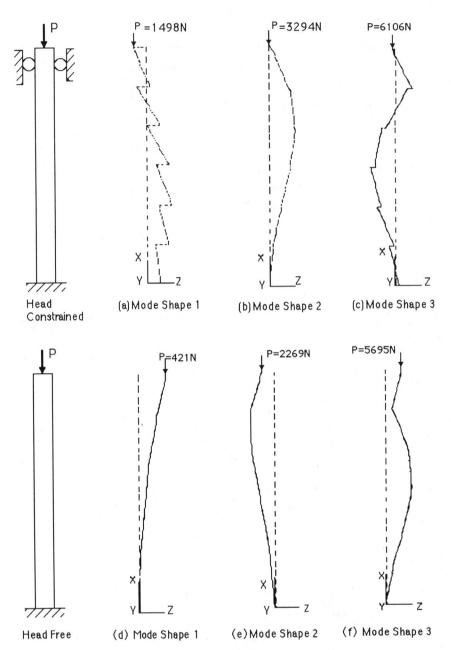

Fig. 2--Sagittal buckling mode shapes and represented failures:
(a) Joint dislocation; (b) Single fracture; (c) Multiple fractures;
(d) Hyperflexion/extension; (e) Single fracture; (f) multiple fractures

TABLE 4--Comparable experimental results

HEAD CONSTRAINED	PEAK FORCE (NECK) (N)	PATHOLOGY
PINTAR [13]	1355-3613	Facet-joint dislocation
PINTAR [16]	1177-6193, Average = 3508	Vertebral body fractures
YOGANANDAN [17]	3300-5600, Average = 4467	Vertebral body fractures
MYERS [18]	Average = 4810 +/- 1290	Vertebral body fractures
HEAD UNCONSTRAINED		
MYERS [18]	Average = 289 +/- 81.4	Specimen intact

DISCUSSIONS AND CONCLUSIONS

Table 4 lists some of the comparable results from in-vitro
cadaveric cervical spine impact experiments. It can be see that the
theoretical buckling loads obtained in this study are in good agreement
with some of the current experimental data. The buckling mode shape of
Figure 2a with the buckling load 1498 N simulates the joint dislocation
type of failure with minimal fractures, as demonstrated by Pintar et al.
[13]. Experimental studies by Hodgson and Thomas show that for axial
loading on the initially straight spine, a peak force of 1420 N was
reached. Stretching of the posterior longitudinal ligament and
interspinous ligaments was observed [14].

The second buckling mode shape of Figure 2b with the buckling load
around .3300 N relates to the compression-flexion type of failure often
involving vertebral body fractures. Yamada summarized compressive
properties of human wet vertebrae according to the specimen's age and
regional differences. The average compressive breaking load for adult
was found to be 3092 N while younger specimens (20-39 years) exhibited
higher breaking load (4101 N) [15]. Clearly, if dislocation between
vertebrae does not occur when the straightened cervical spine is
subjected to axial impact, the compressive stresses can become so high
that vertebral body fractures can result, as demonstrated by the in
vitro cadaveric experiments of Pintar et al. [16], Yoganandan et al.
[17] and Myers et al. [18].

The third buckling mode shape of Figure 2c with a buckling load of
6106 N may also be excited in the case of the straightened cervical
spine subjected to dynamic loading as demonstrated by Pintar et al. [16]
and Yoganandan et al., wherein multiple spinal segments fracture [17].

The model also predicted another possible response of the head-
neck to a head impact, i.e., the head move out of the way of the initial
loading path so that the contact is lost before the force in the neck
becomes high, as noted by Yoganandan et al. in their in vitro
experimental observation [17]. Figure 2d is the mode shape that depicts
this situation with its low buckling load (421 N). This behavior has
also been demonstrated by Myers et al. in their in vitro experimental
result of ligamentous cervical spine, where the head was not constrained
when a compressive load was applied [18]. The measured peak force in
the cervical spine was only an average of 289 N +/- 81 N (Table 4).

A structural column under static loading will buckle into the
first mode shape when the first buckling load is reached. Loading the
column further will only increase the deflection while its mode shape is
essentially unchanged. Hence the higher buckling modes are unlikely to
happen in static loading of a column. In dynamic loading, as in impact
loading, the inertia of the column mass resists transverse movements.
This inertia is greater for the lower buckling modes, and thus, a higher
buckling mode is likely to occur with a correspondingly higher critical
buckling load [19].

The cervical spinal column is in its stiffest configuration under
longitudinal compression when it is straightened (natural lordosis
eliminated). In any other unstraightened configurations, the cervical
spinal column will produce larger deformation under the same load. Liu
and Dai (1989) conceptualized this phenomenon, based on an idealized
continuous beam-column model, and predicted that, for a straightened
cervical spinal column, there exists a unique stiffest axis along which
a compressive force produces no significant deflection of the column
until structural failure takes place, i.e., buckling or material damage
of the column. Their theoretical analysis also predicted that there
exist a set of secondary stiffest axes in a straightened cervical spinal
column when the applied compressive force has an eccentricity to the
stiffest axis [5]. The ligamentous cervical spine consists of 7 bony
vertebral bodies jointed by soft ligamentous tissues making up complex
joints. Between any two adjacent vertebral bodies relative three
translations (longitudinal tension-compression, AP shear, and lateral
shear) and three rotations (flexion-extension, lateral bending, and
torsion) are all possible to some extent, limited by the stiffness and
strength of the joints. The cervical spinal column can thus be
approximated as 7 rigid cylinders connected by elastic joints having
same stiffness characteristics as the cervical intervertebral joints.
This model representation, when under axial compression, is a segmented
beam-column. The segmented beam-column has an additional joint
dislocation buckling mode compared to the continuous beam-column. This
is due to the allowable discontinuity between the segments.

A stiffer structure under dynamic loading has shorter response
time lag between members connected in series. Thus, a stiffer structure
has a tighter dynamic response coupling. The cervical spinal column in
its stiffest configuration behaves like a "tightly-coupled" segmented
beam-column upon impact along its stiffest axis or secondary stiffest
axes. This "segmented beam-column" may buckle when the critical load is
reached, leading to ligamentous injury or spinal joint dislocation
during the post-buckling phase. If the impact speed is high, the
cervical spine may buckle in a higher mode with higher compressive
stresses within the vertebral bodies such that fracture results.

The model used to represent the cervical spine in this study
assumed an axial symmetry and was limited to the two-dimensional
analysis of sagittal plane buckling behavior. The AP shear stiffness
was the same as the PA stiffness, as Table 2 implies. Likewise, the
flexion bending stiffness was the same as the extension bending
stiffness. The stiffness in the lateral plane was not used in this
study. Hence, the model does not differentiate between the AP shear and
PA shear, nor between flexion and extension bending. The buckling mode
shapes shown in Fig. 2 are for illustration only. Any one of the
depicted mode shapes has its equally probable symmetric mode shape, with
the symmetry about the longitudinal axis (x axis).

This study demonstrated that the buckling modal analysis of a
segmented beam-column model for the straightened cervical spine can be
used to approximate the responses of the cervical spine due to "axial"

head impact. Buckling responses of the cervical spine in its stiffest and second stiffest configurations upon head impact may well be the triggering mechanism that causes catastrophic injuries to the cervical spine in many contact sports as well as in motor vehicle accidents.

REFERENCES

(1) Burstein, A.H., Otis, J.C., and Torg, J.S., "Mechanisms and Pathomechanics of Athletic Injuries to the Cervical Spine," Chapter 11, Athletic Injuries to the Head, Neck and Face, Lea & Feliger, Philadelphia, 1982, pp. 139-154.

(2) McElhaney, J., Snyder, R.G., States, J.D., and Gabriesen, M.A., "Biomechanical Analysis of Swimming Pool Injuries," The Human Neck: Anatomy, Injury Mechanisms and Biomechanics, paper No.790137 (SP-438), Society of Automotive Engineers, Warrendale, PA, 1979.

(3) Tator, C.H., and Edmonds, V.E., "National Survey of Spinal Injuries in Hockey Players," Canadian Medical Association Journal, Vol. 130, 1984, pp. 875-880.

(4) Torg, J.S., Truex, R., Quendenfeld, T.C., Burstein, A., Spealman, A., and Nicholas, C., "National Football Head and Neck Injury Registry: Report and Conclusions," Journal of American Medical Association, Vol. 241, 1979, pp. 1477-1479.

(5) Liu, Y.K. and Dai, Q.G., "The Second Stiffest Axis of a Beam-Column: Implications for Cervical Spine Trauma," Journal of Biomechanical Engineering, Vol. 111, No. 2, 1989, pp. 122-127.

(6) Dai, Q.G.,and Liu ,Y.K., "Stiffness Distribution of a Beam-Column as a Model to Assess Cervical Spine Vulnerability," 1992 Conference on Engineering Systems Design and Analysis, Istanbul, Turkey, June 28-July 3, 1992, Vol. 2, pp. 57-65.

(7) Dai, Q.G.,and Liu ,Y.K., "Failure Analysis of a Beam-Column under Oblique-Eccentric Loading: Potential Failure Surfaces for Cervical Spine Trauma," Journal of Biomechanical Engineering, Vol. 114, 1992, pp. 119-128.

(8) Coffee, M.S., Edwards, W.T., Hayes, W.C., and White, A.A. III, "Mechanical Responses and Strength of the Human Cervical spine," Exhibit, American Spinal Injury Association Meeting, Boston, March 1987.

(9) Liu, Y.K., Krieger, K.W., Njus, G., Ueno, K., Connors, M., Wakano,. K., and Thies, D., "Cervical Spine Stiffness and Geometry of the Young Human Male," AFAMRL, Government ordering No. AD-A123535, 1982.

(10) Moroney, S.P., Schultz, A.B., Miller, J.A., and Anderson, G.B., "Load-Displacement Properties of Lower Cervical Spine Motion Segments," Journal of Biomechanics, Vol. 21, No. 9, 1988, pp. 769-779.

(11) Panjabi, M.M., Summers, D.J., Pelker, R.R., Videman, T.,
      Friedlander, G.E., and Southwick, W.O., "Three-Dimensional Load-
      Displacement Curves due to Forces on the Cervical Spine," _Journal
      of Orthopaedic Research_, Vol. 4, No. 2, 1986, pp. 152-161.

(12) Voo, L.M. and Liu, Y.K., "Buckling Analysis of Ligamentous
      Cervical Spine," _Advances in Bioengineering_, American Society of
      Mechanical Engineers 1992, Bed-Vol. 22, pp. 67-69.

(13) Pintar, F.A., Yoganandan, N., Sances Jr., A., Reinartz, J.,
      Harris, G., and Larson, S.J., "Kinematic and Anatomical Analysis
      of the Human Cervical Spinal Column under Axial Loading,"
      Proceedings of the 33rd Stapp Car Crash Conference, Washington,
      D.C., Oct. 4-6, 1989.

(14) Hodgson, V.R., and Thomas, L.M., "Mechanisms of Cervical Spine
      Injury during Impact to the Protected Head," _Proceedings of the
      25th Stapp Car Crash Conference_, Society of Automotive Engineers,
      Warrendale, PA, 1981, Paper No. 801300, pp. 3792-3805.

(15) Yamada, H., _Strength of Biological Materials_, F. G. Evans, Ed.,
      The Williams & Wilkins Company Baltimore, 1970, pp. 76-78

(16) Pintar, F.A., Sances, A. Jr., Yoganandan, N., et al., "Biodynamics
      of the Total Human Cadaveric Cervical Spine," _Proceedings of the
      34th Stapp Car Crash Conference_, Society of Automotive Engineers
      paper No. 902309, 1990.

(17) Yoganandan, N., Pintar, F.A., Sances, A. Jr., Reinartz, J. and
      Larson, S.J., "Strength and Kinematic Response of Dynamic Cervical
      Spine Injuries," _Spine_, Vol. 16, No. 10S, 1991, pp. S511-517.

(18) Myers, B.S., Richardson, W.J., Doherty, B.J., Nightingale, R.W.
      and McElhaney, J.H., "The Role of Head Constraint in the
      Development of Lower Cervical Compression Flexion Injury,"
      Proceedings of the 35th Stapp Car Crash Conference, 1991,
      pp. 391-399.

(19) Macaulay, M.A.: _Introduction to Impact Engineering_, Chapman &
      Hall, 1987, p. 189.

Friedrich J. Unterharnscheidt [1]

30 PLUS YEARS OF HEAD AND NECK INJURIES - PRIMATE AND HUMAN MODELS'
RESPONSES TO ENERGY LOAD AND FORCES

REFERENCE: Unterharnscheidt, F.J., "30 **Plus Years of Head and Neck Injuries - Primate and Human Models' Responses to Energy Load and Forces**," Head and Neck Injuries in Sports. ASTM STP 1229, Earl F. Hoerner, Ed., American Society for Testing and Materials, Philadelphia, 1994.

ABSTRACT: This paper reports on a carefully controlled series of 4 groups of experiments using animal models, examining head and spinal cord injuries. In the first group of experiments, animals were subjected to both direct single and repeated applications of direct controlled impact to the head, using the concussion gun designed by Foltz, et al. causing translational (linear) acceleration. In a second group of experiments controlled nondeforming rotational acceleration was directed through a known path near C7-T1, using Head Acceleration Device II (HADII). The third group consisted of animal experiments using Rhesus monkeys undergoing -Gx impact vector acceleration of the restraint torsi but freely movable head and neck, and in the fourth group the same type of indirect impact acceleration was undertaken using +Gx impact vector acceleration. In each group detailed histological examinations were carried out using a Spielmeyer assortment.

KEYWORDS: animal models, head injuries, spine injuries, spinal cord injuries, direct and indirect impact acceleration, translational (linear) acceleration, rotational acceleration, whiplash

---

The present paper reports on a carefully controlled series of 4 groups of experiments using animal models examining head and spinal cord injuries.

In the first group of experiments animals were subjected to both direct single and repeated applications of controlled impacts to the head, using the concussion gun designed by Foltz, Jenkner and Ward (1953)[1], causing translational (linear) acceleration.

In a second group of experiments concerning the effects of rotational on the central nervous system, controlled nondeforming rotational acceleration was directed through a known path near C7-Th1, using Head Acceleration Device II (HAD-II).

The third group consisted of animal experiments using Rhesus monkeys undergoing indirect -Gx impact vector acceleration of the restrained torsi but freely movable head and neck.

The fourth group of experiments consisted of animal experiments using Rhesus Monkeys undergoing indirect +Gx impact vector acceleration of the restrained torso but freely movable head and neck.

In all experiments a Spielmeyer assortment of tissue blocks for histologic examination was prepared and embedded in celloidin and/or paraplast. Besides such standard staining techniques as hematoxylin-eosin and cresyl-violet (Nissl), additional staining techniques were used.

[1] President, Neuroscience, Inc., 3512 Camp Street, New Orleans, LA 70115

TRANSLATIONAL (LINEAR) ACCELERATION

Translational traumas were studied in an extensive series of experiments
[2-6] in which animals were subjected to both single and repeated
applications of controlled impacts to the head (using the concussion gun
designed by [1], which resulted in severe, permanent brain damage. These
experiments established the subconcussion dose of the individual impact
for cats and rabbits as 7.1 m/s (velocity of impact), producing
approximately 200 g (acceleration of the head). The concussion dose was
established as 8.3-9.4 m/s and 280-400 g.

When discussing brain damage caused by boxing, interest is focused
on the subconcussive dose, for it has been observed that a single
application does not create clinical symptoms. Specifically there is no
loss of consciousness. By contrast, the concussive dose produces
immediate unconsciousness of several seconds or minutes duration,
although after a single application no additional clinical symptom is
observed. Both levels of impact are too low to cause such primary
traumatic lesions as hemorrhages between the enveloping structures of
the brain, so-called cortical contusions, intracranial hematoma, etc.
Higher intensities such as are capable of producing primary traumatic
brain lesions will not be considered here, as they do not have similar
significance for the boxer. However, boxing blows and falls in the ring
do produce lesser primary traumatic lesions, including "cortical
contusions". It was observed during the experiments cited above that the
behavior and the histological findings in cats and rabbits remained
unchanged after the application of a single subconcussive dose. Their
repeated application, however, produced severe permanent brain damage
that was due to circulatory disorders. By repeated applications it is
meant that the blows were delivered at intervals of from 5-20 seconds,
which simulates rather closely the situation in the boxing ring, where a
groggy contender takes an increased number of rapidly succeeding blows.
It is especially noteworthy that animals which were sacrificed
immediately or a few days after the experiment presented no
histopathological findings, and that severe brain lesions were seen only
after prolonged survival times, from several days to weeks. After this
"free interval" the lesions were found in the cerebellum, as
disseminated or total loss of Purkinje cells, principally on the summits
of the vermis, associated with proliferation of Bergmann glia, thinning
of the granular cell layer combined with glial reaction and glial
proliferation in the striae medullares and cerebellar white matter. By
comparison, the pathomorphological changes in the cerebrum were less
pronounced; they consisted of disseminated ischemic nerve cells and
moderate glial proliferation in the white substance.

The significance of successive impacts became apparent after the
application of only 5 blows of subconcussive intensity when the animals
developed parapareses of the forelegs which lasted several hours. It is
of interest to note, keeping in mind observations made of boxers, that
these pareses developed without loss of consciousness. After 10 similar
blows the parapareses of the forelegs persisted for at last several days
and were more often irreversible. After 15 blows of a slightly increased
intensity, the animals developed tetrapareses; their hindlegs showed
only a residual weakness after several days but their forelegs remained
paretic or clearly weakened. A series of impacts, therefore, usually
produced reversible and irreversible pareses; it also seemed that
occurrence of the latter was related to the impact direction of the
blows, which was from above. The initially flaccid pareses were
associated during the first hours (days, if reversible) with severe
muscular hypotony or atony of the affected limbs. The distribution and

quality of the histologic brain lesions resembled the familiar picture
seen in hypoxic lesions. Those areas of the brain that are known to be
especially vulnerable to hypoxic lesions obviously were affected to a
higher degree. After a single impact of concussive strength, no
morphological alterations could be observed in the brain.

The event must be called 'traceless', according to Spatz, and
there are no staining methods available for light microscopy that would
detect such possible alterations. If by contrast, the identical impact
was repeated at 1- or 2-day intervals, the result was apparent - severe
permanent brain damage. Disseminated ischemic nerve cell alterations and
heavy focal and pseudolaminary partial necroses were found throughout
the cerebral cortex. In the Ammon's horn formation the loss of neurons
was either disseminated or occurred as complete destruction of a sector
of the band. The cerebellar alterations were less pronounced, their
quality resembling alterations seen after successive impacts of
subconcussive strength.

It may be concluded from these findings that impacts of the lesser
intensity (as employed in these experiments), when applied in close
succession, caused greater brain damage (several days). It follows that
impact intensities applied at longer intervals (several days), produce
less brain damage. It follows that impact intensity and time interval
are significant pathoplastic factors in relation to the extent of the
permanent brain damage that is produced by blunt blows.

ROTATIONAL ACCELERATION

Very few groups of scientists have studied rotational
acceleration. None of these has controlled the path taken by the head or
the wave form of acceleration used. The experimental designs closest to
our own are those in which the head is caused to move by inertia forces
resulting from whole body acceleration. However, in our setup the head
is moved while encased in a plaster-filled helmet. Hence, the primary
input is to the head and not to the whole body[7,8,].

In experiments concerning the effects of rotational acceleration
on the central nervous system, controlled nondeforming rotational
acceleration was directed through a known path near C7-Th1 of 24
squirrel monkeys [9-11]. The equipment used in these studies was
designed by Higgins and Schmall. The monkeys were subjected to
rotational accelerations ranging from 101 000 -386 000 rad/sec2. The
result was a continuum of clinical effects from no observable signs
through concussion to death.

The lowest rotational accelerations employed (101 000 - 150 000
rad/sec^2) caused apparently no primary or secondary alterations in the
cerebrum. However, the next higher accelerations, up to 1.97 000
rad/sec^2 produced in 10 of 13 animals subarachnoid hemorrhages, combined
in one instance with primary traumatic hemorrhages in the oculomotor
nerve, and tears and avulsions, mainly of veins and capillaries, in
superficial cortical layers in 8 animals. Accelerations of more than 200
000 rad/sec^2 caused severe primary traumatic hemorrhages in the cortex
(in 4 of 6 animals) and white substance (in 3 animals). Rotational
accelerations of more than 300 000 rad/sec^2 were not survived. The 3
animals tested died spontaneously after 8 to 20 minutes. The
histological picture was dominated by subdural and subarachnoid
hemorrhages. In addition, there were rhectic hemorrhages (i.e
hemorrhages caused by tearing of the vessel walls by mechanical force)
of the cerebral hemispheres, of the base of the frontal and/or temporal
lobes, and of the occipital lobes; all hemorrhages were located near the

midline. They presented mostly venous, but also capillary, hemorrhages
in superficial cortical layers. These monkeys were the only animals to
show additional hemorrhages in more central regions of the brain, i.e.
very close to the central pivot. They were found in the hippocampus
formation, associated with a loss of neurons in h2 and h1, and around
the third ventricle; all were caused by overstretching and rupture of
local veins and capillaries. The animals also suffered primary traumatic
lesions in cranial nerves, including the oculomotor nerve, optic chiasm,
and vestibular nerve, caused by vessel tearing due to strain produced by
angular motion of the skull relative to the brain.

Nearly all animals tested showed small rhectic hemorrhages in
various segments of the spinal cord. Capillary and venous hemorrhages
were more frequently found disseminated in the gray substance and were
caused by longitudinal and transverse stretching of ascending and
descending vessel branches. Primary traumatic alterations were seen in
all segments of the cord. These lesions were not fatal and produced no
clinical signs in the animals. In two instances subdural hemorrhages
were found in the cauda equina.

On the whole, it appears that the incidence and severity of
primary traumatic lesions approximately doubled when rotational
accelerations of 174 000 - 386 000 rad/sec^2 were administered, as was
done with 12 of the 24 animals tested.

It must be pointed out that the primary traumatic lesions found in
the cortex do not represent so-called cortical contusions. They are
venorhectic, and occasionally arterious or capillary rhectic hemorrhages
of the more superficial cortical layers, as evidenced by torn vessel
walls. Also, these hemorrhages are always associated with vessel systems
running at right angles to the cortical surface. Pinpoint hemorrhages,
so characteristic of cortical contusions in the first stage, were not
observed.

ANIMAL EXPERIMENTS USING RHESUS MONKEYS UNDERGOING INDIRECT -GX IMPACT VECTOR ACCELERATION

Experimental Equipment

A *225,000 Pound Thrust Horizontal Accelerator* with sled, control
console and enclosed environmentally controlled 700-ft track at NBDL,
New Orleans, Louisiana, was used, This can impart up to 200 G to the
lightweight primate sled for durations of up to 90 ms.

The *Inertial Data Acquisition System* samples 24 channels of
inertial data at 2 000 samples/s/channel, digitizes them, and stores the
digitized data in magnetic discs in real time. After the experiment, the
digitized data are scaled in the computer, using calibration data
resident therein. A digital tape is then made of the scaled digitized
data for further analysis.

The *Physiological Data Acquisition System* is designed to acquire
ECG; EEG, and somatosensory evoked potential for 16 channels via FM/F-
telemetry. The bandwidth of both ECG and EEG is 1.0 Hz to 100 Hz the
somatosensory evoked potential bandwidth is 30.0 Hz to 1 500 Hz

The *Photographic Data Acquisition System* included 3 sled- and
laboratory-mounted cameras, lights, and control console, as well as
phototarget design, which is necessary for obtaining precise three-
dimensional photographic displacement data of primate kinematic
response. A complete description is published elsewhere (Becker [12]).

The *Transducer Mounting System,* which was developed for primates,
permits precise determination of linear and angular acceleration,

velocity, and displacement at the mounting site. Transformation of the data to coordinate systems fixed in the anatomy is accomplished using the results of biplanar x-ray anthropometry that measures the precise three-dimensional spatial position of the instrumentation coordinate system relative to the head anatomical coordinate system (Becker [13]. The head acceleration was measured by a rigidly mounted array of 6 linear accelerometers locked to an implanted pedestal bolted to the calvarium, capable of measuring angular and linear acceleration and velocity in three dimensions [14-16].

Sled Acceleration was also measured.

Restraint Systems of two different types were used; a *rigid molded* one and a *harness vest* There seems to be no difference in the lesions produced with either restraint system, since the head and neck kinematic response is not markedly altered.

In the series of animals subjected to -Gx impact vector direction, before, during, and after the acceleration, epidural EEG interlaced with somatosensory evoked potential and ECGs were recorded. Nonfatal runs were followed periodically with these neurophysiological recordings.

In the series of animals subjected to +Gx impact vector direction, neurophysiological data were not recorded. Such studies are planned in the future.

Pre- and post-run x-rays of the entire spine and skull were performed examining different planes.

All animals were *perfused* with saline and buffered 10 percent formalin via the carotid arteries. Special autopsy procedures for the Gx and +Gx impact vector direction were developed, using a posterior approach (laminectomy) and craniotomy, and performed in two phases (unfixed and formalin fixed material). Detailed data concerning these procedures and the *embedding* and staining techniques used were presented in detail by Unterharnscheidt [17-22].

Experimental Procedures

Twenty-eight rhesus monkeys were subjected to a carefully controlled series of experiments with *whole body -Gx impact acceleration exposures with completely restrained torso but unrestrained head and neck.* That is, the animal was accelerated with the.unrestrained head and neck

Results

The surviving animals were sacrificed after different survival times, ranging from 1 to 27 days.

The results of the -Gx experiments can be expressed in terms of damage to (1) the *Central Nervous System,* (2) the *Vascular System,* (3) the *Skeletal System,* and (4) the *Muscles* and *Ligaments* [17-22].

Traumatic Alterations of the Central Nervous System

Peak sled accelerations ranging from 5.2 -Gx to 63.7 -Gx did not produce clinical or pathomorphological findings on light microscopy. Particularly, they did not produce traumatic transections of the CNS at the atlanto-occipital junction (between lower medulla oblongata and upper cervical spinal cord). It is noteworthy that extensive histological evaluation of the area between lower medulla oblongata and C2 did not reveal any traumatic alterations of the tissue, especially no lesions to the axons or myelin sheaths.

However, in experiments reported by Sances, et al. [23], using slow application of axial forces to the vertebral column with forces that produced an approximate 50 percent reduction in the afferent or efferent evoked potential magnitude, a marked reduction in metabolic activity at the cervico-medullary junction and cervical spinal [24-28]. It is noteworthy that examination with light microscopy in these animals was unremarkable. *Electron microscopic studies* with similar force application demonstrated shrinkage of the axoplasm and disruption of the myelin lamellae in the upper cervical spinal cord, while the thoracic spinal cord and the brain were only minimally altered.

The morphological findings, discussed in the last two paragraphs, show that in -Gx impact vector acceleration further histological studies of the lower medulla oblongata and Cl have to be carried out in the range up to 65 G peak sled acceleration, using electron microscopy and the 14C deoxyglucose method.

The lowest level at which tissue damage occurred was 78.3 G. This animal, which was sacrificed on the same day (and which did not reveal any abnormal radiological findings), showed subarachnoid hemorrhages around the basilar artery and both vertebral arteries. There was no traumatic transection at the atlanto-occipital junction, but a *local indentation* and *brownish discoloration of the tissue at the ventral fissure between lower medulla oblongata and Cl* was seen. The histological examination revealed recent and old traumatic alterations in grey and white matter. Another animal, which was subjected to peak sled acceleration of 87.9 G, showed, radiologically, an incomplete traumatic separation at Cl-C2. The run was fatal; although there was no traumatic transection, a local indentation and brownish discoloration of the ventral surface appeared between lower medulla and upper cervical spinal cord. After dissection, a mostly centrally located hemorrhagic necrosis could be seen in the cord.

One animal subjected to a peak sled acceleration of 123.0 G showed severe clinical findings immediately after the run. This animal was involved in another high-level run (105.5 G) on the same day. The animal was moribund and had to be euthanized after 90 h. There was no traumatic transection, but there was a *thrombosis* of the *right vertebral* and right *inferior posterior cerebellar artery,* with softening of the spinal cord at Cl of the ventral aspect of the lower brainstem and right cerebellar white matter *(Wallenberg syndrome). To* this date, as far as we know from the pertinent literature, there has been no publication of a traumatic Wallenberg syndrome presented in primates.

In 4 animals *incomplete traumatic transections* were seen at 105.3 G, 124.2 G, 126.4 G, and 130.7 G peak sled acceleration.
In 6 animals, *complete traumatic transections* between lower medulla oblongata and upper cervical spinal cord were seen. The lowest level at which a complete traumatic transection occurred was 108.7 G; further complete traumatic transections occurred at peak sled accelerations of 127.4 G, 128.2 G, 131.4 G, 158.4 G, and 162 G. *Complete and incomplete traumatic transections* were found in 10 animals with peak sled accelerations ranging from 105.3 G to 162.8 G.

In the group of animals subjected to high-level -Gx acceleration, 3 revealed no macroscopically visible CNS tissue damage: an animal with 108.6 G peak sled acceleration, an animal with 110.4 G peak sled acceleration, and an animal with 127.3 G peak sled acceleration (which was acutely fatal due to a basilar skull fracture). Of the 15 animals that were subjected to peak sled accelerations of more than 100 G, 12 revealed severe traumatic lesions. In the remaining 3 cases, macroscopic traumatic lesions were excluded.

The two animals that survived peak sled accelerations of more than 100 G, namely 108.6 G and 110.4 G, were subjected to G levels that were near the threshold level. Peak sled acceleration levels, with the restraining conditions stated above, in the -Gx vector between 105 G and 110 G, represent the threshold zone in which traumatic transections may or may not occur. Peak sled accelerations of more than 110.4 G in the -Gx vector were acutely fatal and regularly produced, with one exception, i.e., incomplete or complete traumatic transections between lower medulla oblongata and upper cervical spinal cord.

The histological examination of the acutely fatal monkeys revealed multiple hemorrhages in the direct neighborhood of the transected area. These hemorrhages can be termed primary traumatic or rhectic. They occurred at the moment of impact and were the result of ruptures of vessel walls due to the mechanical forces. These hemorrhages were usually more frequent in the grey substance, but they occurred in the white substance also. These multiple petechial hemorrhages can be so massive that they form a larger hemorrhage due to confluence of the multiple smaller ones. In general, those hemorrhages were seen only in the direct vicinity of the transected area. In some animals, however, they extended proximally into the upper medulla oblongata, the pons, and midbrain, and distally into lower cervical and upper thoracic segments. They decreased in size and number the more distant they were from the transected zone. If the hemorrhages were located in the white substance, these primary traumatic hemorrhages were mainly located near the ventral, and only rarely near the dorsal surface of medulla oblongata, pons, and midbrain. There seemed to be an avulsion of vessels at or near the ventral surface of the described anatomical structures due to overstretching.

There exists a direct relationship between the severity of the applied forces and the severity and distribution of the pathomorphological findings. The higher the mechanical input expressed as peak sled acceleration, the more severe are the hemorrhages and the larger is the involved area; a finding that has been observed in other animal experiments using other vector directions.

The *subdural hemorrhages* of the *spinal cord* seen in the animals with incomplete and complete traumatic transections are large, normally cover the ventral and dorsal aspects of the spinal cord, and extend in some instances into the cauda equina. They are the result of the *rupture of both vertebral arteries* and the *anterior* and *posterior spinal artery.* The hemorrhage therefore extends from proximal to distal, in some cases into the cauda equina, and from distal to proximal into the posterior and middle cerebral fossa.

Examination of the *pituitary gland* revealed no hemorrhages, either macroscopically or microscopically, in any of the animals tested. The stalk was intact and showed no traumatic hemorrhages or disruption.

Traumatic Alterations of the Vascular System

At peak sled accelerations of more than 110 G, complete traumatic transections normally occurred between lower medulla oblongata and upper cervical spinal cord. Above *127.3 G,* these transections occurred regularly. Both vertebral arteries and the anterior spinal artery were ruptured, and subsequent subarachnoid and subdural hemorrhages were found at the base of the brain and around the spinal cord, extending into different levels, in some cases into the cauda equina.

There are two subtypes of rupture of the vertebral arteries .

1. The more frequent injury was that in which both vertebral arteries and, in a few instances, the basilar artery were completely avulsed.

2. The less frequent injury was that in which a separation of the vertebral arteries occurred immediately at the foramen magnum, so that their proximal parts remained intact in the specimen *in situ*.

The vertebral artery that arises commonly from the subclavian artery has 4 segments. The *first* or *prevertebral segment* ascends posterosuperiorly between the longus colli and anterior scalene muscles to enter the transverse foramina of the cervical spine at the level of the sixth cervical vertebra. From this point the artery ascends as the *second* or *cervical segment* through the transverse foramina to become the *third* or *atlantic segment* when it exits from the transverse foramen of the atlas. It then passes posteriorly behind the articular process of the atlas, lying in a groove on the superior surface of the posterior arch of the atlas, and enters the cranial cavity, by piercing the atlanto-occipital membrane and the dura mater to become the *fourth, intracranial,* or intradural *segment.* This segment ascends anteriorly and laterally around the medulla oblongata to reach the midline at the pontomedullary junction, where it unites with the vertebral artery of the opposite side to form the basilar artery.

The rupture of the vertebral arteries occurs at the point where they pierce the atlanto-occipital membrane and dura mater; the rupture takes place between the third and fourth segments. In some cases, the fourth, intracranial, or intradural segment and, in a few instances, the basilar artery were completely avulsed.

Despite peak sled accelerations up to 162.8 G, *no rupture* of a *carotid artery* was observed. The fact that the carotid arteries remained intact and patent could also be deduced from the fact that in some instances subdural hemorrhages developed over both cerebral hemispheres due to ruptured bridging veins. Since the cardiac actions of the animals with a complete traumatic spinal-cord transection continued for about 20 to 30 min, a patent vascular system in the area supported by the internal carotid artery must exist. Since EEG and ECG were recorded in these cases with the developing and expanding hemorrhages, interesting insights into the neurophysiological aspects can be expected from further data analysis.

Traumatic Alterations of the Skeletal System

The lowest peak sled acceleration at which an incomplete traumatic separation of the spinal *column between C1 and C2* occurred was 87.9 G. The run was acutely fatal, but did not result in a traumatic transection. With peak sled accelerations of more than 124.2 G, atlanto-occipital separations, basilar skull fractures, or C1-C2 separation occurred. All these runs were acutely fatal. Between 87.9 G and 123.0 G, radiological findings may or may not occur.

Two types of lesions of the cervical spine occurred: (1) Atlanto-occipital separations with massive dislocation of the segments (7 animals), and (2) *incomplete* and *complete* C1-C2 *separations* (2 animals).

The *only bony fractures* in the entire series were 3 cases of *basilar skull fracture* . The peak sled accelerations of 2 of these animals, 105.3 G and 130.7 G, resulted in an incomplete traumatic transection of the cord. The peak sled acceleration of the third animal, 127.3 C, did not produce a traumatic transection of the cord. It is noteworthy, however, that of the 3 animals with basilar skull fractures, only 2 incomplete traumatic transections of the cord occurred. while the third animal revealed no traumatic transection at all.

These basilar skull fractures occurred at levels of impact acceleration at or above the threshold for atlanto-occipital separation, C 1-C2 separation, and complete traumatic transection. All 3 runs were fatal. The heads of the animals did not impact any structure of the sled; therefore, these fractures cannot be explained by a direct impact of the vertex of the skull and transmission of the force to the base of the skull. These fractures are rarely seen and have not been previously described in the primate literature. We propose to call this injury a 'tension fracture' due to the inertial load of the head. This is of considerable interest because all other lethal injuries were of soft tissue. This indicates that the use of x-rays, in the absence of autopsies, to determine injuries in cadaveric research of this type would not have shown the injuries. Thus, the use of x-rays alone in such research is to be condemned.

Traumatic Alterations of the Dura Mater, Muscles, and Ligaments

A careful anatomical dissection of the ruptured ligaments of the atlanto-occipital junction, using different approaches, allows a quite satisfying description and quantification of the resulting lesions. It was demonstrated that the dura mater near the foramen magnum (the area where the cerebral dura mater is transient into the spinal dura mater) was partially or completely disrupted.

Small to medium sized hemorrhages, probably due to tears and ruptures of muscles near their origin at the posterior margin of the foramen magnum, were seen. Larger hemorrhages existed at the anterior margin of the foramen magnum. The hemorrhages extended into the retropharyngeal space and in some cases perforated into the nasopharynx.

The membrana tectoria and posterior longitudinal ligament in a few cases remained intact, but were completely disrupted in most others. However, after removing these structures, it became evident that the transverse and the proximal parts of the cruciate ligament were ruptured. This led to indentations of the odontoid process of the axis onto a circumscribed area of the ventral portion of the lower medulla oblongata; a lesion that was demonstrated macroscopically and microscopically and that was in some cases survivable, as two of the animals show.

Fractures of the odontoid process of the axis were not observed.

Discussion

Analyzing the local traumatic alterations *(complete transections)* at the area of the *atlanto-occipital junction, three mechanisms* appear to occur during the course of acceleration, simultaneously or consecutively: (1) compression of the spinal cord at the ventral aspect *between lower medulla oblongata and C1 segment,* which leads, in some specimens, to *indentation of tissue* with or without *brownish discoloration or flattening of the specimen in the antero-posterior diameter,* if the threshold is reached. This tissue damage is located at the region of the cord in opposition to the tip of the odontoid process and is, without a doubt, caused by this structure. (2) *Stretch along the longitudinal axis of the medulla oblongata and upper cervical spinal cord,* combined with (3) a *guillotine action* between anterior and/or posterior rim of the foramen magnum on the one side and the anterior arch of the atlas (with the directly posterior located odontoid process of the axis) and the posterior arch of the atlas on the other side, which takes place as the head extends on the neck and then rotates relative to the neck. This results in a succession of tension and shear forces at the head/neck junction. Failure or subluxation of structures at the head/neck junction results in incomplete or complete traumatic transection of the cord tissue.

These experiments lead us to propose a *family of experimental concussion types* in terms of nomenclature:

1. The clinical syndrome of true experimental cerebral concussion due to impact acceleration directly applied to the head, using mainly translational acceleration, which can also be termed experimental cerebral acceleration concussion sui generis.

2. The clinical syndrome of experimental acceleration concussion with extreme neck stretch due to impact acceleration directly applied to the head.

3. The clinical syndrome of experimental acceleration concussion with extreme neck stretch due to whole body -Gx (also +Gx) indirect impact acceleration exposures with completely restrained torso but unrestrained head and neck. In the last case, the impact acceleration is transmitted from the sled to the torso via the restraint system- and then via the vertebral column or neck to the head.

The specific neuropathological injury pattern in - Gx acceleration transmitted indirectly to the head via the neck structures consists of tissue damage at the zone of maximum stretch at the atlanto-occipital junction and, if the threshold is reached, incomplete and complete traumatic transection of the spinal cord and rupture of both vertebral arteries and concomitant basilar and spinal subarachnoid and subdural hemorrhages. Furthermore, at peak sled acceleration levels low enough that neither incomplete nor complete transections occurred, a local indentation of tissue was seen at the ventral fissure, apparently caused by direct impact on the tip of the odontoid process of the axis. This tissue alteration can be considered a spinal contusion.

In some instances, subdural hemorrhages over both cerebral hemispheres due to ruptured bridging veins were seen, probably as the result of rotational acceleration. The ultimate limit for primate survival to -Gx impact vector acceleration for circumstances in which the head and neck are unrestrained is due to failure of the head/ neck junction.

ANIMAL EXPERIMENTS USING RHESUS MONKEYS UNDERGOING INDIRECT +Gx IMPACT VECTOR ACCELERATION

Experimental Equipment

The experimental equipment in the study using +Gx impact vector direction was identical with that applying -Gx impact vector direction.

Experimental Procedures

Fifteen rhesus monkeys were subjected to a total of 34 runs with sled accelerations ranging from 5 G to 141 G in the +Gx vector. One animal was run repeatedly (6 times). Fourteen animals were run only once in order to avoid possible cumulative effects of the multiple runs. It should be mentioned, however, that before each single run, a very low-level run, namely 5 G, was undertaken in order to check the inertial and physiological data systems. This acceleration level is so low that no reversible or irreversible lesions can be expected. In fact, there were 2 runs per animal, but only the second one was significant.

Results

The following *sled parameters* were measured: (1) *peak sled acceleration* (G/max); (2) *end stroke velocity* (m/s); (3) *duration* (ms); and (4) *rate of onset* (m/s^3). The following *peak head parameters* were measured: (1) *angular acceleration (m/s^2)*; (2) *linear acceleration (m/s^2)*; (3) *peak head angular velocity* in Y axis (rad/s); and (4) *angular velocity resultant* (rad/s).

The results of these experiments will be presented in (1) *General Findings*, consisting of a summary of all morphological alterations; (2) *Radiological Findings*; (3) *Pathological Findings*; and (4) *Neuropathological Findings*.

General Findings [29-34]

The results of the living animals subjected to +Gx impact acceleration are arranged in sequence, starting with the lowest peak sled acceleration and continuing to the highest one. The subject number, run number, Julian date, sled parameters, peak head parameters, disposition, radiological findings, pathological findings, and gross neuropathological findings of all animals and runs are summarized.

Six animals were subjected to peak sled accelerations up to 101 G, namely AR538B 83 G peak sled acceleration, AR8862 97 G peak sled acceleration, AR8850 97 G peak sled acceleration, AR8830 100 G peak sled acceleration, AR8800 100 G peak sled acceleration, and AR8754 101 G peak sled acceleration. Four of these animals survived and were sacrificed after a different survival time, ranging from 14 to 17 days. None of these animals was found to have traumatic transection of the cord between lower medulla oblongata and upper cervical spinal cord. The two animals who were involved in a fatal run died after 25 min (AR8850 97 G peak sled acceleration) and 60 min (AR8754 101 G peak sled acceleration). The four animals from this group who survived revealed no radiological, pathological, or gross neuropathological findings. The two animals who died after the run (AR8850 25 min, and AR8754 60 min) had fractures of the spinous processes of the cervical and upper thoracic spine, namely AR8850 97 C peak sled acceleration, C-Th2, and AR8754 101 G peak sled acceleration C3-C4. Additionally, AR8850 97 G peak sled acceleration revealed a dislocation of the Th1-Th2 interspace. The dislocation in the latter two animals occurred at the distally located area of the multiple spinous process fractures.

Four out of the 6 animals in this group that revealed no radiological findings also showed no pathological or gross neuropathological findings. Only the 2 animals with a fatal outcome showed pathological findings. Animal AR8850 97 G peak sled acceleration had extensive hemorrhages in the neck structures around the esophagus and hemorrhages in the upper mediastinum extending into the posterior mediastinum with extensive retropleural and paravertebral hemorrhages of posterior parts of the upper thorax located laterally to the spine. Animal AR8754 101 G peak sled acceleration showed a large hemorrhage originating in the upper mediastinum, extending downward into the pericardium. Death in the latter two animals resulted from dislocation of the interspace of the spine (Th1-Th2, AR8850, and C4-C5, AR8754) and extensive hemorrhages around the esophagus, upper and posterior mediastinum, in AR8754 extending into the pericardium.

It is noteworthy that the first of the animals who died 25 min after the run had an unusually low peak head angular velocity (Y axis), namely 50 rad/s. Examination of high-speed films revealed an interesting phenomenon *(concertina effect)* that will be discussed in detail since its interpretation is vital in comparing lesions in the monkey to similar injuries in man.

The initial position of the head of the monkey in experiments using all impact vector directions is of greatest importance in regard to the resulting lesions; this is especially true in the +Gx vector direction. This will be discussed in detail later in the chapter. Five animals were subjected to peak sled accelerations ranging between 122 C and 123 C, namely ARNR13 122 G peak sled acceleration, AR3944 122 G peak sled acceleration, ARNR12 123 G peak sled acceleration, AR3938 123 G peak sled acceleration, and AR4090 123 C peak sled acceleration. Three animals survived and were sacrificed after a survival time between 15 and 17 days. Two animals were involved in a fatal run (AR3944 survival time 20 min and AR3938 survival time 45 min).

Two of the surviving animals (ARNR13 122 G peak sled acceleration and ARNR12 123 C peak sled acceleration) had no pathological and gross neuropathological findings. The third surviving animal (AR4090 123 G) revealed radiologically a recently fractured right scapula, although the pathological and gross neuropathological findings were normal.

One of the two animals who died after the run (AR3944 122 G peak sled acceleration) revealed radiologically hairline fractures of both scapula and retropleural paravertebral hemorrhages in the upper thorax communicating with the posterior mediastinum. The second animal who died after the run (AR3938 123 G peak sled acceleration) had a fracture dislocation at Th7-Th8; Th8 was pushed anteriorly through the ruptured pleura into the pleural cavity. A complete traumatic transection of the spinal cord resulted.

Four animals were subjected to peak sled accelerations ranging between 139 G and 141 G, namely ARNR22 139 G peak sled acceleration, ARNR08 140 G peak sled acceleration, AR8823 141 G peak sled acceleration, and AR3150 141 G peak sled acceleration. All 4 runs were acutely fatal. Animal ARNR22 died after 3 min, ARNR08 after 5 min, AR8823 after 27 min, and AR3150 after 17 min.

Two of the animals showed extensive, complete traumatic transection of the cord between the medulla oblongata and upper cervical spinal cord, namely ARNR08 and AR3150. One of the 2 other animals that died acutely after the run (ARNR22) was found to have fractures of the spinous processes of C7-Th12. Additionally, there existed paravertebral and intercostal hemorrhages extending from Th1 to Th4 bilaterally, communicating with the posterior mediastinum. Also, there were hemorrhages in anterior and lateral parts of the neck structures, especially in and around the right sternocleidomastoid muscle. The other acutely fatal animal (AR8823) had a thoracic kyphoscoliosis (gibbus) and suffered 5 rib fractures from Th3 to Th7 with hemorrhages in the surrounding tissue. There were no other pathological or gross neuropathological lesions.

The initial position of the head of the monkeys in experiments using all impact vector directions is of greatest importance in regard to the resulting lesions, but especially in the +Gx vector direction. If the monkey has an initial position in which it keeps its head low, i.e., with the chin near the thorax (the cervical spine is more or less flexed), then the early phase of the run results first in (1) compression of the entire cervical spine; (2) with a more or less marked flexion of the cervical spine in the second phase; and (3) rotation of the head in a forward direction. We have termed this phenomenon the concertina effect. A substantial amount of kinetic energy in the initial phase of the acceleration is used up or damped during the compression and flexion of the cervical spine with forward rotation of the head.

After this early phase in the run, the spine then begins a
hyperextension movement with backward rotation of the head.
The concertina effect occurred, too, in other animals of this
experimental project, using +Gx impact vector direction. A pure
experimental design occurs only when applying +Gx impact vector
direction in experiments in which an ideal initial position exists. In
cases of initial positions that are not ideal (they seem to be frequent
in this vector direction!), a *subtype* of acceleration exposures in the
+Gx vector direction occurs with more or less marked compression and
flexion of the cervical spine and forward rotation of the head before
the hyperextension of the cervical spine with backward rotation of the
head begins. In a pure +Gx impact vector acceleration, the
hyperextension of the cervical spine with backward rotation of the head
begins *immediately* in the early phase of the run.

Radiological Findings

   Radiological findings were observed in 9 out of the 15 animals
undergoing +Gx impact vector acceleration. The two animals that were
subjected to the lowest peak sled acceleration, namely AR538B 83 G peak
sled acceleration and AR8862 97 G peak sled acceleration, revealed no
radiological findings. Of the remaining 13 animals with peak sled
accelerations between 97 G and 141 G, 9 revealed radiological findings.
One animal subjected to a peak sled acceleration of 97 G was
radiologically unremarkable (AR8862), while another (AR8850 that was
subjected to the same peak sled acceleration showed radiological
findings. A peak sled acceleration of at least 97 G can be considered
the threshold level for radiological injury in this vector direction.
Lesions of the *bony structures* and *discs* consisted of (1) *spinous
process fractures,* (2) *dislocation* of an *interspace* of the *spine,* (3)
fractures of the *scapula,* and (4) *rib fractures.*

1. Spinous Process Fractures

   Three animals had *spinous process fractures,* namely animal AR8850
97 G peak sled acceleration from C6 to Th2, animal AR8754 101 G peak
sled acceleration from C3 to C4 (multiple runs with 5, 20, 40, 63, 86,
and 101 G peak sled acceleration on the same day), and ARNR22 139 C peak
sled acceleration from C7 to Th2. The spinous process fractures
occurred, therefore, in the middle and lower cervical and upper thoracic
spine.

2. Dislocation of an Interspace of the Spine

   Five out of 15 animals revealed *dislocation* of an *interspace.* The
lowest peak sled acceleration at which a dislocation of the Th1-Th2
interspace occurred was 97 G peak sled acceleration (AR88501. Further
dislocations were seen in animal AR8754 last run 101 G peak sled
acceleration (multiple run animal) at C4-C5, in animal AR3938 123 G peak
sled acceleration at Th7-Th8, and in 2 animals with massive atlanto-
occipital separation, namely ARNR08 140 G peak sled acceleration and
AR3150 141 G peak sled acceleration.
   The first 2 animals with dislocation of an interspace occurred at
Th1-Th2 (AR8050 97 G peak sled acceleration) and at C4-C5 (AR8754 101 G
peak sled acceleration, multiple runs) and in combination with fractures
of spinous processes, always proximally located in regard to the
dislocation. Animal AR3938 123 G peak sled acceleration had a
dislocation of Th7-Th8 with penetration of the lower segment into the

pleural cavity. This massive dislocation in the area between middle and lower thoracic spine was not associated with spinous process fractures.

The two animals with massive atlanto-occipital separations (ARNR08 140 G and AR3150 141 G) were not associated with spinous process fractures. These massive atlanto-occipital separations were similar to those seen in -Gx impact vector acceleration: in general, they seemed to be more massive and extensive.

3. Fractures of the Scapula

Fractures of the scapula were seen in 4 out of 15 animals undergoing +Gx impact vector direction. They can be explained due to posterior-anterior compression of the torso against the seat structure during the run. They occurred at 122 G peak sled acceleration (AR3944), 123 G peak sled acceleration (AR4090), 141 G peak sled acceleration (AR8823), and 141 G peak sled acceleration (AR3150). Fractures of the scapula did not occur in the animals subjected to -Gx impact acceleration. The spinous process fractures in the + Gx impact vector direction must be explained by impact with the seat structure.

4. Rib Fractures

One animal (AR8823 141 G peak sled acceleration) had 5 rib fractures extending from Th3 to Th7 with concomitant hemorrhages and thoracic kyphoscoliosis (gibbus).

Pathological Findings

Two out of 6 animals undergoing peak sled accelerations between 83 G and 101 G showed pathological findings. Animals AR538B 83 G peak sled acceleration and AR8862 97 G peak sled acceleration were unremarkable. Animal AR8850 97 G peak sled acceleration had extensive hemorrhages around the esophagus and aorta, and additional retropleural paravertebral hemorrhages in the upper thorax extending into the posterior mediastinum. Two animals (AR8830 and AR8800) subjected to a peak sled acceleration of 100 G were unremarkable. Animal AR8754 with multiple runs undergoing a peak sled acceleration of 101 G revealed a large hemorrhage originating in the upper mediastinum and extending into the pericardium.

Five animals were subjected to peak sled accelerations ranging from 122 G to 123 G. Three animals (ARNR13, ARNR12, and AR4090) revealed no pathological findings. Two animals of this group showed pathological findings: AR3944 had hemorrhages in the posterior mediastinum communicating with retropleural hemorrhages and AR3938 had extensive paravertebral retropleural hemorrhages extending from Th7 to Th12.

Four animals were subjected to peak sled accelerations ranging between 139 G and 141 G. Three out of these 4 animals showed pathological findings. Animal ARNR22 revealed hemorrhages in anterior and lateral parts of the neck structures, especially around and in the right sternocleidomastoid muscle, and paravertebral and intercostal hemorrhages extending from Th1 to Th4 bilaterally. Animal ARNR08 had extensive hemorrhages in anterior and lateral parts of the neck and minimal retropleural hemorrhages at Th8-Th9. There existed a contusion of the scalp behind the pedestal. Animal AR8823 with thoracic kyphoscoliosis (gibbus) revealed no pathological lesions. Animal AR3150 had paravertebral retropleural hemorrhages extending downward to Th3

left and Th5 right. There were hemorrhages in the upper mediastinum
extending downward into the pericardium.

Neuropathological Findings

Two animals (ARNR08 140 G and AR3150 141 G) had a *complete
traumatic transection* of the *spinal cord* between lower medulla
oblongata and upper cervical spinal cord. These 2 animals revealed
massive *atlanto-occipital separations*. In two animals, transection of
the spinal cord between lower medulla oblongata and C1 with rupture of
both vertebral arteries was identical to transection seen in the animals
subjected to -Gx impact vector direction.

COMPARISON OF ANIMAL DATA OF THE EXPERIMENTS WITH INDIRECT - Gx AND +Gx IMPACT VECTOR ACCELERATION

The *specific neuropathological injury pattern* in -Gx acceleration
transmitted indirectly to the head via the vertebral column consists of
tissue damage at the zone of maximum stretch at the *atlanto-occipital* or
head/neck junction.

Thresholds of Unremarkable Histology

Peak sled accelerations ranging from 5.2 -G to 63.7 G in the -Gx
impact vector direction did not produce clinical or pathomorphological
findings. It is noteworthy that extensive histological examination of
the tissue of the lower medulla oblongata and the cervical spinal cord
did not reveal any traumatic alterations of the tissue, especially no
lesions of the axons or myelin sheaths. However, the postimpact effects
on the average evoked potential were dominated by steady-state changes
in negative-going peaks and positive-going peaks. These effects are
characterized by a stepwise increase in latency of both the negative-
going and the positive-going components. Increases in latency persist
for the duration of the stimulus period in each run. Recovery occurred
some time after the recording was stopped between runs. When
stimulation was restarted in preparation for the next acceleration run,
it was noted that the latency had returned to nearly its previous pre-
run value. Although the magnitude of the latency change is small, it is
significant because the latency variability from average to average is
small [35].

Spinal contusions due to the Odontoid Process of the Axis

The lowest level at which in the -Gx impact vector direction
tissue damage occurred was 78.3 G. This monkey revealed tissue damage at
the ventral aspect of the area between lower medulla oblongata and upper
cervical spinal cord. The indentation of the tissue was the result of a
direct impact of the tip of the odontoid process of the axis on the
tissue. This tissue damage can also be termed a circumscribed contusion
of the spinal cord due to the impacting odontoid process during the run.

The odontoid process of the axis produced, in the -Gx experiments,
a local contusion at the ventral fissure between lower medulla oblongata
and upper cervical spinal cord of a rhesus monkey. The impactor of
Allen's system struck a small surface of posterior aspects of the middle
thoracic spinal cord of dogs or cats [36]. However, the effect in regard
to the quality of tissue damage was the same in both injury mechanisms.

The resulting tissue damage caused by mechanical trauma (tip of odontoid *process* of the axis in our experiments or impactor in the experiments of [36,37]) appears after a free time interval or delayed as a progressive central hemorrhagic necrosis, which extended further proximally and distally and later involved the white matter of the cord, too.

The resulting tissue alteration is not the result of an occlusion of an arterial or venous system; it does not follow an arterial or venous distribution area of a blood vessel. Especially, the tissue damage in our experiments is not caused by an occlusion or thrombosis of the anterior spinal artery. Th same type of lesion produced by the impactor using the method of [36,37] is the result of a mechanical force that was applied at the posterior surface of the spinal cord, a technique that was not likely to lead to an involvement of the anterior spinal artery. These findings are of importance for the interpretation of the pathogenesis of similar lesions in human pathology.

Lesions comparable with those seen in the animals subjected to -Gx impact vector direction at the ventral aspect of the spinal cord between lower medulla oblongata and C1 (indentation and dislocation of tissue, a contusion caused by the odontoid process of the axis did not occur in the +Gx impact vector direction.

Spinal Subdural Hemorrhages

The spinal subdural hemorrhages in the animals undergoing -Gx impact vector direction with transection of the spinal cord between lower medulla oblongata and C1 with rupture of the vertebral arteries were identical to those seen in the animals subjected to +Gx impact vector direction.

Atlanto-Occiputal or C1-C2 Separations with Incomplete And Complete Transections of the Spinal Cord with Bilateral Ruptures of the Vertebral Arteries

The next threshold in the -Gx vector for tissue damage occurring with peak sled accelerations above 105.3 G, were atlanto-occipital or C1-*C2 separations* with *incomplete* and *complete traumatic* transections of the spinal cord between lower medulla oblongata and upper cervical spinal cord. The two animals who survived peak sled accelerations of more than 100 G, namely 108.6 G and 110.4 G, were subjected to G levels that were near the threshold level.

The monkeys with complete transection of the spinal cord showed a bilateral rupture of the vertebral artery. In subtype (1) both vertebral arteries and, in a few instances, the basilar artery were completely avulsed. In subtype (2) the rupture of both vertebral arteries occurred at the foramen magnum, so that their proximal parts remained intact in the specimen *in situ*.

Different Threshold for Atlanto-Occiputal Separations and Traumatic Transections of the Spinal Cord in -Gx and +Gx Impact Vector Experiments

After the experiments subjecting monkeys to -Gx impact vector acceleration were finished and evaluated, and before the experiments subjecting rhesus monkeys to +Gx impact vector accelerations were carried out, the scientific staff was asked whether the threshold levels for cord transections in comparison to -Gx impact vector acceleration were higher or lower or other formulated, would one prefer to be under the same circumstances accelerated or decelerated in the -Gx or +Gx vector direction? The scientific staff answered this question in different ways: The answers were very disparate and sometimes very surprising.

The results of our +Gx experiments show that the threshold for atlanto-occipital separations and traumatic transections of the spinal cord occurred at peak sled accelerations of 140 G and 141 G. The corresponding data for the -Gx vector direction were between 105 G and 110 G. The threshold for atlanto-occipital separation and traumatic transection of the spinal cord in the +Gx vector acceleration is, therefore, about 35 G to 40 G higher than in the -Gx vector. It is noteworthy that in the experiments of Wickström, et al. all primates exposed to acceleration forces developed peak head acceleration forces from 17 Gx to 46 Gx [38]. These peak head acceleration forces were not high enough to produce the local indentations caused by the odontoid process of the axis in ventral aspects of the spinal cord and especially not high enough to produce atlanto-occipital and atlantoaxial separations and spinal-cord transections as in our experiments.

Wickstrom, et al.[38] also noted hyperflexion forces produced significantly greater damage to vertebrae, ligaments, joints, intervertebral discs, and nerve roots than did hyperextension, which in turn tended to produce more damage to the muscle and brain tissue [38]. Our experiments confirm this conclusion, but we want to clarify this. As we have pointed out, our experiments showed that the threshold for atlanto-occipital, atlantoaxial separation, and spinal-cord transection occurs at peak sled accelerations that are in the -Gx impact vector direction about 35 G to 40 G lower than in the +Gx impact vector direction. But it would be wrong to conclude from these findings alone that the -Gx impact vector direction is less dangerous than the +Gx vector direction. As the morphological findings convincingly show, the injury pattern in regard to quality and distribution in both impact vector directions is quite different. In the +Gx impact vector direction, severe bony lesions may occur (they are completely missing in - Gx experiments) when the so-called concertina effect develops in animals with initial positions with flexed neck and forward rotated head.

It is therefore necessary to take the additional tissue alterations into consideration when comparing -Gx and +Gx impact vector direction.

Four out of 6 animals subjected in the +Gx vector direction to peak sled accelerations up to 101 G survived. None of these animals revealed radiological or pathological findings, and none had fractures of the spinous processes of the cervical and upper thoracic spine. The two animals with the fatal outcome revealed pathological findings. They also had extensive hemorrhages in the neck structures around the esophagus and hemorrhages in the upper mediastinum extending into the posterior mediastinum with extensive retropleural and paravertebral hemorrhages of posterior parts of the upper thorax located laterally to the spine. These hemorrhages extended in one animal downward into the pericardium.

Death in the latter 2 animals resulted from the hemorrhages in the neck structures, mediastinum, and pericardium, combined with dislocations of an interspace of the spine at Th1-Th2 and C4-C5, respectively.

Three out of 5 animals subjected to +Gx vector peak sled acceleration ranging between 122 G and 123 G survived. All 4 runs with animals subjected to peak sled accelerations ranging between 139 C and 141 G were acutely fatal.

Hemorrhages in the *upper mediastinum,* descending into the pericardium, were seen only in monkeys subjected to +Gx impact vector acceleration. Further experiments applying serial sections through the structures of the neck and upper thoracic region are under way to determine the exact origin of these hemorrhages, which determine in single cases the fatal outcome of a +Gx impact vector acceleration exposure.

Importance of the Initial Position of the Head in -Gx and +Gx Impact
Vector Acceleration

The threshold in +Gx impact acceleration where fatal outcome may or may not occur is around 100 G. We found it noteworthy that the first of the 2 dead animals had an unusual low peak head angular velocity (Y axis), namely 50 rad/s. The examination of the high-speed films revealed an interesting phenomenon that we termed "concertina effect".
We have pointed out in the discussion of the findings of animals subjected to -Gx impact acceleration that the initial position of the head is very important. It could be shown that a yaw angle of 60 ° or more appeared to significantly reduce the tolerance for head and neck injury for -x whole-body impact acceleration. However, the category or pattern of injury remained the same, namely traumatic lesions at the atlanto-occipital or head/neck junction. It was a quantitative phenomenon and not a qualitative one. However, in animals undergoing +Gx impact acceleration, the initial position of the head is very important. not so much in regard to the yaw angle but in regard to the fact whether the monkey has an initial position in which it keeps its head low, i.e., with the chin near the thorax (the cervical spine is more or less flexed). Then, as we have pointed out earlier, the early phase of the run results in (1) compression of the cervical spine, (2) a more or less marked flexion in the second phase, and (3) rotation of the head in a forward direction. In the term coined by us, concertina effect, a substantial amount of kinetic energy in this initial phase is used up or damped during the compression and flexion of the cervical spine with forward rotation of the head. After this early phase in the run, the cervical spine than begins a hyperextension movement with backward rotation of the head.
The concertina effect occurred, too, in other animals subjected to +Gx impact vector direction. In cases of initial positions that are not ideal (they seem to be frequent in the +Gx vector direction!), a subtype of acceleration in the +Gx impact vector direction occurs with more or less marked initial compression and flexion of the cervical spine and forward rotation of the head before the hyperextension of the cervical spine with backward rotation of the head begins. A "pure" experimental design occurs only when applying +Gx impact vector direction in experiments when an ideal initial position exists. In this case, the hyperextension of the cervical spine with backward rotation of the head begins immediately in the early phase of the run. There is no doubt, in analyzing our findings, that an "impure" initial position leads to a concertina effect that then produces a different pattern or prototype of traumatic lesions in regard to quality and distribution.
This phenomenon must occur in human pathology, too, despite the fact that it is not explicitly mentioned. There exists a discrepancy in the opinions of authors publishing case histories of whiplash injuries. Some authors expressed their opinion that in the initial phase of a "classic" whiplash (+Gx impact vector direction) a hyperflexion occurs before the cervical spine undergoes hyperextension, while other authors categorically rejected this opinion since it would be in contradiction

to the laws of classical physics. It seems to us that both groups of
authors are right: The important point to consider is the initial
position of the head of a driver at the moment his car is hit from the
rear by another car. The driver could have been checking instruments on
his dashboard or changing the program of his auto-radio while keeping
his head down and his cervical spine flexed.

Hawkes [39] made a very, interesting statement:

An explanation of the mechanics of whiplash injury which described
initial flexion occurring as the result of thrust from behind [40,41]
does not seem tenable. It is contrary to the principles of medical
physics as applied to the situation ... Clinical confirmation for the
occurrence of initial hyperextension can be found in the history given
by patients sustaining a whiplash injury while riding in a small truck
struck from the rear. These patients uniformly described the head being
just thrown back against the rear window of the car.

We agree fully with [39] that it is "contrary to the principle of
medical physics as applied to the situation," and we agree fully that
'clinical confirmation for the occurrence of initial hyperextension can
be found in the history given by the patients sustaining a whiplash
injury", but we agree only under the assumption of a perfect or "pure"
initial position of the head and neck of the patient involved in a
whiplash injury. Otherwise the concertina effect occurs, and the
arguments using classical physics are not valid. Another good
observation to substantiate this finding from a clinical standpoint was
presented by Nicholson [42] "A patient with the head and neck slightly
flexed in relaxed position will sustain a more severe injury than a
patient who is braced with the head and neck erect at the time of
impact."

Radiological Findings in Animals Undergoing -Gx and +Gx Impact Vector Acceleration

Radiological findings were observed in 9 out of 15 animals
undergoing +Gx impact vector direction. Peak sled accelerations of up to
97 G did not have radiological findings. they occurred in 9 out of 13
animals with peak sled accelerations between 97 G and 141 G. The highest
peak sled acceleration levels at which no radiological findings occurred
were 122 G and 123 G.

Spinous process fractures occurred in 3 animals subjected to +Gx
impact vector direction; they were seen in the middle and lower cervical
and upper thoracic spine. These spinous fractures were not seen in
monkeys undergoing -Gx impact vector acceleration. The *spinous process
fractures in* the *+Gx vector* must, therefore, be considered and termed
seat and/or restraint system specific lesions.
The spinous process fractures are similar to those described in the
literature as "shoveler's," "creeping," or 'hurling" fracture (also
termed *Schipperfraktur* in the German literature) [43-52].

Marked hypermobility of one or 2 spinous processes of the cervical
vertebra (C7 or C6, or both) was described by Janes and Hooshmand in
patients with whiplash injuries by [53]. This abnormal mobility
apparently represented laxity of the posterior ligaments as well as of
the ligamentous structures surrounding the articular facets of the
cervical spine. Lottes, et al. reported fractures of the spinous process
in whiplash injuries, usually in the lower cervical vertebrae [54].

Spinous process fractures occur, according to Kazarian [55,56], by
abrupt, staccatolike contractions either of the trapezius or of the
rhomboid muscles. They appear primarily at the longest and thinnest
portion of the spinous processes where fragments of bone are avulsed due

to muscle action. The anterior-posterior radiographs may show a double shadow of the spinous process due to downward displacement of the avulsed fragment of bone.

Fractures of the bodies of the vertebrae after whiplash injuries were described by [41,57-59]. They did not occur in our animal experiments subjecting rhesus monkeys to -Gx or +Gx impact acceleration.

In animal experiments using the +Gx vector acceleration, dislocations of an interspace occurred in 5 out of 15 animals, they were seen at 97G peak sled acceleration, 101 G peak sled acceleration, 123 G peak sled acceleration, 140 G peak sled acceleration, and 141 G peak sled acceleration. It is noteworthy that in the first of these three animals, the dislocation was seen at Th1-Th2, C4-C5, and Th7-Th8. Only the two animals with high-level runs of 140 G peak sled acceleration and 141 G peak sled acceleration revealed a massive atlanto-occipital separation. As pointed out, in the -Gx impact acceleration only two types of lesions of the cervical spine occurred: (1) Atlanto-occipital separation with massive dislocation of the segments (7 animals), and (2) incomplete and complete C1-C2 separations (2 animals).

The only bony fractures in the -Gx acceleration series were three cases of *basilar skull fractures* that we proposed to call *tension fractures,* caused by the inertial load of the head. There was no direct impact of the head against other structures with transmission of force to the base of the skull. This is of considerable interest, because all other lethal injuries were of soft tissue. This indicates that the use of x-rays, in the absence of autopsies, to determine injuries in cadaveric research of this type would not have shown the injuries. These basilar skull fractures were not seen in the +Gx impact vector direction.

In addition to peak sled acceleration, initial position of the head relative to the applied acceleration vector appears to be the major contributor to the threshold for fatality, as indicated by Thomas and Jessop [60]. These authors reported that a yaw angle of 60° or more appears to significantly reduce the tolerance for head and neck injury for -Gx whole body impact acceleration. However, the category of injury that occurs— atlanto-occipital separation basilar skull fracture, or first cervical-second cervical vertebral body separation—is independent of the initial position.

One animal, which was subjected in the -Gx vector to a peak sled acceleration of 123.0 G, had to be euthanized in a moribund state 90 h after the run. This monkey had a thrombosis of the right vertebral and right inferior posterior cerebellar artery, with softening of the ventral aspect of the lower brainstem and right cerebellar white matter. This was a *Wallenberg syndrome* of *traumatic origin.*

It is noteworthy that despite peak sled accelerations up to 162.8 G in the -Gx impact vector direction and 141.0 G in the +Gx impact vector direction, *no rupture* of a *carotid artery* was observed.

The accelerator can impart up to 200 G to the lightweight primate sled for durations of up to 90 ms. It is anticipated that, with G levels exceeding 162.8 G in the -Gx and +Gx impact vector direction, ruptures of the carotid arteries and finally decapitation would occur. The decapitation could be considered the end point in these experiments. They were indeed described in single cases after whiplash injuries in humans [61].

Subdural Hemorrhages over the Cerebral Hemispheres

Furthermore, there were no subdural hemorrhages over the cerebral hemispheres in the animals subjected to +GX impact vector direction as seen in some of the monkeys undergoing -Gx impact vector direction. Further experiments have to be carried out to find out whether the absence of subdural hemorrhages over the cerebral hemispheres in +Gx impact vector direction are to be explained by the relatively small number of animals used as compared to 28 used in the -Gx impact vector direction.

Subdural hemorrhages in animal experiments have been described first by Unterharnscheidt and Higgins in squirrel monkeys undergoing *direct impact* with *nondeforming angular acceleration of the head* (using Head Acceleration Device II, HAD-II).

The results of these experiments cannot be used for the interpretation of whiplash injuries. The aim of the HAD-II project was to study the effects of nondeforming angular acceleration of the head. The HAD-II experiments consisted of a nondeforming application of force directly to the head, via a helmet fixed to the animal's head, while the experiments in the -Gx and +Gx vector direction were indirect applications of force to the head from the restrained torso via the neck. The HAD-II experiments had to be considered in 1969 as the first series of animal experiments using direct nondeforming angular acceleration to the head of a monkey; they have to be seen now only in a historic perspective.

In the experiments using Belgian hares, carried out, 92% of the animals exhibited some evidence of injury at necropsy on microscopic examination [38]. More than half of the animals had retro-ocular hemorrhages. "The peculiarity of the structures of the rabbit's brain renders the ophthalmic artery and posterior ciliary artery most vulnerable" [38].

The rabbits in the experiments of Wickström, et al. showed retro-ocular hemorrhages however, these experiments did not reveal retro-ocular hemorrhages in monkeys. The monkeys subjected to -Gx and +Gx impact vector directions in our series also did not show retro-ocular hemorrhages. The *retro-ocular lesions,* therefore, have to be termed *species specific.*

Ocular hemorrhages have been described in humans, not in a single whiplash injury, but in the whiplash shaken infant syndrome. Caffey had remarked that the single shake of an infant may be less forceful and pathogenic than the single whiplash in an automobile accident, and the summation of the injurious effects of the many repeated but less forceful manual shakings may be much more harmful to the brain and internal blood vessels and also to the blood vessels of the eye [62].

COMPARISON OF -GX AND +GX NEUROPATHOLOGY WITH TISSUE ALTERATIONS SEEN IN STATIC STRETCH EXPERIMENTS

It is of interest to compare the pathomorphological findings of the monkeys subjected to -Gx and +Gx impact vector direction with those of animals that were involved in static stretch experiments of the cervical spine carried out by [63,64]. In these experiments, subjecting rhesus monkeys to controlled static axial stretch of the cervical spine *(Note:* this is roughly equivalent of a -Gz acceleration vector), the load bearing and elongation characteristics of the cervical ligaments were examined. Loss of evoked potentials resulting from the in vivo axial loadings of the cervical regions of these monkeys is due to factors other than ligament failure.

The comparison of both injury-producing mechanisms (whole-body -Gx and +Gx impact acceleration exposures with completely restrained torso but unrestrained head and neck, and controlled axial static stretch experiments of the cervical spine) reveals that quality and distribution of the traumatic lesions in both experiments are quite different. This gives proof again that each vector direction produces a typical, well-defined injury pattern.

Further experiments with macaca mulatta monkeys, carried out by [64], using slow application of axial forces to the vertebral column with forces that produced an approximate 50 percent reduction in the afferent or efferent evoked potential magnitude, revealed a marked reduction in metabolic activity at the cervico-medullary junction and cervical spinal cord (using the 14C deoxyglucose method by Sokoloff [24-28], while other levels of the spinal cord were essentially normal. It is noteworthy that examination with light microscopy was unremarkable. However, in a monkey that survived 7 days, damage was observed in the central grey substance at the level between lower medulla oblongata and upper cervical spinal cord. Electron microscopic studies with similar force application demonstrated shrinkage of the axoplasm and disruption of the myelin lamellae in the upper and lower cervical regions, while brain and thoracic spinal cord tissue were only minimally altered. These preliminary findings suggest that the greatest effects in the static stretch experiments occur in the cervical regions with axial distension, and that 14C deoxyglucose and electron microscopy may be valuable for the evaluation of early physiologic tissue alterations following biomechanical trauma to the atlanto-occipital junction .

The tissue alteration in the monkey described above, a progressive central hemorrhagic necrosis, was identical with those lesions described by us after -Gx impact vector acceleration and those described by Osterholm using the Allen's method [37,36]. As we have pointed out before, in both instances, direct impact occurred, namely a spinal contusion, that resulted in this delay,ed tissue-necrotizing, hemorrhagic response that begins in the grey substance of the spinal cord, later engulfs adjacent white structures, and eventually the entire spinal cord. We do not know whether the central hemorrhagic necrosis due to the static stretch experiments carried out by Sances, et al. is the result of local direct impact, is due to temporary local pressure of bony structures of the atlanto-occipital junction against the spinal cord, or whether it is due to overstretching of the tissue of the upper cervical spinal cord with extreme axial loading [64]. But again, it can be demonstrated that an injury to the anterior spinal artery does not play a role in the pathogenesis of this lesion.

It appears, that each injury mechanism and each vector direction of impact acceleration produces a different and predictable type of injury in regard to quality and distribution. This was demonstrated in the experiments where the translational (linear) and rotational acceleration were transferred directly to the head. The second group of experiments reports on a carefully controlled series of experiment with whole body -Gx and +Gx impact acceleration exposures of rhesus monkeys with completely restrained torso but unrestrained head and neck   That is, the animal is accelerated with the unrestrained head and neck undergoing flexion/hyperextension respectively hyperextension/flexion. Thus impact acceleration is transmitted from the sled to the torso by the restraint system, and then via the vertebral column to the head.

Summary

In all 4 series of experiments a continuum from no lesions to severe and lethal ones can be demonstrated, described and quantified. The head-neck and brain-cord systems can be described by input-output relationships.

Each effective mechanical input to the head and neck corresponds to a predictable and typical morphological endstate.

References

[1] Foltz, E.L., Jenkner, F.L. and Ward, A.A. "Experimental cerebral concussion," Journal of Neurosurgery, Vol. 10, 1953, pp. 342-352.

[2] Unterharnscheidt, F. "Experimentelle Untersuchungen über die Schädigung des ZNS durch gehäufte stumpfe Schädeltraumen, Zentralblatt für die gesamte Neurologie ud Psychiatrie, Vol. 147, 1958, p. 14.

[3] Unterharnscheidt, F. Die gedeckten Schäden des Gehirns. Experimentelle Untersuchungen mit einmaliger, wiederholter und gehäufter Gewalteinwirkung auf den Schädel, Monographien aus dem Gesamtgebiete der Neurologie und Psychiatrie, Heft 103, Springer, Berlin Göttingen Heidelberg, 1963.

[4] Sellier, K. and Unterharnscheidt, F. Mechanik und Pathomorphologie der Hirnschäden nach stumpfer Gewalteinwirkung auf den Schädel, Hefte zur Unfallheilkunde, Heft 76, Springer, Berlin Göttingen Heidelberg, 1963.

[5] Unterharnscheidt, F. and Sellier,K. Mechanics and pathomorphology of closed brain injuries, Chapt. 26. In: Cavenes, W.F. and Walker, A.E. (eds) Head Injury, Conference Proceedings, Lippincott, Philadelphia Toronto, 1966.

[6] Unterharnscheidt, F. Discussion, Mechanisms of head injury. In: Gurdjian, E S., Lange, W.A., Patrick, L.M., and Thomas, L.M. (eds) Impact Injury and Crash Protection, Thomas, Springfield, 1970, pp. 43-62.

[7] Higgins, L.S., Schmall, R.A., Cain, C.P., Kielpinski, P.E., Primiano, F.B., Barber, T.W. and Brockway, J.A. The Investigation of Parameters of Head Injury related to Acceleration and Deceleration. Technology Incorporated, Life Sciences Division, San Antonio, TX, T 1-11 8-67-1.

[8] Higgins L.M., and Schmall, R.A. A Device for the Investigation of Head Injury Effected by Nondeforming Head Acceleration, paper No. 679905, Proceedings 11th Stapp Car Crash Conference, Society of Automotive Engineers, Warrendale, PA, pp. 35-46.

[9] Unterharnscheidt, F. and Higgins, L.S. "Traumatic lesions of brain and spinal cord due to non-deforming angular acceleration of the head," Texas Report on Biology and Medicine, Vol. 27, 1969, pp. 127-166.

[10] Unterharnscheidt, F, and Higgins, L.S."Pathomorphology of experimental head injury due to rotational acceleration, Acta Neuropathologica, Vol, 12, 1969, pp. 200-204.

[11] Unterharnscheidt, F. and Higgins, L.S. "Neuropathological effects of translational and rotational acceleration of the head in animal experiments, Chap. 17. In: Walker, A.E., Caveness, W.F. and Critchley, M. (eds) The Late Effets of Head Injury, Thomas, Springfield, 1969, pp. 158-167.

[12] Becker, E. Preliminary discusion of an approach to modeling living human head and neck response to -Gx impact acceleration. In: King, W.F. and Mertz, H.J. (eds) Human Impact Response, Plenum Press, New York, 1973, pp. 321-329.

[13] Becker, E. Stereographic Measurements for Anatomically Mounted Instruments. Proceedings 21th Stapp Car Crash Conference, Society of Automotive Engineers, Warrendale, PA, 1977, pp. 475-505.

[14] Ewing, C.L., and Thomas, D.J. Human Head and Neck Response to Impact Acceleration, Naval Aerospace Medical Research Laboratory Monograph, No. 21, August 1971.
[15] Becker, E. and Willems, G. An Experimentally Validated 3-D Inertial Tracking Package for Application in Biodynamics Research, Proceeding 19th Stapp Car Crash Conference, Society of Automotive Engineers, Warrendale, PA, 1977.
[16] Willems, G. A Detailled Performance Evaluation od Subminiature Piezoresistive Accelerometers, 23th Inernational Instrumentation Symposium, Las Vegas, NEV, May 1-5, 1977, Proceedings of Instrumentation in the Aerospace Industry, Vol. 23, Instrument Society of America, Pittsburgh, PA, 1977, pp. 531-540.
[17] Unterharnscheidt, F., Ewing, C.L., Thomas, D.J., Jessop, M.E., Rogers, J.E. and Willems, G. Premliminary Report on the Neuropathological Findings in Rhesus Monkeys Undergoing Short Duration - Gx Acceleration, paper No. 201, 6th International Congress of Neurological Surgery, Sao Paolo, Brazil, June 19-21, 1977, p.80.
[18] Unterharnscheidt,F. and Ewing, C.L. Potential Relationship between Human Central Nervous System Injury and Impact Forces based on Primate Studies, AGARD Conference Proceedings, No. 253, Models and Analogues for the Evaluation of Human Biodynamics Response, Performance and Protection, Aerospace Medical Specialist's Meeting, Paris, France, November 6-10, 1978, pp. A 18-1 to A 18-8.
[19] Unterharnscheidt, F. Neuropathology of the Rhesus Monkey Undergoing -Gx Impact Acceleration, AGARD Conefernce Proceedings, No. 322, Impact Injury caused by Linear Acceleration: Mechanisms, Prevention and Cost. Aerospace Medical Specialist's Meeting, Cologne, Germany, pp. 17-1 to 17-34.
[20] Unterharnscheidt, F. Neuropathology of the rhesus monkey undergoing -Gx impact acceleration, Chap. 4. In: Ewing, C.L., Thomas, D.J., Sances, A., and Larson, SJ. (eds) Impact Injury of the Head and Spine, Thomas, Springfield,1983, pp. 94-176.
[21] Unterharnscheidt, F. Traumatic Alterations in the Rhesus Monkey Undergoing -Gx Impact Acceleration, Proceedings 6th Meeting, Japanese Society of Neurotraumatology (Tokyo), Vol. 6, 1983, pp. 151-167.
[22] Unterharnscheidt, F. Morphological Findings in Rhesus Monkeys Undergoing -Gx Impact Vector Direction. The Cervical Spine Research Society, December, 7-10, 1983, pp. 26-28.
[23] Sances, A., Myklebust, J., Kostreva, D., Cusick,J.F., Weber, R., Houterman, C., Larson, S.J., Maiman, D., Walsh, P., Ho, K., Saltzberg, B. "Pathophysiology of Cervical Injuries, Proceedings 26th Stapp Car Crash Conference, Society of Automotive Engineers, New York, 1982, pp. 41-70.
[24] Sokoloff, L. "Relation between physiological function and energy metabolism in the Central Nervous System," Journal of Neurochemistry, Vol. 29, 1977, pp. 13-16.
[25] Sokoloff, L. "Mapping of local cerebral functional activity by measurement of local cerebral glucose utilization with (14C) deoxyglucose," Brain, Vol. 102, 1979, pp. 653-668.
[26] Sokoloff, L. "The deoxyglucose method; theory and practice," European Neurology, Vol. 20, 1981, pp. 137-145.
[27] Localization of functional activity in the Central Nervous System by measurement of glucose utilization with radioactive deoxyglucose," Journal of Cerebral Blood Flow and Metabolism, Vol.1, 1981, pp.7-36.
[28] Sokoloff,L., Reivich, M., Kennedy, C. Des-Rosiers, M.H., Patlak, C.S. Pettigrew K.D., Sakurada, O, and Sohara, M. "The (14C) Deoxyglucose

method for the measurement of local cerebral glucose utilization: Theory, procedure, and normal values in the conscious and anesthetized albino rat," Journal of Neurochemistry, Vol. 28, 1977, pp. 897-916.

[29] Unterharnscheidt, F. Morphological Findings in Rhesus Monkeys Undergoing +Gx Acceleration. The Cervical Spine Research Society, paper No. 1, 12th Annual Meeting, New Orleans, LA, 1984, p.15.

[30] Unterharnscheidt, F. Pathological and neuropathological findings in rhesus monkeys subjected to -Gx and +Gx indirect impact acceleration, Chap. 21. In: Sances, A., Thomas, D., Ewing, C.L., Larson, S.J., and Unterharnscheidt, F. (eds) Mechanisms of Head and Spine Trauma, Aloray, New York, 1986, pp. 565-663.

[31] Unterharnscheidt, F. Pathologie des Nervensystems VII, Traumatologie von Hirn- und Rückenmark, Traumatische Schäden von Rückenmark und Wirbelsäule (forensische Pathologie), Springer, Berlin Heidelberg New York, 1992.

[32] Unterharnscheidt, F. Pathologie des Nervensystems VI, Traumatologie von Hirn und Rückenmark, Die traumatischen Schäden des Gehirns, Band 13/VI.A, Springer, Berlin Heidelberg New York, 1993.

[33] Unterharnscheidt, F. Pathologie des Nervensystems VI, Traumatologie von Hirn und Rückenmark, Die traumatischen Schäden des Gehirns, Band 13/VI.B, Springer, Berlin Heidelberg New York, 1993.

[34] Unterharnscheidt, F. Pathologie des Nervensystems VI, Traumatologie von Hirn und Rückenmark, Die traumatischen Schäden des Gehirns, Band 13/VI.C, Springer, Berlin Heidelberg New York, (in press).

[35] Saltzberg, B.W., Burton, M.S., Weiss, M.D., Berger, M., Ewing C.L. Thomas, D., Jessop, E.M., Sances, A., Larson, S.J. Walsh, P.R., Myklebust, J. Dynamic tracking of evoked potential changes in studies of Central Nervous System injury due to impact acceleration, Chap. 10. In: Ewing, C.L., Thomas, D.J., Sances, A., Larson, S.J. (eds.) Impact Injury of the Head and Spine, Thomas, Springfield, 1983, pp. 310-323.

[36] Allen, A.R. "Remarks on the histopathological changes in the spinal cord due to impact, an experimental study," Journal of Nervous and Mental Disease, Vol. 41, 1914, pp. 141-147.

[37] Osterholm, J.L. The Pathophysiology of Spinal Cord Trauma. Thomas, Springfield, 1978.

[38] Wickstrom, J. Martinez, J., and Rodrigues, R. Cervical Spine Syndrome: Experimental Acceleration Injuries of the Head and Neck, Proceedings Prevention of Highway Injury, Highway Safety Research Institute, University of Michigan, Ann Arbor, MI, 1967, pp. 182-187.

[39] Hawkes, C.D. "Whiplash injuries of the head and neck", Archives of Surgery, Vol. 75, 1957, pp. 828-833.

[40] Gay, J.R. and Abbott,K.H. Common whiplash injuries of the neck," Journal of the American Medical Association," Vol. 152, 1953, pp. 1698-1704.

[41] Lipow, E.G. "Whiplash injuries", Southern Medical Journal, Vol. 48, 1955, pp. 1304-1311.

[42] Nicholson, M.W. "Whiplash: Fact, Fantasy, or Fakery, Hawai Medical Journal, Vol. 33, 1974, pp. 168-170.

[43] Lönnerblad, L. "Disruption fracture of spinal processes as a track injury," Acta Chirurgica Scandinavica, Vol. 74, 1934, pp. 434

[44] Matthes, H.G. "Dornfortsatzabrisse, eine typische Verletzung bei schweren Erdarbeiten," Chirurg, Vol. 7, 1935, pp. 665-671.

{45} Lickint, F. "Ein bemerkenswerter Fall von 'Schipperkrankheit,'" Medizinische Welt, Vol. 10, 1936, pp. 965-966.

[46] Bergmann, W. "Über den Arbeitsschaden des Dornfortsatzes," Chirurg, Vol. 9, 1937, pp. 579-581.

[47] Ghormely, R.K. and Hoffman, J.O.E. "Fracturs of the vertebral processes," Mayo Clinic Proceedings, Vol. 17, 1938, p. 617.

[48] Rostock, P. "Die Diagnose des Überlastungsschadens beim Dornfortsatzbruch der Wirbelsäule (Schipperkrankheit)" Bruns Beiträge für klinische Chirurgie. Vol. 169, 1939, pp.15-24.

[49] Canigiani, R. "Gehäuftes Auftreten von Dornfortsatzbrüchen bei Erdarbeitern, Wiener klinische Wochenschrift, Vol. 2, 1940, pp. 892

[50] Hall, R.D.M. "Clay-shoveler's fracture," Journal of Bone and Joint Surgery, Vol. 22, 1940, pp. 63-75.

[51] Kaspar, M. "Ist die Dornfortsatzfraktur der unteren Hals- und oberen Brustwirbelsäule (Schipperkrankheit)) Unfallfolge? Zentralblatt für Chirurgie, Vol. 67, 1940, pp. 898-905.

[52] Snyder, C.H. "Shoveler's fracture ('Schipperkrankheit')," Journal of the Michigan State Medical Society, Vol. 41, 1942, pp. 847-849.

[53] Janes, J.H. and Hooshmand, H. "Severe extension-flexion injuries of the cervical spine," Mayo Clinic Proceedings, Vol. 40, 1965, pp. 353-369.

[54] Lottes, J.A., Luh, A.M., Leydig, S.M., Fries, J.H. and Burst, J.H. "Whiplash injuries of the neck," Missouri Medicine, Vol. 56, 1959, pp. 645-650.

[55] Kazarian, L.E. Classification of simple spinal column injuries, Chapt. 3. In: Ewing, C.L., Thomas, D.L., Sances, A., Larson, S.J. (eds) Impact Injury of the Head and Spine, Thomas, Springfield, 1983, pp. 72-93.

[56] Kazarian, L.E. Upper Cervical Spine Injuries - A Review of Seven Cases, 11th Annual Meeting. The Cervical Spine Research Society, Palm Beach, FLA, December 7-10, 1983, p.29.

[57] Russell, L.W. "Whiplash injuries of the spine, Journal of the Florida Medical Association, Vol. 43, 1957, pp. 1099-1104.

[58] Wright, P.B. and Brady, L.P."An anatomic evaluation of whiplash injuries," Clinical Orthopedics, Vol. 12, 1958, pp. 120-129.

[59] Jackson, R. The Cervical Syndrome, Thomas, Springfield, 1965.

[60] Thomas, D.J. and Jessop, M.E. "Experimental head and neck injury, Chapt 5. In: Ewing, C.L., Thomas, D.J., Sances,A., Larson, S.J. (eds) Impact Injury of the Head and Spine, Thomas, Springfield, 1983, pp. 177-217.

[61] Vernon, S. "Whiplash injury and liability," American Journal of Surgery, Vol. 94, 1957, pp. 535-536.

[62] Caffey, J. "The whiplash shaken infant syndrome: Manual shaking by the extremities with whiplash induced intracranial and intraocular bleedings linked with residual permanent brain damage and mental retardation," Pediatrics, Vol. 54, 1974, pp. 396-403.

[63] Christoffel, T.S. The Effect of Controlled Stretch on the Ligamentous Cervical Spine of the Rhesus Monkey, Master's Thesis, Marquette University, Milwaukee, WIS, June 1980.

[64] Sances, A., Myklebust, J., Kostreva, D., Cusick, J.F., Weber, R., Houterman, C., Larson, S.J., Maiman, D., Walsh, P., Chilbert, M, Unterharnscheidt, F.., Ewing, C,L, Thomas, L, Siegesmund, K. Ho, K. and Saltzberg, B. Pathophysiology of Cervical Injuries, Proceeding 26th Stapp Car Crash Conference, Society of Automotive Engineers, New York, 1982, pp. 41-70.

Frank A. Pintar,[1] Narayan Yoganandan,[2] Anthony Sances, Jr.,[3] and Joseph F. Cusick[4]

EXPERIMENTAL PRODUCTION OF HEAD-NECK INJURIES UNDER DYNAMIC FORCES

REFERENCE: Pintar, F. A., Yoganandan, N., Sances, A. Jr., and Cusick, J. F., **"Experimental Production of Head-Neck Injuries Under Dynamic Forces,"** Head and Neck Injuries in Sports, ASTM STP 1229, Earl F. Hoerner, Ed., American Society for Testing and Materials, Philadelphia, 1994.

ABSTRACT: Compression related mechanisms of injury are common in sports and recreational trauma to the human cervical spine. The purpose of these studies was to experimentally reproduce common clinically seen injuries of the head-neck complex. A total of 19 preparations (8 quasistatic, 11 dynamic) were used to obtain strength and motion information correlated to pathology. The quasistatic studies served to develope a method to kinematically monitor the localized deformations in the tissue as injury occurs. It was observed that significant relaxation of the tissues occur post-traumatically and the kinematic analysis quantified the true extent of the deformations to the cervical spine components. Under dynamic loading, mid to lower cervical spine compression-related trauma occurred. To reproduce these kinds of injuries, the pre-existing lordosis was removed and the head-neck complex was dynamically impacted. Parallel studies on the Hybrid III anthropomorphic manikin head-neck indicated a substantially different response in compression compared to the human cadaver specimens.

KEYWORDS: head-neck, injuries, biomechanics, cervical spine, experimental

[1]Associate Professor and Co-Director, Neuroscience Research Laboratories, Department of Neurosurgery, Medical College of Wisconsin, and the Department of Veterans Affairs Medical Center, Milwaukee, Wisconsin 53295

[2]Associate Professor and Assistant Chief, Biomechanics Research, Department of Neurosurgery, Medical College of Wisconsin, and the Department of Veterans Affairs Medical Center, 9200 West Wisconsin Avenue, Milwaukee, Wisconsin 53226

[3]Professor and Chairman of Biomechanics, Department of Neurosurgery, Medical College of Wisconsin, and the Department of Veterans Affairs Medical Center, 9200 West Wisconsin Avenue, Milwaukee, Wisconsin 53226

[4]Professor, Department of Neurosurgery, Medical College of Wisconsin, and the Department of Veterans Affairs Medical Center, 9200 West Wisconsin Avenue, Milwaukee, Wisconsin 53226

INTRODUCTION

Severe head-neck injuries due to athletic related events continue
to shock and disturb us as well as add to societal costs. The most
common mechanism of sports related injuries to the cervical column are
compression or compression-flexion related [1]. To further understand
these types of injuries and enhance our efforts at prevention, this
trauma must be experimentally reproduced in a controlled laboratory
environment. The majority of previous studies in the cervical region
have been directed towards investigations of elements less than the
total cervical column [2-11]. More recently, studies have been
conducted to determine mechanisms of injury to the total cervical column
[12-25]. The anatomical complexity of the cervical column permits
motion in flexion, extension, rotation, and bending because of its
material properties and architecture. Furthermore, pure motion in any
direction is rarely encountered in the cervical column because of its
articulations and changes in orientation of the facet joints. The
majority of our scientific knowledge regarding injury mechanisms of the
total cervical column have been obtained from retrospective clinical or
biomechanical studies designed to examine tissues following load
relaxation. The relaxation of the injured column following trauma may
obscure the full evaluation of injury mechanisms. Therefore, the goals
of the present study were as follows: 1. To develop a method to
quantify the strength and motion characteristics of the entire human
cadaver cervical spine under axial loading, 2. To reproduce clinically-
relevant cervical spine trauma, and, 3. Correlate resulting injuries
determined from x-rays, computed tomography (CT), and cryosections with
the biomechanical parameters measured during the impact.

MATERIALS AND METHODS

The methodologies used in these studies have been published
previously [21,22]. A brief synopsis is included here for continuity.
To develop a method to determine the strength and motion characteristics
of entire human cadaver cervical spines under axial loading, eight fresh
human cadavers were used. Specimens were evaluated radiographically and
from their medical histories to preclude metastatic disease. The head
and spine were isolated to avoid damage to the ligaments and other soft
tissues. The head-neck complex was separated from the torso at the T2-
T3 junction. Specimens were radiographed in the anteroposterior (AP)
and lateral planes, and CT scans were obtained. Specimens were mounted
in a specially designed apparatus. The distal end of the preparation
was rigidly mounted in polymethylmethacrylate (PMMA) and fixed to a six-
axis load cell. At the proximal end, the cap of the head was removed
with a bone saw through frontal temporal and occipital bones about 5 cm
superior to the Frankfort plane. An aluminum rod with a spherical end
was rigidly fixed into the skull with PMMA. The spherical end of the
rod protruded out of the skull and was used for positioning prior to
test. The cervical column was aligned to remove the lordosis by
adjustment of the spherical end of the rod. The proximal end was then
rigidly attached to a second six-axis load cell and mounted to the
piston of an electrohydraulic piston actuator (MTS Systems, Minneapolis,
MN).

The vertebrae were prepared with retroreflective spherical pin
targets to monitor the motions of the vertebral bodies, facet column
(lateral mass), and spinous processes. Localized kinematic data was
obtained with a video motion analysis system (Motion Analysis
Corporation, Santa Rosa, CA). For this series of tests, the specimens
were compressed at quasistatic rate of 2 mm/sec until noticeable failure
occurred. Failure was defined as a significant dip in the force-time
trace with concomitant fracture or soft tissue tearing. At this point,
the deformation was maintained with the electrohydraulic piston and a

lateral x-ray was taken to document the pathology. The preparation was
also frozen in this state for cryosectioning. The entire frozen
cervical column underwent complete x-ray and CT imaging. The frozen
preparation was then sectioned with a heavy duty cryomicrotome (LKB,
Broma, Sweden). Colored slide photographs of the tissue were taken
every 0.5 to 1 mm intervals to document the anatomic alterations of the
soft and hard tissues.

     The next series of tests were done to dynamically load the human
cadaver cervical column up to 8 m/s. A total of 11 human cadaver head-
neck complexes were dynamically loaded from 2 m/s to 8 m/s. Each
preparation was mounted distally, the same way as described above for
the quasistatic tests. The proximal mounting procedure was modified,
however. The cranium was left intact and not connected to the piston
actuator of the testing device. The head was rigidly mounted in a
neurosurgical stainless steel halo ring with fixation into the skull
using screws. To achieve stability of the head-neck preparation, the
specimen was positioned using a system of pulleys and dead weights in
the anterior and spring tension in the posterior regions of the
preparation. The weights and spring tension were adjusted to be
approximately 30 to 80 N and essentially simulated the neck musculature
that keeps the head erect. By adjusting the spring tension posteriorly
and the anterior dead weight, the head-neck complex was aligned to
remove the cervical lordosis. The vertebrae were prepared with 20 to 30
retroreflective targets as described above.

     Dynamic loading was applied using the electrohydraulic piston
actuator; each preparation was impacted once. A 15 x 15 cm aluminium
plate covered with a 1.5 cm thick ensolite pad served as the impacting
surface and was fixed to the piston actuator. Because of weight
limitations a miniature three-axis force gauge (Kistler Corporation,
Amherst, NY) was attached in series with the piston of the testing
device just above the aluminum plate to record forces along the three
anatomical directions. A uniaxial accelerometer was mounted on the
plate to record z-axis accelerations and served to inertially compensate
the z-axis force. A three-axis accelerometer was fixed into the
temporoparietal bone of the head; a miniature uniaxial accelerometer
(Entran, Model EGA) was glued to the mastoid process of the skull
(approximately the level of the occipital condyles), and another
uniaxial accelerometer was glued to the antero-lateral aspect of the C4
vertebral body. The actuator of the testing device was permitted to
travel two to five cm before contacting the preparation to obtain the
preset constant velocity when the specimen was impacted. The excursion
of the piston after contacting the skull at approximately its vertex was
preset to 2.5 to 4.5 cm. The experiment was filmed using a 16 mm high
speed camera (HyCam II, Red Lake Instruments, Inc., CA). The high speed
camera was synchronized with the digital data acquisition by
electronically coupling the camera, the data acquisition systems, and
electrohydraulic piston so that a single mechanism triggered the entire
system. The transducer data was collected during the event with the
digital data acquisition system sampling at 12.5 kHz. Each specimen was
frozen post-test and CT's, x-rays, and cryomicrotome sections were
obtained. The pathoanatomical images were correlated to the
biomechanical findings by initially identifying the injured component
and analyzing the localized kinematics of the particular area to
determine the time and extent of fracture.

     In the latter four head-neck preparations an instrumented
artificial spinal cord was placed inside the spinal canal of the
cadaveric preparation [26]. This artificial spinal cord models the
physical force-deflection properties of the human spinal cord and the
1mm thick transducers record force experienced by the spinal cord at
seven discrete locations along the column. This transducer system

offers the next step in determining what the spinal cord experiences during these traumatic events.

The Hybrid III head-neck system was similarly tested as above at piston actuator speeds of 0.002 to 7 m/s. The instrumentation was the same as for the specimen tests except that the triaxial accelerometer was mounted at the c.g. of the head, there was no mastoid accelerometer, and a uniaxial accelerometer was glued to the middle ring of the neck to compare with the C4 accelerometer of the cadaver preparation. The Hybrid III head-neck complex was also rigidly mounted to the distal six-axis load cell such that the geometric center of the neck was aligned with the load cell center.

RESULTS

A summary of results is given in Table 1 indicating the maximum values obtained from the measuring transducers during the tests. Some data from the first seven quasistatic tests and the first six dynamic tests were reported previously (21, 22). In general, the off-axis forces and accelerations (x,y) were significantly lower than the vertical (z) forces and accelerations. The F_x shear forces were greater than the F_y forces but less than the compressive forces (F_z). The transverse moment (axial, M_z) were essentially insignificant compared to the flexion-extension moment (sagittal, M_y). Moments in the coronal plane (M_x) were also smaller than M_y. Therefore, with axial compressive loading, flexion or extension moments often with shear were induced into the column. The quasistatic tests (QS1-QS8) demonstrated a force balance between the superior load cell and the inferior load cell. The studies done at higher rates of loading (D1-D11) demonstrated a dynamic effect; the proximal F_z forces were considerably higher than the distal F_z recorded forces. The quasistatic studies demonstrated upper cervical spine pathologies. Often C2 anterior fractures occurred with subluxation between C2-C3 or between C3-C4. It was noted that often multiple injuries occurred with the primary mechanism of injury being either compression-extension or compression-flexion. The kinematic data recorded during these tests revealed the true extent of the displacement of the bony elements relative to each other. Because the preparations were frozen under load the post CT, x-rays, and cryomicrotome images verified the information obtained from the kinematic analysis. For example, in specimen QS2, a C3 vertebral body fracture was evident on CT, x-ray and cryomicrotome images and the kinematic analysis demonstrated 6.3 mm of displacement between the two targets on that vertebral body. These quasistatic studies demonstrated that with four to six targets on each vertebra, the soft and hard tissue injuries could not only be verified with the kinematic information but also quantified.

The high speed loading studies produced mid to lower cervical column compression fractures including wedge compression, burst fractures, and chip fracture). The cadaver head-neck preparations (D1-D11) always indicated at least a 50% decrease between the maximum proximal Z-force and, the maximum distal Z-force. In contrast, there was at most 25% difference between load cell maximums for the three Hybrid III tests. The Z-axis forces recorded on the head of the cadaver preparations were consistently higher than those recorded on the Hybrid III tests. The C4 vertebral body accelerations recorded for the cadaver tests were often similar to the magnitudes recorded at the skull of the same preparation. In contrast, the Hybrid III accelerations recorded at the middle ring of the neck were consistently lower than those accelerations recorded inside the head. Generally for the cadaver tests conducted at high speeds the upper load cell force trace was of greater magnitude but shorter duration than the lower load cell forces, whereas for the Hybrid III tests, the load cell traces were closer in magnitude and duration.

TABLE 1-- Summary of Results

Preparation	Actuator rate (m/s)	Proximal force (kN)	Distal force (kN)	Head accel. (G's)	C4 V.B.* accel. (G's)
QS1	0.002	1.4	1.4	--	--
QS2	0.002	2.2	2.2	--	--
QS3	0.002	1.7	1.7	--	--
QS4	0.002	2.3	2.3	--	--
QS5	0.002	3.6	3.6	--	--
QS6	0.002	2.3	2.3	--	--
QS7	0.002	2.6	2.6	--	--
QS8	0.002	1.9	1.9	--	--
D1	3.0	5.9	1.6	--	--
D2	4.5	8.4	3.6	--	--
D3	5.5	7.6	1.2	281	266
D4	8.1	11.2	5.1	450	412
D5	7.1	18.5	6.2	489	467
D6	7.1	19.2	3.3	354	351
D7	8.3	12.9	4.6	--	--
D8	5.1	10.4	5.0	450	260
D9	2.3	12.5	5.7	460	342
D10	4.3	11.3	3.8	560	330
D11	5.3	14.5	4.8	630	539
Hybrid III	0.002	6.9	6.9	--	--
Hybrid III	0.03	6.7	6.7	--	--
Hybrid III	1.3	8.6	7.0	--	--
Hybrid III	4.0	8.5	7.8	129	70
Hybrid III	4.8	7.5	6.9	111	61
Hybrid III	6.8	12.9	9.7	243	135

Notes: Values for forces, moments, and accelerations are maximums and not necessarily time coincident. Head accelerations are from the resultant. Proximal and distal forces given are in the Z (vertical) direction.

*V.B. indicates vertebral body for specimen tests; C4 accelerations on the Hybrid III tests are from the middle ring.

Also, the actuator force curves for the specimen tests were single short duration pulses, whereas the Hybrid III actuator force curves were multiple, longer duration pulses. The distal load cell recorded multiple peaks for the specimen tests whereas the Hybrid III tests demonstrated single peaked traces inferiorly. This is most likely due to the failure of one or more cervical spine components in the specimen tests whereas the Hybrid III is nonfrangible.

The kinematic analysis revealed the temporal order of multiple injuries and often direct quantitative data regarding the failure of a particular spinal component. For example, in specimen D2 where a burst fracture of the C5 vertebral body took place, the kinematic analysis revealed at least 11 mm of local compression which took place in approximately 3 msec. This is equivalent to more than 60% compression of the C5 body. A wedge compression fracture recorded in specimen D3 occurred over a longer time duration, approximately 5-6 msec. The film analysis also revealed continued compression of the spine after the actuator was unloaded due to the inertia imparted to the head. Additional injury would often occur at this time and spine compressions from the target analysis became greater than the applied actuator displacement. The Hybrid III tests did not experience additional spine compressions; the preparation followed the movement of the actuator.

DISCUSSION

Sports and athletic related injuries to the head-neck complex often incorporate compressive forces transmitted through the occipital condyles of the cranium to the neck of the person. The present series of experiments were conducted to simulate this event of vertex loading to the head-neck complex. The piston actuator used in the testing offers controlled velocity inputs from quasistatic to dynamic rates. This simulates the often seen mechanism in sports related neck trauma of the head becoming trapped and the body of the athlete following up to compress the neck between the head and the torso. This scenario often results in mid to lower cervical vertebral body fractures including burst, wedge, or chip compression fractures. In the present series of experiments, mid to lower cervical vertebral body compression fractures were produced consistently in the dynamic (high rates of loading) studies. The quasistatic studies produced upper level injuries with often multiple levels of trauma. Even though the prealignment of the head-neck complex was consistent between quasistatic and dynamic studies, different types of injuries occurred between the two series of tests.

It was observed in the quasistatic series of tests that the vertebral segments in the column would shift and realign as the head was displaced downward. This shifting often caused subluxations and ligamentous injuries. In the dynamic series of tests the cervical column demonstrated its viscoelastic effects and could not shift and realign as the piston proceeded downward. This loading scenario produced more bony trauma to the mid and lower cervical spine. Ligamentous damage occurred in the high speed tests, but only after the initial compressions of the vertebral bodies occurred under the compressive loading. Therefore, to replicate the types of injuries commonly experienced by survivors of sports and athletic related neck trauma, one must use the entire head-neck complex, carefully prealigned to remove the lordosis, and apply compressive loading at high rates. This finding has been confirmed by a more recent theoretical model [27].

A unique feature of the present series of experiments is that the motions of the components of the vertebral column were measured using retroreflective pin targets. Because multiple targets were used, from four to six targets per vertebral level, localized component motions were measured even when failure of one or multiple components occurred. This unique method offers not only quantification of localized deformations of the structures, but also tracks the temporal occurrence of multiple fractures to the cervical spine. The kinematic data also reveals the full extent of the deformations that occur during traumatic events. Clinical x-rays taken of patients that have experienced these severe trauma reveal only a retrospective look of the injury after a degree of recovery has occurred. The kinematic analysis in the present experimental series demonstrates that 50% or more recovery can take place after the initial injury. It was also determined that a burst fracture can occur almost twice as fast as a wedge or other type of compression fracture. We have also observed that often the primary injury (e.g., burst fracture) will subsequently affect the neighboring segments with additional deformations. However, after recovery and retrospective x-ray, only the burst fracture is clearly seen. These results may suggest that for these severe types of injuries the clinician may suspect the stability of the adjacent tissues.

Evaluation of the forces recorded from the distal load cell for the specimen tests demonstrated lower magnitude and longer duration pulses than the upper load cell. Also, the head accelerations were roughly equivalent to the C4 accelerations. These finding suggest a substantial decoupling between the head and spinal column. The high magnitude and short duration pulses recorded on the upper load cell are indicative of the force needed to overcome the inertia of the head with little resistance offered by the spine. The distal load cell records the force transmitted through the spine as the fracture is occurring, evidenced by multiple peaks on the curve. The Hybrid III anthropomorphic head-neck complex demonstrated quite different properties than the human cadaver spines. It has been demonstrated in previous studies that the axial compressive stiffness of the Hybrid III neck is from five to ten times stiffer than the cadaver neck [25,28]. The Hybrid III tests indicated similar magnitude and duration for upper and lower load cells. Further, the evaluation of the high speed films demonstrated that the Hybrid III head followed the actuator excursion, both downwards and upwards. These finding suggest a more rigid coupling between the Hybrid III head and neck than those observed for the human specimen tests. This study implies that when the Hybrid III anthropomorphic dummy is evaluated under axial loading conditions to the vertex of the head, careful interpretation should be done when analyzing the results.

Our future studies in this area are directed toward a greater understanding of what the spinal cord experiences during these types of trauma. A seven sensor instrumented artificial spinal cord has been designed and constructed for use in these specimen tests. The instrumented artificial spinal cord is inserted into the spinal canal of the human cadaver preparation. The location of the sensors are documented using x-rays. Each sensor is designed to measure a force transmitted parallel to the axial plane. In other words, as a burst fracture or subluxation occurs under dynamic loading that would cause constriction of the spinal cord, these small one millimeter thick sensors measure the force directed in that area of the cord. A series of preliminary tests have been done using this sensor in the cadaver head-neck complex. The results demonstrate higher magnitudes of force in the regions of the spine that demonstrate the greatest trauma. These studies will lead to greater preventative measures for accidents that occur during sports and recreational activities.

ACKNOWLEDGMENT

This study was supported in part by PHS CDC Grant R49CCR507370 and The Department of Veterans Affairs Medical Center Research Service. The material presented in this manuscript does not necessarily reflect the opinions of the sponsoring institutions.

REFERENCES

[1]   Torg, T. S., _Athletic Injuries to the Head, Neck, and Face_, 2nd Edition, Mosby - Year Book, Inc., St. Louis, MO, 1991, 694 pp.

[2]   Cusick, J. F., Yoganandan, N., Pintar, F., Myklebust, J., and Hussain, H., "Biomechanics of Cervical Spine Facetectomy and Fixation Techniques," _Spine,_ Vol. 13, No. 7, 1988, pp 808-812.

[3]   Goel, V. K., Clark, C., McGowan, D., and Goyal S., "An _in vitro_ Study of the Kinematics of the Normal, Injured and Stabilized Cervical Spine," _Journal of Biomechanics_, Vol. 17, 1984, pp 363-376.

[4]   Liu, Y. K., Krieger, K. W., Jnus, G. O., Connors, M. P., Wakano, P., and Thies, D., "Cervical Spine Stiffness and Geometry of the Young Human Male," Wright Patterson AFB, Dayton, OH, _AFAMRL-TR-80-138_, 1983.

[5]   Moroney, S., Schultz, A., Miller, J., Gunnar, B., and Andersson, J., "Load-displacement Properties of Lower Cervical Spine Motion Segments," _Journal of Biomechanics_, Vol. 21, No. 9, 1988, pp 767-779.

[6]   Panjabi, M. M., White, A. A., and Johnson, R. M., "Cervical Spine Mechanics as a Function of Transection of Components," _Journal of Biomechanics_, Vol. 8, 1975, pp 327-336.

[7]   Pintar, F. A., Myklebust, J. B., Yoganandan, N., Maiman, D. J., and Sances, A. Jr., "Biomechanics of Human Spinal Ligaments." In _Mechanisms of Head and Spine Trauma_, A. Sances, Jr., D. J. Thomas, C. L. Ewing, S. J. Larson, F. Unterharnscheidt, Eds., Aloray Publisher, Goshen, New York, 1986, pp 505-527.

[8]   Sances, A. Jr., Myklebust, J. B., Maiman, D. J., Larson, S. J., Cusick, J. F., and Jodat, R., "Biomechanics of Spinal Injuries," _CRC Critical Reviews in Bioengineering_, Vol. 11, No. 1, 1984, pp 1-76.

[9]   Sances, A. Jr., Thomas, D. J., Ewing, C. L., Larson, S. J., Unterharnscheidt, F., Eds. _Mechanisms of Head and Spine Trauma_, Aloray Publisher, Goshen, NY, 1986, 746 pp.

[10]   White, A. A. and Panjabi, M. M., _Clinical Biomechanics of the Spine_, 2nd Edition, J. B. Lippincott Company, Philadelphia, PA, 1990, 722 pp.

[11]   Yoganandan, N., Pintar, F., Butler, J., Reinartz, J., Sances, A. Jr., and Larson, S. J., "Dynamic Response of Human Cervical Spine Ligaments," _Spine,_ Vol. 14, No. 10, 1989, pp 1102-1110.

[12]   Alem, N. M., Nusholtz, G. S., and Melvin, J. W., "Head and Neck Response to Axial Impacts," _Proceedings of the 28th Stapp Car Crash Conference_, Society of Automotive Engineers, Paper No. 841667, Warrendale, PA, 1984, pp 275-288.

[13]   Hodgson, V. R. and Thomas, L. M., "Mechanisms of Cervical Spine Injury During Impact to the Protected Head," _Proceedings of the 24th Stapp Car Crash Conference_, Society of Automotive Engineers, Paper No. 801300, Warrendale, PA, 1980, pp 15-42.

[14]   Hodgson, V. R. and Thomas, L. M., "A Model to Study Cervical Spine Injury Mechanisms Due to Head Impact," _Institution of Mechanical Engineering_, London, 1980, pp 89-96.

[15] McElhaney, J. H., Paver, J.G., McCrackin, J. H., and Maxwell, G. M., "Cervical Spine Compression Responses," Proceedings of the 27th Stapp Car Crash Conference, Society of Automotive Engineers, Paper No. 831615, Warrendale, PA, 1983, pp 163-178.

[16] McElhaney, J. H., Doherty, B. J., Paver, J. G., and Myers, B. S., "Combined Bending and Axial Loading Responses of the Human Cervical Spine," Proceedings of the 32nd Stapp Car Crash Conference, Society Automotive Engineers, Paper No. 881709, Warrendale, PA, 1988, pp 21-28.

[17] Mertz, H. J. and Patrick, L. M., "Strength and Response of the Human Neck," Proceedings of the 15th Stapp Car Crash Conference, Society of Automotive Engineers, Paper No. 710855, New York, NY, 1971, pp 207-255.

[18] Myers, B. S., McElhaney, J. H., Doherty, B. J., Paver, J. G., Nightingale, R. W., Ladd, T. P., and Gray, L., "Responses of the Human Cervical Spine to Torsion," Proceedings of the 33rd Stapp Car Crash Conference, Society of Automotive Engineers, Paper No. 892437, Warrendale, PA, 1989, pp 215-222.

[19] Nusholtz, G. S., Melvin, J. W., Huelke, D. F., Alem, N. M., and Blank, J. G., "Response of the Cervical Spine to Superior-Inferior Head Impact," Proceedings of the 25th Stapp Car Crash Conference, Society of Automotive Engineers, Paper No. 811005, Warrendale, PA, 1981, pp 197-237.

[20] Nusholtz, G. S., Huelke, D. E., Lux, P., Alem, N. M., and Montalvo, F., "Cervical Spine Injury Mechanisms," Proceedings of the 27th Stapp Car Crash Conference, Society of Automotive Engineers, Paper No. 831616, Warrendale, PA, 1983, pp 179-197.

[21] Pintar, F. A., Yoganandan, N., Sances, A. Jr., Reinartz, J., Harris, G., and Larson, S. J., "Kinematic and Anatomical Analysis of the Human Cervical Spinal Column Under Axial Loading," Proceedings of the 33rd Stapp Car Crash Conference, Society of Automotive Engineers, Paper No. 892436, Warrendale, PA, 1989, pp 191-214.

[22] Pintar, F. A., Sances, A. Jr., Yoganandan, N., Reinartz, J., Maiman, D. J., and Suh, J. K., "Biodynamics of the Total Human Cadaveric Cervical Spine," Proceedings of the 34th Stapp Car Crash Conference, .Society of Automotive Engineers, Paper No. 902309, Warrendale, PA, 1990, pp 55-72.

[23] Prasad, P., King, A. L., and Ewing, C. L., "The Role of Articular Facets During +Gz Acceleration," Applied Mechanics, June 1974, pp 321-326.

[24] Yoganandan, N., Sances, A. Jr., Maiman, D. J., Myklebust, J. B., Pech, P., and Larson, S. J., "Experimental Spinal Injuries With Vertical Impact," Spine, Vol. 11, No. 9, 1986, pp 855-860.

[25] Yoganandan. N., Sances, A. Jr., and Pintar, F. A., "Biomechanical Evaluation of the Axial Compressive Responses of the Human Cadaveric and Manikin Necks," Journal of Biomechanical Engineering, Vol. 111, No. 3, 1989, pp 250-255.

[26] Schlick, M. B., Pintar, F. A., Yoganandan, N., Maiman, D. J., and Sances, A. Jr., "An Instrumented Physical Spinal Cord Model for In Situ Pressure Measurement," Proceedings of the 15th Annual Meeting of the American Society of Biomechanics, Oct. 16-18, 1991, pp 102-103.

[27] Liu, Y. K. and Dai, Q. G., "The Second Stiffest Axis of a Beam-column: Implications for Cervical Spine Trauma," Journal of Biomechanical Engineering, Vol. 111, No. 2, May 1989, pp 122-127.

[28] Myers, B. S., McElhaney, J. H., Richardson, W. J., Nightingale, R. W., and Doherty, B. J., "The Influence of End Condition on Human Cervical Spine Injury Mechanisms," Proceedings of the 35th Stapp Car Crash Conference, Society of Automative Engineers, Paper No. 912915, Warrendale, PA, 1991, pp 391-400.

Nathaniel R. Ordway[1], W. Thomas Edwards[1], Ronald G. Donelson[2], Mary Bosco[3]

THE EFFECT OF HEAD POSITION ON THE ANALYSIS OF CERVICAL MOTION

REFERENCE: Ordway, N. R., Edwards, W. T., Donelson, R. G., Bosco, M. E., "The Effect of Head Position on the Analysis of Cervical Motion," Head and Neck Injuries in Sports, ASTM STP 1229, Earl F. Hoerner, Ed., American Society for Testing and Materials, Philadelphia, 1994.

ABSTRACT: The motion of the head and neck until injury, or the threshold of injury is normally limited by the tension of soft tissues along the cervical spine and by any obstruction. The relative range of motion (ROM) available during loading until injury is dependent partially upon the initial starting position and the combinations of motions. In this study, an electromagnetic six degree of freedom digitizer was used to quantitatively assess the effect of head position on cervical spine ROM measurements for a group of 25 subjects with no known cervical symptoms. Forward sagittal translation of the head with respect to the thorax (protrusion) diminished the amount of extension motion available by $4.6°/cm$. Backward sagittal translation of the head (retraction) diminished the amount of flexion motion available by $6.1°/cm$. In addition, when the head was axially rotated losses of approximately 50% were displayed for measurements of flexion, extension, and lateral bending. This paper illustrates the importance of a defined starting head position when measuring cervical motion and the effects of combined motions. Accurate cervical ROM measurements will be influential in the design of sports equipment and in determining mechanisms of injury.

KEYWORDS: cervical spine, motion analysis, range of motion, injury

Athletic injuries to the cervical spine have been well documented for a variety of sports such as tackle football, basketball, ice

[1]Research Instructor and Associate Professor, respectively, Orthopedic Research Laboratory, Department of Orthopedics, 750 E. Adams St., Syracuse, NY 13210.

[2]M.D., Assistant Professor, Department of Orthopedics, 750 E. Adams St., Syracuse, NY 13210.

[3]Physical Therapist, Department of Physical Therapy, 550 Harrison Center, Syracuse, NY 13210.

hockey, gymnastics, and water sports [1,2]. These injuries range from
simple sprains to fracture-dislocations with quadriplegia. The response
of the cervical spine under extreme loading conditions is determined by
the magnitude and rate of the applied load, the point of load
application, the direction of the load, and the initial position of the
head relative to the thorax. All of these factors influence the amount
of displacement (rotation or translation) for the range of motion (ROM)
until an injury occurs.

   A number of studies have examined the loading conditions involved
with cervical injuries. Mechanisms and classifications of injury have
been hypothesized from clinical observations [3,4,5,6]. Epidemio-
logically, the most severe injuries (dislocation/burst fractures
resulting in quadriplegia) to the cervical spine occur with low velocity
pure compressive impacts when the neck is partially flexed [3,7,8,9].
Less severe injuries have resulted if the neck is not in a columnar
position or if the impact is not axial [3]. Roaf produced various spinal
injuries by a combination of compression and/or flexion-rotation loads
[10]. These previous studies show the importance of and have
concentrated on the loading aspects of injury. Although catastrophic
cervical spine injuries result from axial loads when the cervical spine
is in a columnar position, many other injuries result from the head and
neck translating and/or rotating beyond the injury threshold limit. The
earlier studies do not show the effect of head position on the ROM
available before loading. The ROM of the head and neck until injury, or
the threshold of injury is normally limited by the tension of soft
tissues along the cervical spine and by obstruction (eg. the chin
touching the chest).

   Normative ROM measurements are helpful for determining the
thresholds of pain and/or injury as well as the nature and cause of an
injury. Many times during sport the head deviates from its normal
position and the cervical spine is exposed to combined motions of
translation and rotation. Normative values have been reported in the
literature for uniaxial rotations - sagittal flexion/extension, lateral
bending, and axial rotation by Ferlic [11], and Alund and Larsson
[12]. In addition, a number of articles on uniaxial measurements have
been summarized by White and Panjabi [13]. In terms of sagittal head
translation or gliding movement of the head with respect to the torso in
the sagittal plane, Hanten has reported on values for men and women for
ranges of translation [14]. These studies do not quantify the effect of
combined motions or how uniaxial rotations are affected by initial head
position.

   Since the cervical spine is so mobile, the starting head position
can have an effect on the measured ROM. In addition, the orientation of
the head at the time of impact during sport will have an effect on the
motion available until injury. The objective of this study was to
quantitatively assess the effect of head orientation on cervical spine
ROM measurements. Uniaxial rotations with the head starting from a
defined reference position were measured followed by measurement of
uniaxial rotations with the starting head position sagittally translated
or axially rotated.

EXPERIMENTAL METHOD

Subject Group

   The sample consisted of 25 healthy volunteers (12 women and 13
men) with no known cervical disorders. The sample was collected from the

Departments of Orthopedics and Physical Therapy and consisted of
students and employees. Their mean age was 32.8 years and the range was
from 21 to 49 years.

Instrumentation

An electromagnetic six degree of freedom digitizer (3Space
Isotrak, developed by Polhemus Navigation Sciences Division, McDonnel
Douglas Electronics Company) was used to collect the motion analysis
data of the head and neck relative to the trunk. The system consists of
a source that emits electromagnetic fields and a sensor. The position of
the sensor with respect to the source within the field is described
completely with three translations and three rotations. In this study,
the sensor was attached to the top of the head with a velcro strap and
the source was attached to an outrigger on a fixing vest. The fixing
vest was adapted from a Halo-vest (Levtech Cervical-Thoracic Orthosis
Carbon One, Levtech Inc.) and was attached only at the torso. The vest
is light weight and unemcumbering and has been shown to have low
mobility [15]. This fixing vest helped to exclude flexion and extension
of the thoracic spine from the measurements during the various
maneuvers. The digitizing system was hardwired to a personal computer
for data collection.

The data in this study consisted of translations and rotations of
the head and neck with respect to the torso. With the source attached to
the fixing vest (therefore limiting the amount of upper thoracic motion)
and the sensor attached to the top of the head, the data collected
represented the motion between the center of the head and T1.

Procedure

Each subject was fitted with the fixing vest and the head strap
and were seated in a straight back chair. A lumbar roll was placed just
above the buttocks to assist in standardizing the sitting position among
subjects. Next, all subjects were instructed on the various maneuvers
listed below:

Reference position--trunk upright, ear lobes centered over
shoulders, and face vertical.

Uniaxial rotations--these motions were chosen for comparison
purposes with the existing literature and consisted of sagittal flexion
and extension, left and right lateral flexion (or bending), left and
right axial rotation.

Sagittal translation--a gliding movement of the head either
forward (protrusion) or backward (retraction).

Combined rotations--from a fully left and right axially rotated
position, another component of rotation was performed (e.g., flexion,
extension, lateral bending).

Three groups of measurements were collected after the subjects
were educated on and practiced the positions. The first group consisted
of the uniaxial rotations performed from the reference position. For the
second group, the head started in three different sagittally translated
positions (fully protruded, partially protruded or relaxed, and fully
retracted) and at each position the uniaxial rotations were repeated.
The last group of measurements examined the effects of combined

rotations whereby the head was first axially rotated from the reference position and then the movements of flexion, extension, and lateral bending were repeated. For each group of measurements, the data were collected at end range of motion and each movement was repeated three times for statistical purposes.

Data Analysis

The translations and rotations from the electromagnetic digitizer are given in terms of millimeters and degrees, respectively, and require no manipulation once created and stored into a computer file. Although both the rotational and translational components were collected for three dimensions, only the primary rotational component was analyzed for the rotational positions. For the sagittally translated positions, the primary rotational component along with the starting horizontal translational component was analyzed. Finally, for the combined rotations, the primary rotational component along with the starting axial rotated component was analyzed. Descriptive statistics were calculated for the three trials and for the entire subject group. Statistical comparisons of the data were done with StatView 512+ software (BrainPower, Inc. and Abacus Concepts, Inc.).

RESULTS

Uniaxial Rotations

Starting from the reference position, total range of motion (ROM) for sagittal flexion-extension, lateral bending, and rotation was determined for the 25 subject group (Table 1).

TABLE 1--Total range of motion (mean and S.D.) for the uniaxial rotations

Uniaxial Rotation	Mean, °	Standard Deviation, °
Flexion/Extension	118.5	22.9
Lateral Bending	82.5	14.8
Axial Rotation	140.2	17.3

Effects of Sagittal Translation

The total amount of sagittal head translation (retracted to protruded) averaged 8.7 cm (±3.2 cm) and ranged from 5.9 to 14.1 cm. When the head deviated from the starting reference position by either translation or rotation, losses in ROM for the uniaxial rotations were observed. Axial rotation and lateral bending were slightly diminished, but not significantly, when the head was held in either the retracted, relaxed, or protruded positions. Flexion and extension were significantly effected by altering the starting sagittal head position. A statistically significant difference resulted when comparing the amount of flexion starting from the retracted position and the amount of flexion starting from the reference position (t-test, p<0.01). Neither the protruded nor relaxed starting positions had a significant effect on the amount of flexion measured from the reference starting position. Another statistically significant difference resulted when comparing the amount of extension starting from the protruded position and the amount of extension starting from the reference position (t-test, p<0.01). Neither the retracted nor relaxed starting positions had a significant effect on the amount of extension measured from the reference starting position.

Based on the previous results and the variation in the amount of motion among subjects, it was thought that a relationship between the starting head position and the amount of flexion or extension available may exist. To examine the relationship between the starting sagittal head position and its effect on the amount of motion, flexion and extension were plotted against the amount of sagittal translation. Since extension was only significantly effected by protrusion, the amount of extension was plotted against the amount of protrusion. Additionally, flexion was only significantly effected by retraction, so the amount of flexion was plotted against the amount of retraction. A linear regression showed a moderate correlation between head protrusion and the amount of extension available, 4.6°/cm (R^2=0.66, Fig. 1). Similarly, the amount of available flexion diminished by 6.1°/cm when the head was retracted and shows a weak correlation (R^2=0.32, Fig. 2). The reference position in Figures 1 and 2 is represented by 0cm.

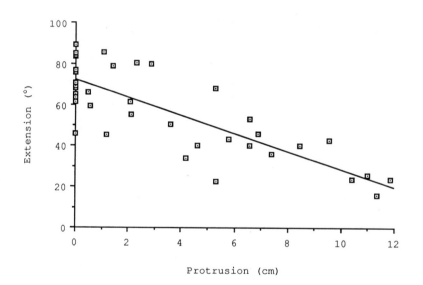

FIG. 1--Effect of protrusion on the amount of extension available.

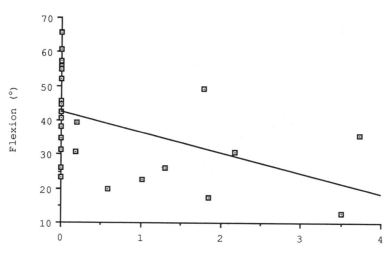

FIG. 2--Effect of retraction on the amount of flexion available.

Effects of Combined Rotations

The ROM for flexion, extension, and lateral bending was plotted for the head starting in either the reference, left, or right rotated position (Fig. 3). Decreases in flexion, extension, and lateral bend measurements were statistically significant (t-test, $p < 0.01$) when the head started with a rotated position.

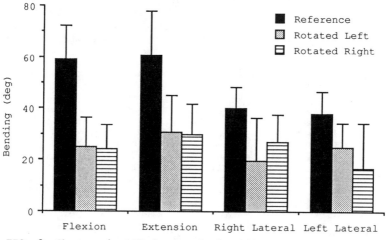

FIG. 3--Changes in ROM due to the head fully rotated with respect to the neck.

DISCUSSION

This study quantified the loss in cervical spine ROM when uniaxial rotations were measured from various starting head positions. Uniaxial rotations measured from the reference position compared well with previously published literature (Table 2). Hanten et al.[14] reported values of 10.7±3.0cm for total range of sagittal head translation. These papers do not address how the motion was affected when the head did not start from a reference position. Deviations from the reference position can be either a translation or a rotation. Consideration must be given to the reference head position used in quantifying cervical motion for results to be meaningful.

TABLE 2--Comparison of normative values for uniaxial
rotations with the literature

Author	Age Range	Flexion/ Extension,°	Lateral Bend,°	Axial Rotation,°
White & Panjabi[13]	—	127	114	150
Ferlic [11]	25–34	127±21	74±14	143±20
Alund [12]	24–58	140±18	91±12	153±16
Ordway	21–49	119±23	83±15	140±17

The ROM of the cervical spine describes limits of motion due to increased tension in the soft tissues, obstruction of motion, or discomfort. Our study demonstrates that sagittal flexion/extension, lateral bending, and axial rotation measurements are reduced by combinations of head and neck translations and rotations. In the protruded head position, the lower cervical segments are required to flex thus reducing the available range of extension. Conversely, with the head fully retracted, the available range of flexion is diminished since the lower cervical segments remain in extension. When the head is axially rotated, flexion, extension, and lateral bending are all diminished because of tightening of the underlying cervical musculature and ligaments. Earlier cadaver studies have shown that spine segments fail at lower loads when combinations of motion (sagittal and axial rotation) are applied [16]. Our findings suggest that for such conditions the threshold of injury is greatly reduced because the available ROM is reduced by approximately 50%, if for example, axial rotation is maintained during extreme flexion-extension motion.

The speed, strength, and size in athletes continue to increase in order to achieve a higher performance. With this higher performance there comes a higher demand on the musculo-skeletal system and equipment. Because of the physical nature of sport, athletes are subjected to conditions of combined motions of the head and neck at the time of contact. Neck injuries result from excessive cervical motion above the injury threshold. Although rule changes and equipment have helped to decrease the number of injuries, cases still persist in a variety of sports. In order to avoid disastrous injuries, equipment or methods will have to be further developed by examining the position of the head and the available ROM. There may be positions of the head and neck that are optimal for reducing the risk of severe injury which could be incorporated in injury prevention stratagies. Range of motion measurements are invaluable to the design of equipment and in the study of cervical injuries. The measurements presented in this paper are among the first to examine the maximum voluntary motion available from a starting reference position, and the limitations when translation and rotation maneuvers combine.

REFERENCES

[1]   J. Torg, J. Vegso, B. Sennett and M. Das, "The National Football head and neck injury registry," JAMA, 254, 24, 1985, 3439-3443.

[2]   J. S. Torg, "Epidemiology, pathomechanics, and prevention of athletic injuries to the cervical spine," Medicine and Science in Sports and Exercise, 17, 3, 1985, 295-303.

[3]   A. Burstein, J. Otis and J. Torg, Athletic injuries to the head, neck, and face, Lee & Febiger, 1982, 139-154.

[4]   J. Melvin, The human neck: Anatomy, injury mechanisms and biomechanics. (SP-438), Society of Automotive Engineers (SAE), 1979.

[5]   J. Sances A., J. Myklebust, C. Houterman, R. Weber, J. Lepkowski, J. Cusick, S. Larson, C. Ewing, D. Thomas, M. Weiss, M. Berger, M. E. Jessop and B. Saltzman, Conference Proc. on Impact Injury Caused by Linear Acceleration-Mechanism, Prevention, and Cost, AGARD , 1982.

[6]   J. Sances A, J. Myklebust, J. Maiman, S. Larson, J. Cusick and R. Jodat, "The biomechanics of spinal injuries," CRC Critical Reviews of Biomedical Engineering, 11, 1984, 1-76.

[7]   E. R. Gonza and I. J. Harrington, Biomechanics of Musculoskeletal Injury, Williams and Wilkins, 1982.

[8]   J. H. McElhaney, J. G. Paver and H. J. McCracklin, Proc. of the 27th STAPP Car Crash Conference, Soc. of Automotive Engineers, 1983, 163.

[9]   J. McElhaney, R. Snyder and J. States, "Cervical Spine Compression Respones," The human neck: Anatomy, injury mechanisms and biomechanics. (SP-438), Society of Automotive Engineers (SAE), 1979.

[10]   R. Roaf, "A Study of the Mechanics of Spinal Injuries," J. Bone Joint Surg., 42-B, 1960, 810-823.

[11]   D. Ferlic, "Range of motion in 'normal' cervical spine," Bulletine of John Hopkins Hospital, 110, 1962, 59-65.

[12]   M. Alund and S.-E. Larsson, "Three-dimensional analysis of neck motion. A clinical method," Spine, 15, 2, 1990, 87-91.

[13]   A. White III and M. Panjabi, Clinical biomechanics of the
        spine, J.B. Lippincott Company, 1990.

[14]   W. P. Hanten, R. M. Lucio, J. L. Russell and D. Brunt,
        "Assessment of Total Head Excursion and Resting Head
        Posture," Archives of Physical Medicine and Rehabilitation,
        72, 1991, 877-880.

[15]   M. Krag and B. Beynnon, "A new halo-vest: rationale, design
        and biomechanical comparison to standard halo-vest designs,"
        Spine, 13, 3, 1988, 228-235.

[16]   M. Shea, W. T. Edwards, A. A. White and W. C. Hayes,
        "Variations of stiffness and strength along the human
        cervical spine," J. Biomechanics, 24, 2, 1991, 95-107.

Mechanism of Injury

J.H. Heald,[1] and D.A. Pass[2]

BALL STANDARDS RELEVANT TO RISK OF HEAD INJURY

REFERENCE: Heald, J.H., Pass, D.A., **"Ball Standards Relevant to Risk of Head Injury"**, Head and Neck Injuries in Sports. ASTM STP 1229, Earl F. Hoerner, Ed., American Society for Testing and Materials, Philadelphia, 1994.

ABSTRACT: Several baseball and softball physical properties relate directly or indirectly to the risk of head injury, namely size, weight, hardness, and liveliness. Rule book specifications for the official game balls in baseball and softball specify the size and weight. Ball liveliness is sometimes specified. This study has evaluated the effects of ball hardness and liveliness on the risk of head injury in impact studies with humanoid head models, rigid head forms, and actual cadaver impact tests. The Severity Index (SI) and Head Injury Criteria (HIC) were both measured over a wide range of ball hardness and impact speeds. The risk of head injury was determined using the Prasad-Mertz risk curves. The results reveal a very strong relationship between ball hardness and head injury risk, ranging from 80% risk at 28.6 m/s (60 mph) for popular hard baseballs and softballs, down to 1% risk for softer balls now being used in some youth league programs. The cadaver impact tests confirmed that the humanoid head model and Severity Index injury criteria are well suited for the prediction of head injury risk for highly focal (concentrated in small area) blows from baseballs and softballs to the side of the unprotected head. Field test injury statistics show that the use of softer type baseballs in youth league play can reduce the incidence of ball impact injuries by about 70%.

KEYWORDS: head injury, baseball injury, baseball standards, injury standards, baseball injury standards, ball impact injuries

---

[1]Director, Research and Development Division, Worth, Inc., Tullahoma, Tennessee, 37388

[2]Manager, Research and Development Division, Worth, Inc., Tullahoma, Tennessee, 37388

Injury statistics in the sports of baseball and softball [1,2,3] make it clear that ball impact is the leading cause of injury, and the most frequently occurring injury is head injury from ball impact. To manufacture baseballs and softballs designed to meet rule book specifications which also reduce the risk of head injuries requires information on the effects of ball hardness and liveliness on the risk of head injury over a wide range of ball speeds. Additionally, an appropriate test system is required to evaluate with assurance the potential for injury from ball impact to the unprotected head. Previous studies [4,5,6] conclude that ball impact to the unprotected head at speeds commonly encountered in youth league play pose a high risk for head injury. However, these same studies raise questions as to the most appropriate test system for evaluating the risk of head injury from ball impact. The humanoid head model and Severity Index (SI) injury criteria are used in the athletic goods industry to assess such risks, while the auto industry uses the rigid head form on the Hybrid III dummy with the Head Injury Criteria (HIC). The primary objective of the studies reported herein was to ascertain the most appropriate test system to assess the risk of head injury from baseball/softball impact and then to determine how ball standards could be set to reduce this risk.

EXPERIMENTAL METHOD

Test Procedure

An experimental array of both baseballs and softballs covering a wide range of hardness and liveliness was used in a series of impact tests to determine the relationship between these properties and the risk of head injury. Two balls of each type were tested. All test balls are commercially available and meet rule book specifications for various levels of play.

Test ball properties--The test balls were all categorized by ball hardness as defined by a compression strength measurement. The pressure required to compress the ball 0.63 cm (0.25 inches) between two flat plates was measured and used to differentiate the balls during all the subsequent tests (Table 1).

Ball liveliness was defined by a measurement of Coefficient of Restitution (COR). All test balls were propelled against a rigid concrete wall at 28.6 m/s (60 mph) and the velocity measured before and after impact using a light screen timer. The COR was then calculated as the ratio of the velocity after impact to the velocity before impact (Table 1).

TABLE 1--Test ball properties

Ball No.	Description	Compression Strength newtons/cm(lbf/in.)	COR At 28.6 m/s (60 mph)	Impact Area At 28.6 m/s(60 mph) cm²	(in²)	Impact Pressure At 28.6 m/s(60 mph) newtons/cm²	(psi)
	Baseballs						
1.	Synthetic Yarn Wound	770 (440)	0.54	...	...	...	...
2.	Molded Cork Core	735 (420)	0.44	...	...	...	...
3.	Molded Poly-U. Core	889 (508)	0.53	...	...	...	...
4.	Major League Wool Wound	714 (408)	0.56	20.25	(3.14)	2450	(3550)
5.	Synthetic Yarn Wound	889 (508)	0.54	...	...	...	...
6.	Molded Poly-U. Core	175 (100)	0.52	30.90	(4.79)	1075	(1560)
7.	Molded Poly-U. Core	350 (200)	0.53	...	...	...	...
8.	Molded Poly-U. Core	112 (64)	0.50	40.0	(6.20)	586	(850)
14.	Molded Poly-U. Core	481 (275)	0.52	...	...	...	...
15.	Molded Poly-U. Core	437 (250)	0.52	...	...	...	...
16.	Synthetic Yarn Wound	1015 (580)	0.54	...	...	...	...
	Softballs						
9.	Molded Poly-U. Core	952 (544)	0.50	22.90	(3.55)	2050	(2980)
10.	Molded Cork Core	735 (420)	0.45	...	...	...	...
11.	Molded Eva Core	875 (500)	0.50	...	...	...	...
12.	Molded Poly-U. Core	511 (292)	0.47	49.47	(7.67)	460	(670)
13.	Molded Poly-U. Core	161 (92)	0.47	59.92	(9.29)	370	(540)

Note: Poly-U. is an abbreviation for polyurethane foam

To compare the balls in terms of the area and pressure of impact as a function of ball compression strength, pressure sensitive film was mounted on the wall during some of the flat wall impact tests. The resulting area of impact and approximate pressure was calculated (Table 1).

Head model impact tests--Two types of head models were used to measure the impact forces for a wide range of ball hardness and speed. The humanoid head model used in the athletic goods industry for evaluation and certification under the National Operating Committee for Standards in Athletic Equipment (NOCSAE) standards [7,8] was used to measure the force of impact at the model center of mass, and in turn used to calculate the Severity Index. The Prasad-Mertz risk curves [7] were used to translate the Severity Index measurements to risk factors for serious head injury. All ball impacts were in the prescribed temple area of the unprotected head model. Each ball was impacted six times at each speed.

The Hybrid III dummy head model was used in a series of tests along with the Head Injury Criteria (HIC) calculations to compare the results using this rigid head form to those from the more flexible humanoid head model. Ball impacts covered a wide range of speeds and ball hardness and impacts were in the temple area of the unprotected dummy head form.

Cadaver head impact tests--In order to determine which head model and injury criteria were best suited for measuring the risk of ball impact to the unprotected head for balls of different hardness, a series of cadaver tests was conducted on a contract basis with Wayne State University [9]. Four cadavers were instrumented with accelerometers to give acceleration-time readings during each impact for calculation of both the SI and HIC. The cadavers were impacted on one side with test ball type number 4 (hard major league baseball) and on the other side with test ball type number 6. Impact speeds were increased until skull fracture occurred.

Hit ball speed calculations--The measured ball COR values were used to theoretically calculate hit ball speed [10]. These speeds were then used with the measured effects of ball speed on head injury risk to determine the level of influence of ball liveliness on the risk of head injury for the batted ball.

Ball hardness effects on injury statistics--Two recent studies of injuries in youth league baseball involved the use of slightly softer balls similar to those used in these tests [11,12]. The results of these tests make possible the estimation of the reduction of injuries which could result from widespread use of lower compression balls.

RESULTS

Head model impact tests--The results of impacting the humanoid head model with the 16 test balls (Table 1) at 28.6 m/s (60 mph) are plotted on Fig. (1). Standard deviation was 10%. The Severity Index increases exponentially with the ball compression, in an approximate power of 2 relationship. That is, doubling the ball compression raises the Severity Index by a factor of 4. For balls with compression strengths over 700 newtons/cm (350 lbf/in.) the risk of head injury exceeds 50% for a 28.6 m/s (60 mph) blow to the unprotected temple area. All "traditional" yarn wound baseballs and most popular softballs fall above this compression strength level.

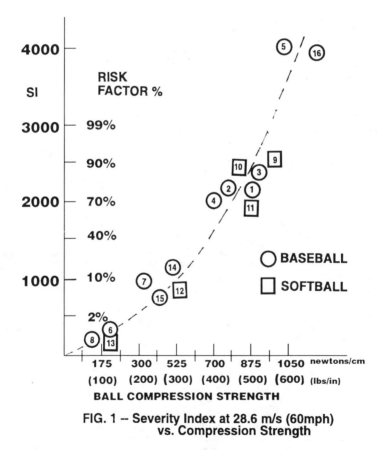

FIG. 1 -- Severity Index at 28.6 m/s (60mph)
vs. Compression Strength

When the test balls were impacted on the humanoid head model over a wide range of speeds, a family of curves was generated for each level of ball compression strength (Fig. 2). The severity index level was quite sensitive to ball

speed. For the major league baseball, increasing ball speed
from 14.3 m/s (30 mph) to 28.6 m/s (60 mph) increased the
severity index from 1000 to 2000 and the resulting risk
factor for head injury from 10% to 80%. Balls with
compression strengths below 525 newtons/cm (300 lbf/in.)
have relatively low risk factors for speeds under 28.6 m/s
(60 mph). Conversely the balls with compression strengths
greater than major league baseballs produce extremely high
risk factors at speeds above 14.3 m/s (30 mph).

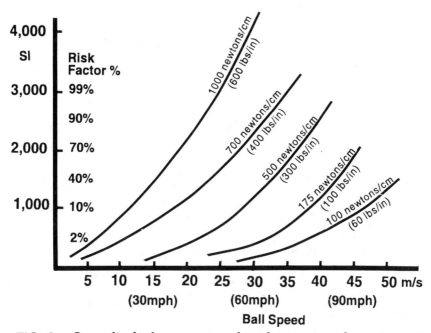

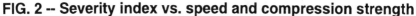

FIG. 2 -- Severity index vs. speed and compression strength

In the tests comparing results from the humanoid head
model to those from the Hybrid III dummy there were
similarities, but also distinct differences (Fig. 3,4,5).
The results for the three different baseballs in Fig. (3)
show that the Severity Index levels for the harder ball are
higher but not as high as the readings from the humanoid
head model. As the ball hardness is decreased, the
measurements from the two models are in closer agreement.
For the softest ball used in these tests, the readings are
in good agreement over a wide speed range (Fig. 5). The
Hybrid III does not show as much sensitivity for harder ball
impacts as the humanoid head model, and therefore does not
predict as high a risk factor.

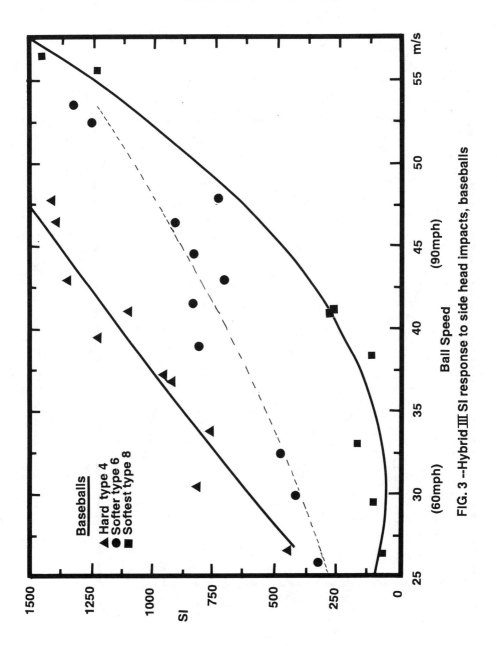

FIG. 3 --Hybrid III SI response to side head impacts, baseballs

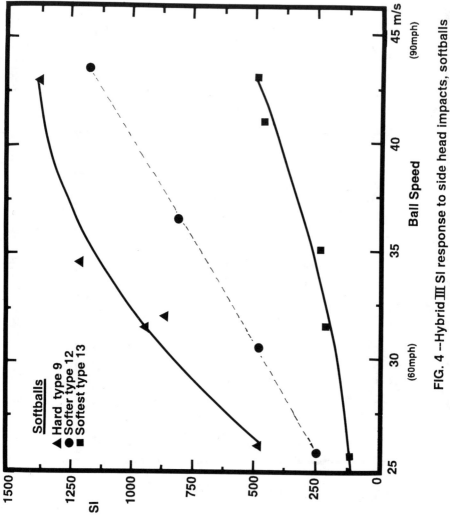

FIG. 4 —Hybrid III SI response to side head impacts, softballs

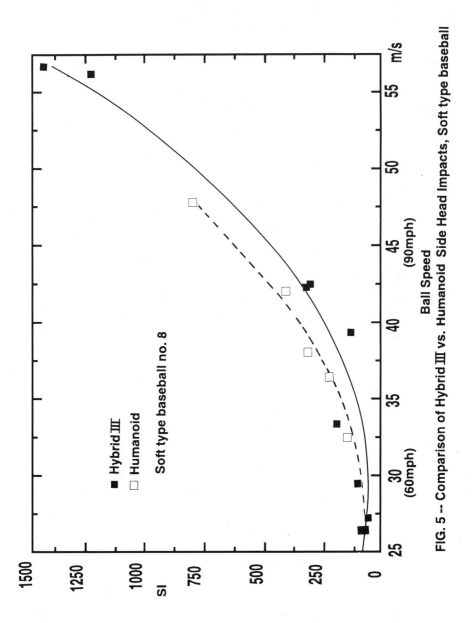

FIG. 5 -- Comparison of Hybrid III vs. Humanoid Side Head Impacts, Soft type baseball

Some of the Hybrid III impacts were analyzed using both the HIC and SI injury criteria (Table 2). In all cases, the use of the SI resulted in higher readings by 13 to 20%.

TABLE 2--<u>Hybrid III side head impact; SI, HIC comparison</u>

Ball type (From table 1)	Speed m/s	(mph)	HIC	SI	Peak G
4	19.7	(41.4)	138	156	134
6	21.7	(45.4)	75	85	84
4	23.4	(49.0)	211	240	165
6	23.8	(49.8)	83	94	88
4	29.1	(61.1)	425	490	233
6	30.4	(63.8)	140	158	110
4	34.3	(71.9)	1137	1362	367
6	35.2	(73.8)	326	368	166

<u>Cadaver head impact tests</u>--The four instrumented cadaver impact tests produced measurements of peak forces (G), SI, HIC and fracture speeds for the two different test balls, type number 4 (hard major league) and type number 6 (softer polyurethane core). Measurements taken at impact speeds closest to 28.6 m/s (60 mph) are listed in Table (3).

TABLE 3--Cadaver side head impact; SI, HIC comparison

Ball type (From table 1)	Speed m/s	(mph)	HIC	SI	Peak G
4	35.2	(73.7)	1711	2087	415
4	29.1	(61.0)	1516	2144	507
4	28.8	(60.4)	1846	2507	476
4	26.6	(55.7)	1525	2011	471
6	28.8	(60.4)	385	557	261
6	28.2	(59.2)	214	309	176
6	28.5	(59.8)	755	885	289
6	28.5	(59.8)	498	569	225
6	26.9	(56.3)	133	156	148

Values of SI over the range of test speeds for the two balls are plotted on Fig. (6) along with Prasad-Mertz risk factors. The impact speeds at which skull fracture generally occurred were 28 m/s (60 mph) or less for the harder baseball, and over 38 m/s (80 mph) for the softer ball. In one cadaver test the fracture speed exceeded 48 m/s (100 mph) for the softer ball, and occurred at 26 m/s (55 mph) for the harder ball. Tabulations of all cadaver impact measurements are available from Worth, Inc. [9].

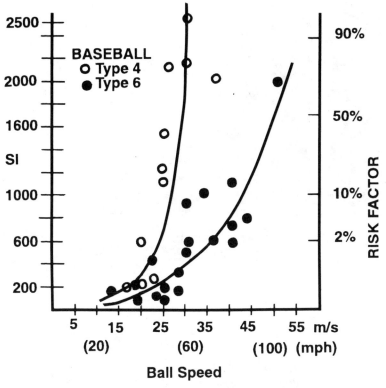

FIG. 6 -- Cadaver side head Response

The cadaver impact tests results make possible a comparison of the effectiveness of the two different head models and injury criteria for predicting injury to the unprotected side head for balls of different compression strength, (Figs. 7 8). For the harder ball, (Fig. 7), the humanoid model using the SI injury criteria predicts very closely the conditions for skull fracture when compared to the cadaver measurements. The closer agreement for the different systems with the slightly softer ball (Fig. 8) suggest that the humanoid head model predicts more accurately the risk for more focal blows, and as the impact area increases (becomes more diffuse) the different systems produce measurements in closer agreement.

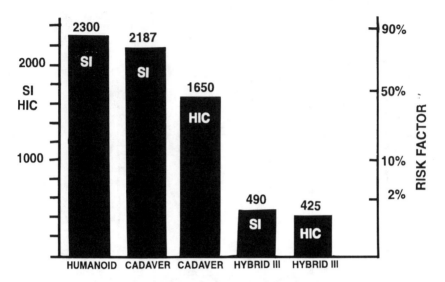

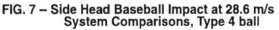

**FIG. 7 – Side Head Baseball Impact at 28.6 m/s
System Comparisons, Type 4 ball**

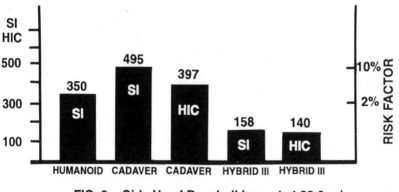

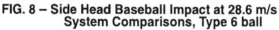

**FIG. 8 – Side Head Baseball Impact at 28.6 m/s
System Comparisons, Type 6 ball**

<u>Hit ball speed calculations</u>--Values of ball Coefficient of Restitution (COR) over a wide speed range for test baseball type 4 (major league), and a popular slow pitch softball (test ball type 9) are plotted on Fig. (9). Over the speed range from 19 to 43 m/s (40 to 90 mph) the COR for both the baseball and softball decrease by approximately 30%.

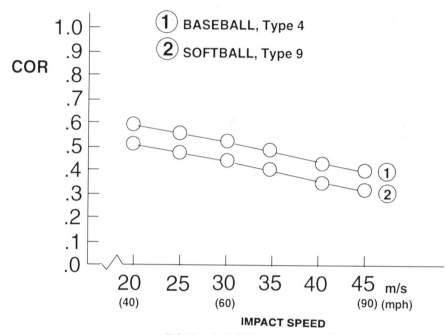

FIG. 9 -- Ball COR. vs. Speed of Impact

The experimentally determined values of COR were used in the theoritical calculation of hit ball speed [10] for a typical bat speed and pitch ball speed encountered at the adult level (Fig. 10). The range of ball COR values from Table (1) are marked on Fig. (10). This range of COR values relates to a range of hit ball speeds of 6 m/s (12 mph) for the example given. Based on the SI data of Fig. (2), this range of hit ball speeds from variations in ball liveliness could result in a change in SI on impact by as much as 1000 for the harder balls and approximately 500 for the softer balls.

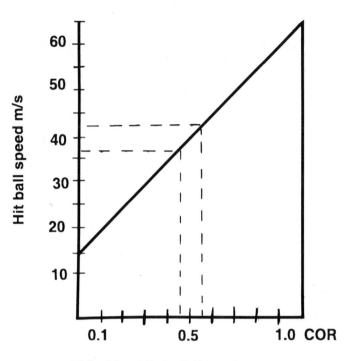

FIG. 10 -- Hit ball Speed vs. ball COR

Injury statistics evaluation--The effects of ball hardness on the frequency of ball impact injuries were reported in two recent studies. In Japan, the use of softer baseballs (similar in compression to test ball type 6) have been mandated in youth league play up to age 14 for over 50 years. According to a four year study of four million participants [11] no ball impact deaths occurred and the percentage of impact injuries was 75% lower than U.S. reports [1,2].

The 1992 Youth Sports Institute Study [12] compared the injuries which occurred with 100 youth league teams using traditional harder type baseballs (test ball type 1) to the injuries from 100 teams using softer type baseballs (test ball types 6,7,8). In game conditions for an eight week season, the number of ball impact injuries with the softer type baseballs was 70% lower than the number occurring with the harder ball.

CONCLUSIONS

1.   The relationship between ball hardness and the risk of head injury has been established over the range of ball speeds commonly encountered in the sports of baseball and softball.

2.   The humanoid head model and Severity Index (SI) test system are well suited for assessing the risk of head injury for the more focal blows of baseballs and softballs to the side of the unprotected head. The Hybrid III dummy and HIC system respond with much less sensitivity for focal blows covering an impact area less than 31 cm^2 (4.8 in.^{2}), which equates to balls with compression strength greater than 175 newtons/cm (100 lbf/in.).

3.   Ball liveliness (COR) can influence the risk of impact injury for the batted ball by a significant amount for balls at the livelier end of the range in common use (0.55 COR) compared to those at the lower end (0.45 COR). The measured severity index (SI) can be 500-1000 greater for the livelier balls.

4.   Recent injury statistics indicate that the use of slightly softer baseballs and softballs can reduce the incidence of ball impact injury by 70%.

5.   The evidence of these studies supports the need to establish hardness and liveliness standards for official baseballs and softballs.

REFERENCES

[1]   Rutherford, G., Kennedy, J., McGhee, L., "Hazard Analysis; Baseball and Softball Related Injuries," U.S. Consumer Product Safety Commission, 1984.

[2]   Hale, C.J., "Protective Equipment for Baseball," The Physician and Sportsmedicine, Vol. 7, Nov. 7, July 1979.

[3]   Heald, J.H., "Summary of Baseball/Softball Injuries," Worth, Inc., Tullahoma, TN, 1991.

[4]   Stolmaker, R., Rojinavonick, V., "A Practical Application of the Translational Energy Criteria: Evaluation of Baseball and Softball Head Impact Injury Potentials," 1990 International IRCOBI Conference on the Biomechanics of Impacts, Sept. 12-14, Bron-Lyon, France.

[5] Melvin, J.W., "Baseball Impacts to Dummy Heads," Final
     Report, UMTR1-84-36, Oct. 1984, University of Michigan
     Transportation Research Institute.

[6] Saczolski, K.J., States, J.D., Wagar, I.J., Richardson,
     E.Q., "A Critical Assessment of the Use of Non-Human
     Responding Surrogates for Safety System Evaluation,"
     Twentieth STAPP Car Crash Conference, 1976, Society of
     Automotive Engineers, New York.

[7] Standard Method of Impact Test and Performance
     Requirements for Baseball and Baseball Batter's
     Helmets," National Operating Committee on Standards for
     Athletic Equipment, Kansas City, MO.

[8] Hodgson, V.R., "Impact Standards for Protective
     Equipment," Athletic Injuries to the Head, Neck and
     Face, 2nd Edition, Mosby-Year Book, 1991.

[9] Hodgson, V., King, A., "Comparison of the Effect of RIF
     and Major League Baseball Impacts on the Acceleration
     Response and Skull Fracture Patterns of Cadaver Heads,"
     unpublished report available from Worth, Inc.,
     Tullahoma, TN, 1992.

[10] Watts, R.G., Bayhill, A.T., Keep Your Eye on the Ball,
     W.H. Freeman and Co., New York, 1990.

[11] "Comprehensive Injury Research During Sports Activities
     1984-87", Sports Safety Association of Japan, copies
     available from Worth, Inc., Tullahoma, TN.

[12] Seefeldt, V., Brown, W., "Injury in Youth Baseball,"
     Institute for the Study of Youth Sports, Michigan State
     University, 1993.

Jonathan F. Heck -1

THE INCIDENCE OF SPEARING BY BALL CARRIERS AND THEIR TACKLERS DURING A HIGH SCHOOL FOOTBALL SEASON.

REFERENCE: Heck, J.F., "The Incidence of Spearing by Ball Carriers and Their Tacklers During a High School Football Season," Head and Neck Injuries in Sports, ASTM STP 1229, Earl F. Hoerner, Ed., American Society for Testing and Materials, Philadelphia, 1994.

ABSTRACT: This study established the cumulative incidence per season of ball carrier spearing and concurrent defensive spearing by tacklers for a New Jersey high school football season. Spearing (flexing the neck and initiating contact with the top of the helmet) is a significant cause of injury to the head and neck in football. To reduce the risk of head and neck injuries in football all types of spearing must be explored. Nine game films from the 1989 football season were viewed to determine the incidence of ball carrier spearing and concurrent defensive spearing. There were 167 incidents of ball carrier spearing (1 per 5.1 plays) and 72 incidents of concurrent defensive spearing (1 per 2.3 ball carrier spears). Officials can now penalize any player who initiates contact with his head. However, there were no spearing penalties called throughout the 1989 season. This study detected a surprisingly high cumulative incidence of ball carrier spearing and concurrent defensive spearing, along with poor enforcement of the spearing rule. To further reduce the risk of head and neck injuries officials should acknowledge ball carrier spearing as a rule infraction and enforce existing spearing rules during the tackling process. Coaches also should teach and drill correct technique with ball carriers, tacklers, and blockers throughout the season.

KEYWORDS: ball carrier spearing, concurrent defensive spearing, head down, spearing, tackling process.

Catastrophic head and neck injuries are among the most devastating injuries in sports. Because the damage from these injuries is often permanent and limits rehabilitation, prevention of these injuries is the only acceptable management plan. Even the few catastrophic injuries that have occurred each season are too many (1).

1- Head Athletic Trainer, Stockton State College, Pomona NJ 08240.

The National Federation of State High School Associations (NFSHSA) and the National Collegiate Athletic Association (NCAA) changed their football rules in 1976, making the deliberate use of the helmet to ram or punish (spear) an opponent illegal (2). The NFSHSA and the NCAA did this in an effort to reduce the number of head and cervical spine injuries occurring in football . Head and neck injuries in high school and college football have declined since 1976 (3,4,5,6,7). The rule change (3,4,6,8,9) and subsequent changes in the way coaches teach their players to tackle are believed responsible for this reduction (3,4,10).

Injuries to tacklers (defensive backs and linebackers) account for the largest percentage of cervical spine injuries (4,6). The contact techniques of these players have received the majority of attention and corrective coaching. Consequently, it seems that coaches and officials have overlooked ball carrier spearing.

This lack of instructional technique, overlooking ball carrier spearing as a rule infraction, and poor enforcement of the spearing rule during tackling have allowed ball carrier spearing to become an unquestioned aspect of football. Therefore, the purpose of this study was to determine the cumulative incidence per season of ball carrier spearing and concurrent defensive spearing during a high school football season.

METHODS

In this study, spearing was defined as the lowering of the head, either on purpose or as a reflex action, during the tackling process. A ball carrier was defined as any player who runs with the football-- running back, kick-returner, receiver, any player who advances a fumble, or any player who returns an interception. Ball carrier spearing was defined as spearing by the ball carrier while being tackled. Concurrent defensive spearing was defined as a head- first technique used by the tackler of a spearing ball carrier.

Incidents of ball carrier spearing were tabulated if the ball carrier lowered his head before contact and initiated or attempted to initiate contact with the tackler using the crown or top of his helmet. Incidents of concurrent defensive spearing were tabulated if the ball carrier speared on the particular play and his tackler lowered his head before contact and initiated contact using the top or crown portion of his helmet.

Offensively, incidents of ball carrier spearing were only tabulated during the tackling process. Incidents of spearing by any offensive player other than the ball carrier were excluded.

Concurrent defensive spearing was counted only if a tackler used a head first technique while tackling a spearing ball carrier. Or concurrent defensive spearing only occurred simultaneously with ball carrier spearing as defined for this study. Therefore, incidents of concurrent defensive spearing were considered only after ball carrier spearing had been established. This study excluded all other types of defensive spearing.

Data were obtained from the observation of a New Jersey high school varsity football team. Nine regular season game films were reviewed from the 1989 season on a 16mm Kodak projector with standard reverse mode and slow motion capabilities. Each game was graded individually on its own score sheet. The score sheet consisted of: total plays, un-viewable plays, ball carrier spearing, and concurrent defensive spearing --for both teams.

In viewing the game films, total plays only included plays in which a ball was carried. These included: returned kick-offs, returned punts, interceptions, plays with a fumble, running plays, passes, and plays that included a penalty which allowed the play to continue, such as clipping or holding. A play was considered un-viewable when contact by the ball carrier and the tackler(s) could not be seen on the game film.

RESULTS

The totals for the nine observed games are shown in table 1. Ninety seven percent of the plays were viewable. There were an average of 94.9 (+/-8.7) total plays per game. The mean score for incidents of ball carrier spearing was 18.6 (SD 3.0) per game. The mean score for incidents of concurrent defensive spearing per game was 8 (SD 2.3).

TABLE 1-- The Number of Total Plays (TP), Un-viewable Plays (UP), Ball Carrier Spears (BCS), Concurrent Defensive Spears (CDS) and the Incidence of Ball Carrier Spearing and Concurrent Defensive Spearing per Game.

					GAME					
	1	2	3	4	5	6	7	8	9	TOTAL
TP	88	87	102	107	101	105	89	90	85	854
UP	1	6	1	4	3	2	1	4	5	27
BCS	20	22	18	20	18	22	13	15	19	167
CDS	7	11	5	8	7	10	8	5	11	72
BCS/ PLAY	1/ 4.4	1/ 4.0	1/ 5.7	1/ 5.4	1/ 5.6	1/ 4.8	1/ 6.9	1/ 6.0	1/ 4.5	1/ 5.1
CDS/ BCS	1/ 2.9	1/ 2.0	1/ 3.6	1/ 2.5	1/ 2.6	1/ 2.2	1/ 1.6	1/ 3.0	1/ 1.7	1/ 2.3

There was an incident of ball carrier spearing in 20% of the total plays. In 43% of the plays that involved ball carrier spearing, there was also an incident of concurrent defensive spearing. The cumulative incidence per season of ball carrier spearing was 1 per 5.1 plays. The cumulative incidence per season of concurrent defensive spearing was 1 per 2.3 ball carrier spears. The incidence of ball carrier spearing and concurrent defensive spearing per game are also shown in table 1.

A total of 239 incidents of spearing were found for the year. The selected team accounted for 92 (55%) of the total ball carrier spearing incidents. The nine opponents accounted for 75 (45%) of the 167 incidents of ball carrier spearing. The opponents were responsible for 39 (54%) of the 72 incidents of concurrent defensive spearing, while the selected team's tacklers were responsible for 33 (46%) of concurrent defensive spears.

DISCUSSION

<u>Ball</u> <u>Carrier</u> <u>Spearing</u>

Only in three games were there less than seven ball carrier spears for a team. Two factors that possibly could have caused a lower number of ball carrier spears were a high number of passing attempts or poor performance by the offense.

When an incomplete pass was thrown, there was no ball carrier as defined in this study. Also, when a receiver caught a pass, he often was tackled immediately and from behind. These situations would have eliminated the possibility for ball carrier spearing. Therefore, a high number of passing attempts could have lowered the incidence of ball carrier spearing.

If the offense was not sustaining "drives" and making first downs (a poor performance) there would be fewer plays involving a ball carrier for that game. This could also result in a lower incidence of ball carrier spearing, because spearing opportunities would have decreased.

Ball carrier spearing is dangerous for two reasons. First spearing and the use of the head as an offensive weapon have an inherent risk of quadriplegia (11). Second, forces generated through running followed by head-first contact are sufficient to cause a concussion (12). Ball carrier spearing has been an overlooked hazard of being a ball carrier.

According to Hodgson and Thomas (1) the rule changes, the rule book warnings, and the helmet warnings have not eliminated head-first hitting in football. The incidence of ball carrier and concurrent defensive spearing found in this study support that opinion.

Concurrent Defensive Spearing

For every two incidents of ball carrier spearing there was one incident of concurrent defensive spearing. The cumulative incidence per game of concurrent defensive spearing also was consistent. A possible explanation for this may be that, generally, the defense reacts to the offense (12), and the tackler reacts to the ball carrier when attempting to make a tackle. Often what the ball carrier does will determine how the tackler brings him down (shirt tackle, arm tackle, etc.) The situation for concurrent defensive spearing arises when a ball carrier decides to break a tackle or to run over a tackler by lowering his head.

When a tackler has a spearing ball carrier running directly toward him, he has three basic options. He can remain upright and attempt to make the tackle with a helmet stuck in his abdomen or chest. He can attempt to get lower than the ball carrier and consequently lower his head into the spearing position. Or, he can choose to take on the ball carrier in a similar position, often initiating helmet-to-helmet or shoulder pad-to-helmet contact. Tacklers chose the latter two options 43% of the time in this study.

I believe that there is a relationship between incidents of ball carrier spearing and concurrent defensive spearing, although this study cannot substantiate that opinion. Further research needs to be done comparing the incidence of general defensive spearing to the incidence of concurrent defensive spearing.

Reducing The Risk Of Head And Neck Injuries

Spearing greatly increases the risk of head and neck injuries to defensive players while tackling (3,4,8,9,11,12,13,14). But, for some reason, this has not been applied to spearing by ball carriers. The literature mentions the danger of spearing in relation to tacklers and blockers, but neglects ball carriers. Each time a ball carrier lowers his head at contact, he increases the risk of head and neck injury. Head and neck injuries are far more common to defensive players, but ball carriers are not exempt from these injuries.

Mueller and Blyth (3) found that being tackled was one of the leading activities responsible for head and neck fatalities. Also between 1977 and 1987, being tackled was the activity associated with seven cases of quadriplegia (4). The exact mechanisms for these injuries were not reported in these studies. Although we cannot conclude that spearing caused the above injuries, this study does demonstrate that possibility. One study reported being tackled with the head down was the activity associated with a paralyzed ball carrier in 1982 (1).

The head-first technique has been shown to cause cervical spine injuries in tacklers (5,6,10,14). It seems that it would be potentially dangerous to all players who spear. Albright et al (8) partially attributed the decrease in non-fatal head and neck injures in his 8- year study to the teaching of blocking and tackling techniques that avoid the use of the head as a major weapon. Buckley (12) found that wide receivers and quarterbacks had a greater risk of receiving a concussion when being tackled than when blocking. Being tackled and blocking were found to be equal risk activities for running backs. Head-to-head and head-to-knee contact with tacklers was postulated as a cause of concussions for running backs.

The number of paralyzed players does not come close to exposing the risk of hitting with the head down. There is also far more energy generated in a football collision than is required to break the neck of a player hitting with his head down (1). The Prevention of these injuries starts with decreasing the use of the head as a weapon (11). This information is also applicable to ball carriers.

No Spearing Penalties Called

Officials are now able to penalize any player who uses his head as a primary point of contact (15). However, these officials did not exercise that power because there were no spearing penalties called throughout the 1989 season. In the limited spearing scope of this study there were 239 incidents of spearing identified. This demonstrates both an extremely poor enforcement level of the spearing rule and the officials of these games were not using the spearing flag as a deterrent to players.

The spearing rule is the single most important rule in football in terms of consequences (paralysis) and yet may be the least enforced. This may be because the spearing rule is the only rule in football that penalizes a player's action for his own protection. The majority of football infractions protect one player from the actions of another (clip, face mask, hold, etc.). The NFSHSA and the NCAA adopted the spearing rule to deter and therefore protect the player who spears. Its primary function is not to protect the player getting speared. It is the only action penalty in football that protects a player from himself.

It is my observation that the spearing flag is thrown exclusively in the pile-on-situation-- that is, a defender coming late and head- first into a pile of players who are already down. It would appear in this situation the officials are trying to protect the player getting speared. I believe this is a misinterpretation of the spearing rule. Officials should deter and thereby protect the player who is spearing. Officials need to begin to acknowledge spearing during the tackling process, when most injuries occur (3,4,5,6,10,13,14,16), to further reduce the risk of head and neck injures.

The spearing rule is stated in a way that includes all players (tacklers, ball carriers, blockers) and needs to be interpreted as

such. Officials need to enforce existing spearing rules, and they
should be educated about the mechanisms of serious head and neck
injuries that occur to football players (9). According to Dr. Robert
C. Cantu (17), Chief of Neurosurgery at Emerson Hospital in Concord,
Mass., "Referees and umpires of games who are not calling the rules
as they are written should be held responsible for injuries and
deaths."

Safest Position At Contact

     Making contact with the head up greatly reduces the risk of
serious head and neck injury (1,3). When the neck is extended (and
in neutral) the force is absorbed by the neck musculature, the
intervertebral discs, and the cervical facet joints. With the head
up, the tackler or ball carrier can see when and how impact is about
to occur and can prepare the neck musculature for impact. Both are
important factors in reducing the risk of head and neck injury.
Leidholt (18) emphasized the importance of ball carriers and tacklers
keeping their necks in extension at contact.

     This does not indicate contact should be initiated with the
head even if the neck is extended. Contact should be initiated with
the shoulder while keeping the neck extended. This places the
head and cervical spine in the least amount of danger by focusing the
impact force on the shoulder. But this technique must be practiced
until a player overcomes the powerful instinct to protect his eyes
and face by lowering his head at contact.

Recommendations

     The athletes should be educated about the mechanisms of head and
cervical spine injuries. The athletic trainer is in the ideal
position to accomplish this task. In a classroom, the athletic
trainer should instruct the players on spearing's relationship to
head and/or neck injuries and how they can reduce the risks of these
injuries. The athletic trainer should do this before contact begins,
repeat it halfway through the season, and have the athletes sign
attendance sheets at each meeting.

     The coaching staff must teach, demonstrate, and practice proper
tackling, blocking, and ball carrier contact techniques throughout
the season. They should put specific emphasis on each of these
techniques at least four times a season: before contact begins, at
game 2, at game 5, and at game 7. The coaching staff or the athletic
trainer also should document each time this topic is covered. Virgin
(19) believed that proper coaching techniques are imperative for the
prevention of injury. Teaching contact skills that protect the neck
will do far more to prevent injuries than exercises will (18).

     Coaches and athletic trainers should design drills for ball
carriers, tacklers, and blockers. The coaches should focus each
drill or session solely on keeping the head up and initiating contact

with the shoulder. The progression should be from slow walk through skills to full- speed contact. The technique has to be drilled in game like situations. They should also include the types of collisions Torg (7) identified with quadriplegia. These include two athletes colliding while moving in opposite directions and athletes meeting at an oblique angle.

It is also extremely important for the coaching staff to have a strict enforcement policy for dealing with spearing during practice. Spearing at any time should not elude the coach's or athletic trainer's attention without their attempting to correct the player's technique.

CONCLUSION

The incidence of ball carrier spearing and concurrent defensive spearing were surprisingly high. Spearing increases the risk of head and neck injury to all players including ball carriers. This study also revealed the spearing penalty was not enforced during this season. To further reduce the risk of injury, officials should recognize all types of spearing and enforce the spearing penalty during the tackling process. They should also use the spearing flag as a deterrent to protect the player who spears, including ball carriers, tacklers, and blockers. The athletes should be educated to the mechanisms of head and neck injuries. The coaching staff should increase practice time on correct contact techniques throughout the season in game like situations.

ACKNOWLEDGMENTS

I thank and credit Toby Barboza, M.Ed., ATC, for suggesting the idea of offensive spearing to me about 6 years ago. Also, Thanks to the Millville football program for their cooperation and allowing me the extended use of their equipment.

REFERENCES

(1) Hodgson VR, Thomas LM. Play head-up football. National Federation News. 1985; 2:24-27.

(2) National Collegiate Athletic Association, NCAA Football rules and/or modifications, Rule 2, Section 24; Rule 9, Section 1, Article 2-L; Rule 9, Section 1, Article 2-N. Jan 23, 1976.

(3) Mueller FO. Blyth CS. Fatalities from head and cervical spine injuries occurring in tackle football: 40 years' experience. Clinics in Sports Medicine. 1987; 6:185-196.

(4) Mueller FO, Blyth CS, Cantu RC. Catastrophic spine injuries in football. Physician and Sportsmedicine. October 1989-17:51-53.

(5) Torg JS, Quedenfeld TC, Moyer RA. Truex R, Spealman AD, Nichols CE. Severe catastrophic neck injuries resulting from tackle football. Journal of the American College Health Association. 1977; 25:224-266.

(6) Torg JS, Vegso JJ, Sennett B. The national football head and neck injury registry: 14 year report on cervical quadriplegia. Clinics in Sports Medicine. 1987; 6:61-72.

(7) Torg JS. Epidemiology, pathomechanics, and prevention of football- induced cervical spinal cord trauma. Exercise and Sport Sciences Reviews. 1992; 20: 321-338.

(8) Albright JP, Mcauley E. Martin RK, Crowley ET, Foster DT. Head and neck injuries in college football: an eight-year analysis. American journal of Sports Medicine. 1985; 13:147-152.

(9) Football related spinal cord injuries among high school players- Louisiana, 1989. Morbidity and Mortality Weekly Report. 1990; 39:586-587.

(10) Torg JS, Sennett B, Vegso JJ. Spinal injury at the third and fourth cervical vertebrae resulting from the axial loading mechanism: an analysis and classification. Clinics in Sports Medicine. 1987; 6:159-185.

(11) Watkins RG: Neck injuries in football players. Clinics in Sports Medicine. 1986; 5:215-247.

(12) Buckley WE. Concussions in college football. American Journal of Sports Medicine. 1988; 16:51-56.

(13) Torg JS. Epidemiology, pathomechanics, and prevention of athletic injuries to the cervical spine. Medicine and Science in Sports and Exercise. 1985;17:295-303.

(14) Torg JS. The epidemiologic, biomechanical and cinematographic analysis of football induced cervical spine trauma. Athletic Training, Journal of the National Athletic Trainers Association. 1990; 25:147-159.

(15) Kuland KN. The Injured Athlete. 2nd ed. Philadelphia, PA: Lippincott Co.: 1988:288.

(16) Saal JA, Sontag MJ. Head injuries in contact sports: sideline decision making. Physical Medicine and Rehabilitation. 1987; 1: 649-657.

(17) Ramotar JE. New briefs: no direct deaths in high school football. Physician and Sportsmedicine. September 1991; 19: 48-50.

(18) Leidholt JD. Spinal injuries in athletes: be prepared. Orthopaedic Clinics of North America. 1973; 4:691-707.

(19) Virgin H: Cineradiographic study of football helmets and the cervical spine. American Journal of Sports Medicine. 1980; 8: 310-317.

Robert C. Cantu,[1] *M.D.*

How to Make Professional Boxing Safer—The American Medical Association Controversy

REFERENCE: Cantu, R. C., **"How to Make Professional Boxing Safer—The American Medical Association Controversy,"** *Head and Neck Injuries in Sports, ASTM STP 1229,* Earl F. Hoerner, Ed., American Society for Testing and Materials, Philadelphia, 1994.

ABSTRACT: Cerebral concussions occur frequently in contact sports; more than 250 000 concussions occur annually in football alone. Definitions and classifications of severity of concussions vary, which makes evaluation of data extremely difficult. By combining elements of various definitions, the author has developed a practical, on-the-field grading scheme for identifying concussions in contact sports (grade 1: mild, with no loss of consciousness; grade 2: moderate, with less than five minutes of unconsciousness or more than 30 minutes of post-traumatic amnesia; grade 3: severe, with five or more minutes of unconsciousness or 24 or more hours of post-traumatic amnesia.) Also discussed are management of concussions and guidelines for determining when an athlete may safely return to play.

Boxing has been criticized as a brutal sport, and many have called for its abolition. The author reviewed the literature on the health hazards of boxing and found that it has a lower fatality rate than several other sports, including horseracing and parachuting. The most serious health effect of boxing is chronic encephalopathy that affects the pyramidal, extrapyramidal, and cerebellar systems. Often called punchdrunk syndrome, it appears to be directly related to skill level and frequency of participation. Symptoms usually do not appear until after the boxer has retired. The boxing council and a medical surveillance program are necessary to enforce uniform licensing and medical standards and to generate data for research.

KEYWORDS: boxing, injuries, safety, American Medical Association (AMA)

Through the 1962 statement of the AMA Committee on the Medical Aspects of Sports "Statement on Boxing," the AMA had long ago addressed the issue of the medical risks of boxing [1]. It was the January 14, 1983 issue of JAMA that sparked a debate that resulted in extensive major network television coverage, newspaper articles and editorials, magazine stories, an AMA sponsored conference on the medical aspects of boxing, a Congressional hearing on boxing, and the embarrassing position of the AMA appearing to support both sides of the debate simultaneously.

In that issue of JAMA, two major articles on boxing were published [2,3], neither calling for its abolition, and two impassioned editorials each calling for the abolition of boxing based on moral, ethical, and medical grounds [4,5]. It is ironic that the AMA's council on scientific affairs study on the safety issue of boxing, a study and recommendations already approved by the house of delegates at the 1982 annual meeting and thus the official policy of the AMA, appears in the same issue as the conflicting editorial opinion. The council, after deliberation of the medical evidence, concluded that "boxing is a dangerous sport and can

---

[1]Department of Neurosurgery, Emerson Hospital, Concord, MA 01742.

result in death or long-term brain injury" but to ban boxing would not be a "realistic solution to the problem of brain injury." It called for establishing a national registry for all amateur and professional boxers, mandating the use of uniform protective equipment and standardizing ringside safety and medical procedures.

At odds with these recommendations was the editorial of Lundberg who concluded "Boxing seems to me to be less sport than is cockfighting; boxing is an obscenity. Uncivilized man may have been bloodthirsty. Boxing, as a throwback to uncivilized man, should not be sanctioned by any civilized country" [4]. Furthermore a second editorial by Van Allen chimed in "is now not the time to suppress exposure of this fragment of our savagery by the mass media and leave boxing to those who enjoy privately staged dogfights" [5].

While the controversy raged sparked by the January 14, 1983 JAMA issue, in February of 1983 the AMA conference on the medical aspects of boxing was held. The panel, which included among others professors of neurology and neurosurgery, after reviewing all the medical evidence did not call for a ban on boxing, but instead made eight recommendations to improve boxing safety.

At the June 1983 AMA annual meeting in Chicago the 351 member house of delegates by voice vote adopted a resolution calling for the "elimination of boxing from amateur scholastic, intercollegiate, and government athletic programs" because it is deleterious to health. This June resolution represents the first time the AMA officially opposed boxing and does conflict with previous endorsement of the council report. The AMA, apparently not for the first time, was endorsing conflicting policies. When asked of this dilemma, AMA spokesperson Mike Cherskov responded "he didn't know whether the June resolution accurately represented the feelings of most physicians . . . and that the board of trustees traditionally endorses reports of its scientific committee."

A review of the eight proposals for the improvement of safety in (especially professional) boxing of the AMA's panel of experts follows.

1. Establishment of a National Registry of All Professional Boxers

Just as is true for amateur boxing where there is a passport registry system that includes all the pertinent medical and boxing exposure of the athlete, a similar registry is sorely needed in professional boxing. The medical obligations concerning eligibility to box must also become uniform nationally. This would eliminate the present practice of a fighter who is medically barred in one state fighting in another state under an assumed name.

We believe we also need a national boxing registry or commission, and a strong willed National Boxing Commissioner comparable to Commissioners in other major sports.

Others in professional boxing agree. To quote nationally recognized trainer Teddy Atlas, "We need a national commission or some way of having consistent blanket control and knowledge of all fighters, so as to avoid fighters K.O.'d one night in a city fighting two nights later in another. It's not the commissioners fault they don't have the money or have the means to handle the situation with Federal money. What of course scares me is a National Federally subsidized commission means political cronies that know nothing and don't care but maybe that's the nature of the beast when you venture into national commissions."

The first attempt to introduce a federal boxing bill was in 1961 by then Senator Estes Kefauver. Through the years other attempts have been made but the 1992 bills by Senator William Roth and William Richardson and backed by Senator John Glenn (Bill #S2852) is gaining momentum. The salient features of the Professional Boxing Corporation Act of 1992 include establishing a Professional Boxing Corporation to help:

(1) create a universal set of rules and regulations governing boxing.

(2) eliminate exploitation, conflicts of interest, questionable judging, corruption and the influence of organized crime.
(3) safeguard the health and welfare of boxers and establish the sport's credibility.

An executive director will be appointed by the President of the United States. The director will name a professional boxing board of five members who will establish a Congress of State Boxing Administrators. Some of the corporate functions would be

(1) establish a national registry and licensing data base,
(2) issue certificates of licensing and registration,
(3) prescribe regulations to ensure safety of participants,
(4) establish standards,
(5) encourage insurance funds for the boxing community, and
(6) prescribe regulations prohibiting conflicts of interest.

In the words of Steve Acunto, who with Rocky Marciano co-founded The American Association for the Improvement of Boxing (AAIB), "The P.B.C. Bill sponsored by this committee has the best potential to date to solve the problem of sound regulation, especially since it will be self-supporting and portends no cost to the taxpayer."

It is ludicrous and reprehensible to think that our great country has not been able to regulate boxing and restore public confidence through an organization that would place it on the same plane as other major sports in America. This undertaking will not succeed unless individuals appointed to P.B.C. are truly knowledgeable, competent, and dedicated to achieving the purposes of the bills. The primary purpose should be the physical safety and financial security of the pugilists who are now victims of poor regulations.

All of us here should be inspired by the magnificent mosaic of the Olympic athletes who exemplify the true integrity of the sport. We cannot let them down by permitting unscrupulous individuals to prevail on the American boxing scene.

Boxing is at the crossroads. Today, the world's oldest sport is fighting to survive a seemingly endless chain of corruption, fragmentation, and disarray that has left it at a hopeless impasse. That's why new legislation proposed by Senators William Roth and William Richardson and backed by Senator John Glenn is of vital importance and deserves the support of everyone concerned with the survival of the game.

The Roth bill would create a non-profit Professional Boxing Corporation, while Richardson's legislation would establish a U.S. Boxing Commission under the U.S. Department of Labor.

The resulting Professional Boxing Corp (PBC) will be completely self-supporting except for an initial start-up loan, which will be paid back with interest—at absolutely no cost to the taxpayer. Further, the PBC will not supplement any state boxing regulations nor will it attempt to micromanage professional boxing. Boxing will be, as it should be, left to boxing.

The proposed Professional Boxing Act of 1992 has been carefully screened by the AAIB, and we would like to state unequivocally that the Roth-Richardson bills are the best yet devised as a permanent solution to upgrading boxing and placing it on the level of other major professional sports.

For skeptics who say, "I've heard that song before," we understand your cynicism. Since the first boxing bill was introduced in 1961, there has been no less than eight bills or hearings designed for the same purpose with an almost identical litany: *Hearings, Testimonies of champions, promoters and ring participants. . . .* followed by a universal clarion call for "*Cleaning up boxing,*" and *establishing a national governing body.* But, in the end, the result has always been to paraphrase the Great Bard, "full of sound and fury, and signifying nothing."

Despite this past history, this new legislation may indeed be the breakthrough, but it won't be a reality without the support of everyone concerned with the survival of Boxing. We urge everyone connected with the sport including boxers, managers, trainers, sports writers, and publishers of ring publications to join us in expressing support for Bill #S2852 which will establish the Professional Boxing Corporation.

There never was a better time to say "enough" to boxing's corruption, inadequate protection for the ring combatants and lack of confidence in the fight game. Public support coupled with the boxing writers of America will make this bill a reality.

2. Authorize the Ring Physician to Stop a Bout at Anytime to Examine a Boxer and to Terminate the Contest if He/She Feels It Is Indicated

Presently in most states it is up to the discretion of the referee to suspend action to seek the ringside physicians opinion as well as up to the referee to terminate a contest short of one side or the other throwing in the towel. In my opinion, the ringside physician should also have those powers and if there is disagreement the physician should be empowered to override the referee. Who best should know when to suspend or terminate action, a properly trained experienced ringside physician or a well intended but not necessarily medically trained layman.

3. Frequent Medical Training Seminars Should be Held for *All* Ring Personnel

In many states, to become a ringside physician requires only a license to practice medicine. It doesn't require that you be a neurologist, neurosurgeon, or have had extensive experience dealing with head injuries. This is wrong as all ringside physicians should be experienced in the recognition and initial assessment of especially head in addition to other injuries. All ringside personnel should be instructed in Basic Life Support (BCLS) and the physician ideally in Advanced Life Support (ACLS).

4. Provide Adequate Ringside Life Support Systems and Evacuation Plans

State of the art emergency medical technician (EMT) personnel and equipment should be at ringside as well as evacuation plans to a neurosurgical facility where a neurosurgeon is on duty and available.

5. Boxing Matches Should Be Held Only When Proper Neurosurgical Facilities Are Nearby

Matches should not be held in remote locations where full neuroradiologic and neurosurgical capabilities are not immediately available. To do otherwise is to needlessly risk fatal injury before diagnostic medical care can be rendered. Some have advocated the ringside attendance of a neurosurgeon. To me this is like a priest at a hanging, it may provide comfort but it will not alter the outcome. No a neurosurgeon is only of value where he or she works, in the hospital, and no match should occur without immediate proximity to neurosurgical care. This is especially true when we reflect on the second impact syndrome as well as acute subdural hematoma, which can place the athlete in a life threatening situation within minutes.

6. Establish Mandatory Safety Standards for Ringside Equipment

Boxers may not only receive a brain injury from an opponent's direct blow, but also indirectly from their head striking a ring post or the floor. Uniform safety standards regarding all ring equipment, the padded floor surface, tension and number of ring ropes, and padding on ring posts should be established and adopted for uniform use.

7. The Medical Evaluation of Boxers by State Boxing Commissions Must Be Upgraded and Enforced

Just as is true for amateur boxing in this country there should be for professionals standardized periods of enforced inactivity after bouts terminated by head blows. As is true in New York State there should be periodic examinations and criteria for when a head CT or MRI scan should be done.

It is also suggested that each professional boxer have his own psychological profile established with a battery of psychological tests. The need for such standardized testing on a national basis is imperative. If deterioration is determined consistent with brain injury, a boxer should be withheld from the ring, both sparring and contests. Neither boxing fans nor boxers themselves wish professional boxers to sustain permanent and progressive brain injury, and it is apparent today that such injury can usually be detected by neuropsychological tests before atrophy or other chronic traumatic brain injury is seen on head CT or MRI scans.

8. Eliminate *All* "Tough Man" Contests

Already illegal in many states, this activity should be banned in all states so opinioned the AMA's panel of experts and so argues this author. This activity is not boxing and does not sufficiently protect the safety of the combatants to be allowed. To this author, it is analogous to the state of affairs the AMA editors falsely ascribed to professional boxing.

Although embellished by the author's opinions, these eight proposals were all recommended by the AMA's panel of experts. Additional suggestions to further enhance the safety of boxing, especially at the professional level where it is most sorely needed, follow.

9. Selection of Ring Physicians

In most states the selection of ringside physicians is a largely political process, more a question of who you know rather than what you know. Often ringside physicians have no special training in the immediate assessment and care of head injuries, the most life threatening condition they are likely to face. This is just plain wrong.

Boxing physicians should be selected from the elite of sportsmedicine physicians and all must have specialized training and experience in the recognition of head injuries, especially mild concussions. They must fully understand far short of a boxer being absolutely "out on his feet" when it is prudent to stop a contest due to head blows.

10. The Round-Ending Bell Should Not Be Allowed to Save a Boxer from a Knockout

If a boxer is rendered unconscious or is still stunned (grade I concussion) and unable to continue with less than 10 seconds left in a round, the referee's knockout or "standing" count should continue and if it reaches ten the fight should be over. Boxers should not be able to be "saved by the bell."

This is especially important when we reflect on the fact that the second impact syndrome is not only more common than previously thought, but occurs not just in football, but in all contact and collision sports especially boxing. Thus all ringside physicians must be acutely aware of this condition.

Though first described by Richard Schneider in his book on head and neck injuries [6] it was Saunders and Harbaugh in their 1984 JAMA article [7] that used the term second impact for what has since been called the second impact syndrome of catastrophic head injury. With this syndrome an athlete receives an initial head injury, often a concussion or possibly worse such as a cerebral contusion. After this first head injury the athlete suffers post concussive symptoms, i.e. headache, difficulty with thought processes, memory, visual, vestibular (balance) motor, or sensory symptoms. Prior to all of these symptoms clearing, be it minutes, days or weeks later, the athlete returns to competition. Following a second head blow which may be remarkably minor, say being hit on the chest, side, or back snapping the head and imparting acceleration forces to the brain, this syndrome may occur.

What happens pathologically with the SIS is a loss of autoregulation of blood supply to the brain leading to vascular engorgement within the cranium [8]. This in turn produces markedly increased intracranial pressure, which leads to either herniation of the medial surface (uncus) of the temporal lobe or lobes below the tentorium or herniation of the cerebellar tonsils through the foramen magnum. The usual time course is rapid, 10 to 20 seconds to a few minutes, and with brain herniation and brainstem compromise with coma, ocular, and respiratory failure rapidly ensuing.

With such a castastrophic condition where the mortality rate may approach 50% and the chance of morbidity nearly 100%, prevention takes on the utmost importance. Prevention is clearly the key.

To allow a boxer who has already sustained a concussion to continue because the "bell saved him," is to invite this condition.

11. A Boxer Rendered Unconscious or a Bout Terminated Due to Head Blows is Suspended for a Specified Period and Must be Medically Cleared Before Return to Competition

This is especially important because of the concerns of the second impact syndrome. Suspensions such as those for amateur boxing would be prudent, that is,

a) 30 days suspension: The contest is stopped due to minor head blows—excessive standing eight counts.
b) 90 days suspension:
   1) unresponsive for less than 2 minutes.
   2) multiple 30 day suspensions in the same year.
c) 180 days suspension: The boxer has been unresponsive for over a 2 minute period of time.

Before resuming boxing after a restriction, the boxer must be free of all postconcussion symptoms and have a physicians examination and clearance to return. Furthermore a boxer may be required to have an EEG or CT scan at the examining physicians discretion.

As you may read in Dr. Jordan's chapter, in New York State presently a professional boxer stopped by a TKO is suspended 45–60 days and 90 days for a K.O. All boxers must have a CT scan or EEG before they can be reinstated.

12. The Same Suspensions and Medical Clearance Restrictions Recommended for Competition Should Pertain to Sparring in the Gym

Obviously in terms of especially the second impact syndrome, the brain does not respond differently to injuries sustained in the gym versus a formal contest. Thus the rules regarding suspension after head injury should be the same.

It is interesting to reflect on the words of trainer Teddy Atlas. "It has been my experience and the feeling of my teacher Cus D'Amato who spent 50 years in the sport that many times when there is a serious injury such as hemorrhaging of the brain automatically it is assumed that the condition was the result of those punches from the immediate fight. Cus' feeling was that in his investigations of these incidents he found that many of the fights were boring, uneventful fights where few punches were landed yet the tragic result. His findings were that the fighters had suffered a previous undisclosed injury that went unreported or possibly a cerebral aneurysm was present. But without the benefit of an autopsy in the tragic cases where death occurred the conclusion that punches in the fight caused the condition was unfair and inaccurate" [9].

Ted goes on to say regarding the risk of injury to a boxer: "If there is injury risk it is obviously to a great extent during his sparring in the gym since he's doing much more sparring than rounds of fighting. So there should be some commission supervision (if you can find qualified people). If a guy is hurt or K.O.'d in the gym it should be known" [9].

13. Better Teaching of Boxers and Perhaps Certification of Trainers and Managers

Foremost at the top of the list to improve safety in the sport for Teddy Atlas is "better coaching so the fighters are taught what the real approach of the sport is suppose to be— *hit and don't get hit* as much as possible. I don't know how practical it really can be but *screen* and *rate* and *test* the coaches and get rid of the unqualified—they're dangerous."

I believe these are very cogent words whose time has come. It doesn't require great prescience to realize that improper coaching of a boxer invites injury.

14. Improvement and Certification of Boxing Equipment

Everything that was mentioned in recommendation number six regarding ring equipment, can also be stated for the boxers equipment. It is ridiculous to think the bicycle, hockey, motorcycle, and football gear worn by children must pass rigid certification standards before they can be sold. Yet there is no certification standards or process for the boxing headgear worn in sparring by professionals, and the gym and competition alike by amateur boxers. An offshore country can produce boxing headgear under no standards or controls, import to this country where an American label may be stuck on, and the product sold. This is wrong! The same comprehensive research that was followed in the certification process for football helmets for example, should be followed for protective boxing headgear.

Boxing gloves, just like headgear, are presently archaic and much in need of "space age" materials and technology. Presently their weight can be significantly increased by sweat and water absorbed by the leather. The padding can also remold during the course of a fight and provide less of an impact cushion over the knuckles as the fight progresses.

15. Continued Research On Chronic Brain Injury

A final recommendation regarding improving boxing safety would also pertain to other contact/collision sports as well. The research started by the John's Hopkin study on amateur boxing should be continued and extended to other sports where head contact is common. Presently articles have appeared regarding chronic brain injury in soccer, football, rugby, and the equestrian sports to name a few. Other sports where the overall risk of head injury is low, have unique positions or events (ie: the goalie in soccer or the pole vaulter in track) where the risk of head injury may be high. All studies in other sports presently lack the controls true of all the boxing studies prior to the John's Hopkin study.

We need more sophisticated neuropsychiatric tests that hopefully can be administered within a fifteen minute time period. We also must develop more accurate brain scanning devices that will detect not only yearly structural but also physiological changes.

Therefore to make not only boxing but all sports with a risk of head injury safer, significant research challenges lie ahead for the sports medicine/sports science community.

References

[1] AMA Committee on the Medical Aspects of Sports, "Statement on Boxing" *Journal of the American Medical Association,* Vol. 181, 1962, p. 242.
[2] Ross, R. J., Cole, M. et al., "Boxers—Computed tomography, EEG and Neurological Evaluation," *Journal of the American Medical Association,* Vol. 249, 1983, pp. 211–213.
[3] Council on Scientific Affairs Report, "Brain Injury in Boxing," *Journal of the American Medical Association,* Vol. 249, 1983, pp. 242–257.
[4] Lundberg, G. C., "Boxing Should Be Banned in Civilized Countries," *Journal of the American Medical Association,* Vol. 249, 1983, p. 250.
[5] Van Allen, M. W., "The Deadly Degrading Sport," *Journal of the American Medical Association,* Vol. 249, 1983, p. 250–251.
[6] Schneider, R. D., *Head and Neck Injuries in Football: Mechanisms, Treatment and Prevention,* Baltimore, Williams & Wilkins Co., 1973.
[7] Saunders, R. L. and Harbaugh, R. E., "The Second Impact in Catastrophic Contact Sports Head Trauma," *Journal of the American Medical Association,* Vol. 252, 1984, pp. 538–539.
[8] Cantu, R. C., "Second Impact Syndrome," *The Physician and Sports Medicine.* September, 1992.
[9] Atlas, T: Personal Communication.

Friedrich J. Unterharnscheidt [1]

THE HISTORICAL AND MEDICAL ASPECTS - BOXING

REFERENCE: Unterharnscheidt, F.J., "The Historical and Medical Aspects - Boxing," Head and Neck Injuries in Sports. ASTM STP 1229, Earl F. Hoerner, Ed., American Society for Testing and Materials, Philadelphia, 1994.

ABSTRACT: This paper presents a survey of historical and biomechanical aspects of boxing, acute and chronic clinical findings and acute and chronic morphological findings of body organs, and the central nervous system of boxers. The historical section begins with the development of fistfighting in Greece and Rome. The impact mechanics of boxing blows against the head is discussed. Successive sections describe facial injuries, eye injuries, hearing impairment, injuries to the hand and wrist, cardiac injuries, acute renal change, and the different knock-down and knock-out mechanisms. Also discussed are the oculecardiac reflex, boxing blows against the lateral region of the neck, the chronic clinical findings, and the acute and pathomorphological findings in the brain. It is shown that boxing leads to a severe permanent brain damage, in amateur and professional boxers, which depends mainly on the number of bouts and the weight class of the boxer.

KEYWORDS: boxing injuries, historical aspects of boxing, acute and clinical findings, acute and classic pathomorphological findings, knock-out mechanisms, biomechanics of impact

---

INTRODUCTION

When the question of the dangers of boxing is raised in either scientific or journalistic publications, its supporters fervently plead for the *"noble art of self-defense"*, the *"fist-fencing"* which is wholesome to the body and the mind. Just as fervent, however, are the detractors of boxing, who demand the prohibition of both amateur and professional boxing which they call the "only legal way of killing...The moment has come that boxing should no longer be officially encouraged, but generally prohibited. A way of acting that in everyday life is punished by prison, hard labor, and even death, is rewarded in boxing with publicity, gold medals, and money"[1]. A person who seeks to justify boxing as the noble art of self-defense seems to be "blindfolded in the use of an inapposite phrase"[2].

Boxing is different from all other athletic endeavors in that the nature of the sport causes injury by intention rather than by accident. Injuries are coincidental in other sports, "but in boxing the aim and object - explicit or implied - is to render the opponent hors de combat. Traumata are therefore not so much regretted as regrettable"[3]. Boxing is a "medical experiment for the study of traumatic head injury"[4].

The accident rate of 2.0% often quoted in defense of boxing is

---

[1] President, Neuroscience, Inc., 3512 Camp Street, New Orleans, LA 70115

misleading; it covers such relatively inconsequential lesions as skin abrasions, bruises, hematomas, distortions, fractures, and the like, but does not reflect the number of serious injuries causing permanent or late damage to the Central Nervous System. It is therefore, essential that the dangers of boxing be re-evaluated in the light of results obtained during the last decade, through investigation into the origin and significance of closed traumatic injuries to the CNS as caused by blunt blows to the head.

Monographic treatments of the medical aspects of boxing have been published[1,5,6,7,8,9,10,11,12,13].

HISTORICAL ASPECTS

Boxing, or fistfighting, was included in the 4 celebrated Greek holy festivals: the Olympian Games in Olympia, the Pythian Games in Delphi, the Isthmian Games in Corinth, and the Nemean Games in Nemea. They occurred periodically and were called the *periodos*. The winner of one of these periodos was awarded a wreath, and his name inscribed with honor on a permanent roll.

Boxing was first introduced in the 23rd games in Olympia, 688 B.C., followed 40 years later by competition in pankration, a combination of boxing and wrestling, in the 33rd games, 648 B.C. There were only 2 classes of athletes in the Olympian and Pythian games: boys - those under 18 years of age - and men - those over 18. Weight did not enter in. At the Isthmian and Nemean festival, there was a third class, the beardless - boys from 16 to 18 - and the boys' class were those under 16 years old. The rules were flexible enough, however, to allow an especially well-developed boy to compete in a higher age group. Boys were not allowed to take part in the boxing competitions until 616 B.C. (Olympia 41) and in pankration until 200 B.C. (Olympia 145).

The competitors simply drew lots; they were not matched by weight. Because there was often an odd number of fighters, one drew a blank, and so got to enter the second bout without winning the first. He was called "ephedros", "he who merely sits beside the ring". This fighter had the obvious advantage of starting his bout fresh. "Akoniti" meant "without dust", and such a man was so formidable an athlete that nobody dared to fight him. At each festival only one winner was honored - the man who triumphed over all other contestants.

In ancient Greece and Rome, we can distinguish 3 periods in the history of boxing: First, the period of the soft thongs, himas malakoteros, extending from Homeric times to the close of the fifth century, second, that of the sharp thongs, himas oxys, from the fourth century B.C. to Roman Empire times; third, that of the Roman caestus. We shall see how, as the form of the glove changed, the style of boxing became more brutal.

The transition from fighting with bare fists to boxing with thong-covered hands occurred before Homeric times, for in the games held in honor of the dead Patroclus, thongs were used [14]. The thongs were approximately 9 feet long and according to Pausanias [15,16] were made, "ek boeas omaes", "of untanned oxhide". However, Jüthner states that since they were not stiff, they were probably made of tanned oxhide [17,18]. Scholars are also uncertain as to whether the fighter himself put on the thongs after his companions presented them to him [19], or whether his companions actually wrapped the leather strips around the fighter's hands [20]. At any rate, the thongs were wound several times around the knuckles and wrist and the lower part of the forearm. The fingers remained free. From vase painting we know that the fighters used their teeth, to secure the final knot. Originally, the thongs served to protect the hands, especially the knuckles, and not to intensify the effect of the blow.

About 400 B.C., the long, flat thongs, which had to be wound on the hand before every bout, were replaced by a prefabricated form into which the fighter could simply slip his hand. This forerunner to a glove had a thickened and hard hump over the knuckles.

Jüthner [17,18] thinks that between the development of the soft thongs and the sharp thongs came the stage of the prefabricated sphairai. While training, the fighter placed soft glove, "episphairai" [21], over the sphairai to soften the force of the blows.

Later the Greeks used sharp thongs. They consisted of two parts – a glove and a hard leather ring encircling the knuckles. The glove extended almost to the elbow and ended in a thick strip of fleece to protect the arm, which might be easily injured by a blow from so formidable a weapon. The glove itself appears to have been padded, with the ends of the fingers cut off and an opening on the inside. On the knuckles was a thick pad which prevented the ring from slipping. The ring was formed of 3 to 5 stripes of hard stiff leather, bound together by small strips and held in place by thongs around the wrist. These sharp gloves remained in use until at least the 2nd century A.D.

From the sharp thongs the Romans later developed the caestus. At first, they reinforced the humps over the knuckles with hard leather, not only to protect the knuckles but also to increase the effectiveness of the blow. To protect the arm from opponents' blows, the Romans padded the caestus and extended this protection up the lower arm with a cuff of padding or fur. Later, to make the caestus more dangerous, the Romans added lead to the glove and metal spikes over the knuckles. No Greek writers mention the masses of lead and iron with which, according to Roman poets, the caestus was loaded. Because of the brutality of a fight with the caestus and the callousness a person would need in order to enjoy or participate in such a fight, Gardiner [22] believes that the caestus did not originate in Greece. Rudolph [19] corroborates this opinion, calling the caestus an unsporting tool for murdering.

Philostratos [23] states that the boxer Onomastos from Smyrna, the winner in Olympia 23, defined the rules for boxing, but unfortunately those have been lost. We do know, however, that there was no ring nor limitation of fighting time. The contestants fought without rounds or pauses until one was defeated, unless both fighters agreed to take a break. Only in the older literature are there statements that blows were directed against all parts of the body. Later, only the head was the target of the blows.

A floored fighter was given no grace, and Schröder [24] believes that kicking was even allowed. However, Gardiner [22] does not agree. Instead, he believes the Greek word "prosbainein", means advancing close to and clinching the opponent. A fighter won not by accruing a certain number of points, but by disabling his opponent – in most cases, apparently a knock-out. A fighter could acknowledge defeat by raising his hand with an extended index finger, apagoreuein [15,16]. Boxers of good defensive technique are known from literature: "syn technae malista", "with excellent technique". One celebrated fighter, Melankomas, who was himself rarely hit in fights, could bring his opponent to concede without ever hitting them [20,25]. Competitions were open to all comers and under the conditions described, weight had perhaps a greater advantage than it has today, Consequently, boxing tended to become the monopoly of the heavy-weight. Vase paintings illustrate blows to the chin, while Homer [26] describes blows against the ears in the fight between Odysseus and the beggar Iros. "Cauliflower ears", the result of ear lesions, are frequently found on statues (for example, Boxer of Apollonius from the Thermen Museum in Rome), but not in vase paintings because of the difficulty of painting such detail on the small figures.

Dodging with the head is found in vase paintings [19], but no ducking. Shadow boxing, "skiamachein", is known. The sandbag, "korykos", is described in literature [15,16] and in engraving on the Ficeronic Ciste - first half of the 3rd century B.C.

Pankration

Pankration, a combination of wrestling and boxing, was introduced in Olympia 33 [23,27]. It seems to have derived from war training, yet it appears quite late in Olympia; other sports evolving from war training appeared quite early. More wrestling than boxing [19], , pankration was held in great esteem by the people of the times. The boxing part of this discipline was done with bare hands. There is, however, an exception - two athletes with thong-covered hands pictured on a drinking vessel in a wild struggle [28].

Although begun in the standing position, pankration continued on the ground. The end of the fight occurs not as in wrestling after 3 floorings, but when one fighter declared himself defeated by knocking, "apagoreuein", upon the trunk of the winner, because speech was often impossible when the victor was strangling his opponent in a strong grip. The pankratiasts, like Thai boxer, used their knees and feet in attack and defense maneuvers. All was acceptable except biting, scratching, gouging, pocking, and digging with the fingers. However, these exceptions were strictly enforced by the trainers or officials with a rod. Pankration finds its modern counterpart in jiujitsu and catch-as-catch-can. Serious injuries and indeed fatal accidents did occur.

Gardiner [22] does not agree with the translation "digging with the fingers". Rather, he interprets the original Greek to mean banning "boring the fingers in the eyes, mouth, other orifices, or any parts of the body". He relates this to 2 quotations in Aristophanes [29], where this concept has an obscene connotation. Gardiner's [22] quotation also reveals that the Greeks considered boxing more dangerous than pankration.

During the Middle Ages, interest in boxing virtually died, and it experienced no revival until the 17th century in Great Britain and somewhat later in the United States. A summary of the historical development of fistfighting and boxing in Great Britain and the United States will be presented in another publication, space does not permit it in this paper.

IMPACT MECHANICS

General Aspects

The violence of a blow to the head is related to the velocity of the fist and the masses involved. If further depends on the mechanical properties of the colliding bodies, namely glove and head[30-33]. On impact, a force is induced on both the gloved fist and the head; it accelerates the head and decelerates the fist. During contact, the two bodies are deformed by the force of this impact.

A better knowledge of the process of collision between two given bodies with elastic surfaces may be obtained using the following analogous model: the masses of the colliding partners are represented by two rigid spheres of corresponding mass, connected by a spring. The spring is chosen to possess the stiffness that is required to achieve the same collision time as in the real situation. The stiffness (c) of a spring is expressed in kp/cm, indicating the weight (kp) required to compress the spring by 1 cm: the higher the value of c, the stiffer the spring. Often several springs participate in the collision. For example, in a blow dealt with the gloved fist, one would count the effects of the compressible lining of the glove, the tissue overlying the bony skull, the compressibility of the wrist and possibly that of the elbow as behaving in a spring-like manner. With regard to our problem, the compressibility of the glove is so much greater than that of all other elastic elements in the system, such as the skin and bones, that it can be ignored.

The accurate assessment of the striking mass is also a problem, since it is composed of the masses of the glove, hand, forearm and upper arm, and to a certain degree that of the chest. Moreover, the total mass involved in a blow differs not only with the individual but also with his technique, depending on how much body weight is thrown into the blow.

Translational and Rotational Acceleration [30-33]

There are two kinds of impact to be considered - central and oblique. In the first case, the projected impact axis passes through the center of gravity of the skull. The resulting head motion is simply a translational (linear) acceleration, exemplified by a straight blow into the face. In the second case, however, the axis is not centered, and the resulting motion is combined translational and rotational acceleration of the head. This occurs in swinging blows to the head, uppercuts, or hooks. The degree to which both motions participate in the acceleration depends on the obliquity of the blow; e.g. tangential impact, such as an uppercut to the chin, produces practically pure rotational acceleration. Initially the skull alone begins to rotate, while the brain, by reason of its inertia, does not follow the motion immediately and therefore pulls at its suspensions. This relative displacement distends the bridging veins between brain and superior sagittal sinus, and may eventually cause tearing. The effect of force on the brain is always transmitted by the skull; the effect of the impact on the brain depends on the nature of the acceleration. In translational acceleration, the skull is set in motion before the brain can overcome its inertia. It follows that, at the impact point, the distance between the inner surface of the skull and that of the brain is reduced and increased in pressure develops. At the point opposite the impact pole this distance is slightly increased, thus giving rise to the development of a decrease in pressure. The pressure gradient thus produced in the brain has been found to be approximately linear.

In boxing, the majority of blows hit the head either straight on, slightly obliquely into the face, or from below. The soft tissue of the face reduces the acceleration to some extent, by reason of its compressibility. The same blow directed to the unprotected chin or the angle of the mandible bone will consequently generate a higher acceleration of the head.

Translational Acceleration

Blunt impact may produce brain injury by the stress waves it induces in the brain or by the acceleration which it imparts to the head, or by a combination of both. In general it has been found that the force of an impact on the head has such a slow rise time, due to the cushioning effect of the skin and the scalp, that the action produced is essentially quasi-atactic in nature. As a result, the stress waves

generated by the impact are not important. Thus the injuries which
result from a blunt impact must be attributable to both the
accelerations imparted to the head and to the internal forces which must
be developed if each part of the system is to accelerate at the same
rate.

The simplest action, from an analytical standpoint, develops if
the head is given pure translational acceleration. Such an acceleration
is produced if the head is free of all constraints and the force of the
impact is directed through the center of gravity of the head. Since the
brain is comparatively uniform in density (all of the elements, nerve
tissue, blood, and cerebrospinal tissue have about the same density as
water) and is encased in a skull which is very rigid in comparison to
the rigidity of the brain, the entire system, for analytical purposes,
where translational acceleration is involved, can be regarded as a thin-
walled spherical shell filled with water. It may be readily shown that
if a skull is given a translational acceleration, a pressure gradient
will develop across the skull in the direction of the acceleration with
the maximum pressure occurring at the point of impact and the minimum at
the point opposite the impact, the antipole. The pressure at any point
is essentially hydrostatic, i.e., no shearing stresses develop. At the
impact point the pressure is positive (above ambient) while at the
antipole the pressure is negative (below ambient). Consequently there is
some intermediate point at which no pressure change has occurred. This
is referred to as the "nodal" point. For an incompressible fluid and an
inextensible skull the nodal point is at the center of the shell. If the
fluid is compressible and the shell extensible the pressure variation is
linear but the position of the nodal point shifts.

The positive pressure does no damage as far as we now know.
However, the negative pressure may cause damage if the pressure at any
point below the vapor pressure and hence therefore produces cavitation.
The injuries which result from this type of action are described in
detail in a later section which deals with the so-called contre-coup
injuries.

Rotational Acceleration

If the force of a blunt impact is not directed through the center
of gravity of the head, or if the head is constrained to rotate about
some fixed point, a rotational acceleration is imparted in addition to a
translational acceleration. For a purely rotational acceleration to
develop, the impact would have to be in the form of a couple, or pure
momentum. Such an impact is not very probable, but it is helpful to
consider the action which results if a purely rotational acceleration
is imparted to the head. The action may be compared to that which occurs
when a rigid container filled with water is given an angular
acceleration. The container moves and the water remains essentially at
rest. If a more viscous liquid is substitutes for the water the relative
motion between the container and the liquid is reduced. The force
necessary to accelerate the fluid is developed as a result of the
shearing action between the container and the fluid and between adjacent
layers of fluid. Obviously conditions can exist in which very large
shearing deformations will develop. The brain and skull form a much more
complicated system than the container and the liquid inasmuch as there
are blood vessels and nerves passing into the brain from openings in the
skull, there are protuberances from the skull, and there are membranes
and other supporting structures which help to maintain the position of
the brain relative to the skull. As a result of the relative motion
between the brain and the skull and between the different parts of the

brain, which must take place before sufficient force is developed to accelerate the brain along with the skull, the weaker elements of the system will be injured. Blood vessels will be torn, axons may be torn, and lesions will be produced at points of greatest stress throughout the brain,

Combined Acceleration and Rotation

In actuality one type of acceleration rarely occurs to the total exclusion of the other. The head is constrained by its support system so that it must rotate about some point in space. Consequently even a force directed through the center of gravity will produce angular acceleration as well as linear translation. In some impacts one type of acceleration may predominate initially, with the other type predominating later, or both types of acceleration may be present and of comparable amplitude throughout the impact. In any event it may be supposed that a superposition of effects occurs. That is, any injuries which might be produced by the translational acceleration acting alone, will also be produced if the translation is accompanied by rotational acceleration, and vice versa. Direct evidence on this point is not available, but comparisons of the pathomorphology of head injuries produced by pure rotational accelerations and those produced by more general types of impacts seem to support this assumption.

Relationship between Weight of Gloves and Severity of Impact

When attempting to quantitatively assess the violence exerted on the head during boxing matches, the properties of boxing gloves of (6 to 16 oz) and of various types of ring canvas were examined with regard to their influence on the impact. Leather and padding of gloves are of equal weight: an 8 oz glove of 228 g consists of 114 g leather and 114 g padding.

A simple experimental device which consisted of two pendulums representing the striking fist and the unrestrained head was employed [34,35]. The first pendulum was a metal tube carrying at its free end a wooden hand covered with the test glove. The second pendulum carried a wooden block with plain surfaces; the side facing the gloved pendulum was covered by a piece of woolen fabric about 1.5 mm thick, the opposite side carried an accelerometer. Naturally, the magnitude and the velocity of the impacting masses are important factors in the successful simulation of real fight conditions. One of the author's first concern's however, was to obtain comparable values of the violence generated with boxing gloves of different weights.

The experiments were carried out on the basis of the following values: (1) Head model, 3.1 kp; and (2) model hand without glove, 2.6 kp (the inertia of the metal tube was taken into account).

The velocity achieved with a glove of 6 oz. was found to be about 2.7 times greater than that achieved with a 16 oz. glove. Strangely enough, two supposedly identical gloves of 8 oz. produced different acceleration values that were well outside our other experimental data. Repeated measurements showed the same deviation. Further, it was observed that on the average, higher accelerations were registered from the last blow of a series of 3 or 4 consecutive blows. This indicated that the material slightly 'faded' or retained its deformation, an effect that may be observed in regular fights [35].

Measurement of Acceleration in Boxers

To measure the intensity of the blows in an actual bout, two physical education students, who were unskilled in boxing, fought for 10 minutes (using 12 oz. gloves) with accelerometers bandaged to their heads. The measurements obtained indicated that 21 blows accelerated the head by 0-5 g, 12 blows by 6-10 g, 3 blows by 11-15 g, 3 blows by 16-20 g, and two blows by 21-25 g (the first group of 21 blows certainly included some defensive movements of the head that had the same effect as blows). If the students had used 6 oz. gloves, as in professional contests, these values would have been at least twice as high, since the results correspond to those obtained for 16 oz. gloves in the model experiments. Had the subjects been professional boxers who could deliver more effective blows, the values would certainly have been higher. If in a 10-minute fight (equivalent to little more than 3 rounds) this many blows had hit the head, it can be safely concluded that their number must be multiplied when a complete bout of 12 to 15 rounds is to be considered [34,35].

The impressive impact intensity of the boxing blow is recorded not only in the measurements of clinical and morphological injuries to boxers, but is directly reflected in photographs of the moment a boxer is struck. The tremendous force of the blow deforms and displaces the soft parts of the face. This selection of press photographs demonstrates the effects of deformation, acceleration and inertia on the facial features which, at times, are hardly recognizable. It is obvious that blows of such distorting power do indeed damage the brain. Although it has been argued that like effects are seen only among professional boxers, the blows dealt by amateurs are generally damaging enough to produce similar results. Blows of such intensities as those depicted are by no means rare events, as a random search through the illustrative material of press archives will prove. (Compare with papers [7,10,11,13]).

INJURIES APART FROM CENTRAL NERVOUS SYSTEM DAMAGE

Facial Injuries

Facial injuries occur frequently in amateur and professional boxing because the face is all that lies between the gloved fist and its destination, the skull and brain. The existence of a laceration is self-evident. Coexisting injuries to the facial nerve and separation of the parotid duct must be considered.

Craniofacial lesions in boxers were described by [36] with reference to the different types of boxing blows and their typical lesions.

In the so-called *uppercut* against the mandible, this structure presses against the maxilla with great intensity. The upper teeth can be damaged severely. Fracture of the mandible and maxilla are possible complications. The effect of an uppercut is less severe when the boxer keeps his mandible in occlusion with maxilla, so that both parts form a block. PALAZZI (1925) [36] saw a boxer who was hit by an uppercut and succumbed a few hours later in hospital due to a fracture of the base of the skull.

Swinging blows which connect with the horizontal ramus of the mandible may lead to sudden dislocations of the mandible to the contralateral side, which can be complicated by ruptured ligaments, especially the spheno-maxilllar ligament and the capsular ligament.

A *straight blow* against the tip of the chin produces an abrupt retropulsion of the mandible against the dorsal wall of the cavum articulare glenoidale with frequent fracture of the anterior wall of the meatus auditivus; those boxers show not infrequent hemorrhages out of the ear.

A *straight blow against the mouth* impacts against the frontal areas of maxilla and mandible simultaneously and causes more or less severe damage to the incisors, with possible loss of one or several teeth.

The *most common facial injuries* are: (1) *Bruises, abrasions, or cuts*; (2) *bruises, lacerations, or cuts around the eye, eyebrows or eyelids*, (3) *cuts of the lips*, (4) *"cauliflower" ears*, (5) *fractures of the mandible*, (6) *injuries to and loss of teeth*; and (7) *injuries and fractures of the nose.*

(1) The general *bruises* and *abrasions of the face* can be the result of multiple repetitive impacts. The skin may be swollen ("puffy") or there may be "lumps" of swollen tissue due to edema and hemorrhages.

(2) The skin around the eye lids has an abundant blood supply, is thin and slides easily. *Periorbital hematomas ("black eyes")* may reach so large a dimension that the eye is completely closed. They are the result of injuries to blood vessels, which can be severed by a blow by which the vessel is "cut" by the more or less sharp edge of the orbital rim or ruptured due to the displaceable thin skin in this area. Some individuals are especially predisposed to these types of injuries. Application of ice bags or the administration of adstringentia or raw meat will not influence the swelling at all.

Many of these cuts around the eye are the result of a clash or butt of the head of the opponent, and can to a certain degree be avoided by a scrupulous and attentive referee. If a boxer has a cut eye and the fight is not stopped by the referee, the injured area is subjected to more blows which increase the damage. Cuts around the eyes have to be treated with great care by a physician in order to achieve a first intention healing; they should be treated in an emergency room or hospital, with good lighting and with aseptic conditions. Untrained cornermen or "cut men" should not attempt to treat these injuries between rounds, especially as their emergency treatment often consists of daubing at wounds with a dirty towel the second had carried draped around his neck, using quack remedies, or covering the edges of skin cuts with carpenters' glue, or rubbing adrenalin into open cuts to stop the bleeding (sometimes in a dosage sufficient to affect the boxer's pulse, blood pressure, etc.).

The following experience was described, [37]: "In the Albert Hall in London, I once watched a boxer whose left eye became totally closed by a large hemorrhage into the eyelids, caused by punches. Consequently he was unable to aim properly, and his punches often missed their objective by more than a foot. He seemed to be doomed, when during the next interval, his second took a knife, made a small incision underneath the brow and sucked the blood out of the wound with his mouth. The swelling immediately subsided, the boxer was able to see again, and won the fight".

If the same boxer had been treated by a physician in this manner, he would most certainly have sought a malpractice suit against him.

MILLARD (1963) is of the opinion that it is quite possible to close the laceration of the eyelid-eyebrow region with one or more sutures during a one-minute corner rest period and, if all other factors are favorable, the contest could be allowed to continue [38].

Suturing should always be done, as we have stated above, in an emergency room or hospital with good lighting and sterile conditions and not in the boxing ring. Exceptions may include suturing in *life-threatening situations* as in battlefield environments or in similar situations in civilian emergencies. Whether this procedure is available in "National or Olympic quests for glory,"in "professional fights where not only pride but the purse is important," or is "possibly...limited to world title fights" is here irrelevant; general basic principles of medicine have priority. For this reason, therefore, this practice must be unconditionally condemned.

(3) *Lip injuries* are frequent in boxing, but *cuts of the lips* are relatively rare, although they do occur despite properly fitted gum-shields. Larger cuts have to be sewn with fine stitches under local anesthesia.

(4) *Injuries of the tongue* are frequently due to bites.

(5) *"Cauliflower" ears,* resulting in the deformation of the auricle, are relatively frequent in boxers. Typical ear injuries are the result of a tangential blow against the ear with the skin sliding across the perichondrium *(Decollement traumatique),* or fracture of the cartilage of the ear which may occur when the ear is folded against the skull by a blow. In such a case blood collects on both sides of the cartilage.This leads to an isolation of the cartilage from the soft tissue, which is important for its metabolism. First an othematoma exists, then when the damage is not corrected, a necrotic chondritis follows. The so-called *"cauliflower" ear* is the result. The auricle is grossly distorted and thickened, and the concha and the auditory meatus are filled with hyperplastic cartilaginous masses of almost the density of bone. The process can be diagnosed as *hyperplastic chondritis* or *perichondritis.* The treatment consists, in early phases, of aspiration of the fluid from both sides of the cartilage and the prevention of new fluid deposits by compresses.

(6) Fracture of the mandible is a relatively rare occurrence in boxing, but may occur at the condyle neck or at the angle of the mandible. [39-41].

(7) *Injuries to and loss of the teeth* occur despite properly fitted gum-shields. These also must be treated by a specialist.

(8) *Injuries and fractures of the nose* occur frequently. They can be identified by displacement and crepitus on palpitation. The inferior half or three-fifths of the septum is unprotected by the nasal bones and is vulnerable to direct trauma [42]. Laterally applied force may dislocate the septum from its seat on the maxilla, pushing it to one side. Sometimes the cartilage cracks along the line of curvature into which it is bent by the blow, and occasionally the ethmoidal plate will also snap across vertically. More direct frontal violence may produce a number of different deformities, all based on the production of crumbling injuries [42]. The bony portion of the septum, chiefly the ethmoid and vomer, snaps across in varying places depending on the direction and force of the blow, while the cartilage may buckle or break if its elasticity is exceeded. The fragments sometimes slide alongside one another producing a thickened septum, whilst at other times they become angulated.

When the blow has been sufficiently strong to break the nasal bones, the septum is invariably fractured at the same time and the fragments are dragged into positions governed by the final positions of the nasal bones.

The net result of these various injuries ranges from virtually nothing on the one hand to severe cosmetic deformity on the other. Sometimes, however, when neither the appearance nor the function are affected, epistaxis may later occur with the slightest trauma.

Compound fractures, which can occur when the nose strikes against the rope-supporting poles, the floor of the ring, or against the opponent's head, are also mentioned [23].

On at least two occasions, fractures of the perpendicular plate of the ethmoid following a severe frontal blow to the face, with penetration of the cubiform plate and consequent injury to the brain substance were reported.

In boxers who have had as many as 50 or more bouts, there is seldom any notable bleeding from the nose. Repeated injuries have so destroyed the septum and the normal nasal lining with replacement by dense scars of corrective tissue, that either vascularity is reduced or the vessel walls are so thickened as to be less vulnerable. This is not a hard and fast rule, however; the blood vessels may remain thin and elastic.

In rare cases there may be no external deformity in early injury to the boxer's nose, but on examination with the speculum the various sign are plainly evident.

After repeated fights, the tip of the nose always appears rounded and bulbous as a result of blows on the lower lateral cartilages, by which they may be repeatedly fractured (especially about the angle).

SELTZER (1967)[42] concluded his excellent review of the surgery of the pugilist's nose with the statement, "An important point for the surgeon before performing a reconstructive operation of the nose of a professional boxer is to have it conclusively understood that his pugilistic life must be given up if he wishes to preserve a normal appearing nose, since the operation cannot be repeated with success and a nose once reconstructed is particularly vulnerable."

It should be remembered with regard to facial injuries that in general boxers suffer not only an altered visage, but also an irreversibly altered brain and mind.

Eye Injuries

Ocular injuries due to boxing were discussed by [43-58].

"Although retinal detachment is rightly dreaded as one of the most devastating ocular hazards of the ring, it is only one among a formidable array " [43].

In 1952, ALBAUGH [44] reported on his experience as a consulting physician to the Athletic Commission of the State of California for the previous 6 years. This included 154 injured or allegedly injured eyes in 92 cases.

This author noted that: "Although similarities exist between the types of eye injury resulting from boxing and those resulting from other occupations, some important differences must be noted. Eye injuries resulting from boxing are confined to a definite age group. Boxers, for example, are licensed in California only between the ages of 18 and 36. Exceptions are extremely rare... Damage to the eye is almost always the result of a direct blow upon the eyeball, and is usually severe enough to cause profound pathologic changes... He also notes that, "because of fear of disqualification, many severe injuries are not reported until so long after they occur that healing processes have become well established and it is much too late for adequate constructive treatment." In some cases the injured men retire from fighting before asking for help... One of the tragic features of eye injuries sustained in boxing is that all too often they are bilateral... Of the 154 injured eyes, 38 had cataracts, and in 10 instances this was bilateral. Other structures besides the lens frequently were damaged. In the only operative case, the results were excellent - 20/20 vision (corrected). In 4 the cataracts cleared spontaneously (taking from one month to two years), and in the remaining 33 cases no follow-up was possible.

Of the one 154 injured eyes, 29 showed retinal separation, and in 2 this was bilateral. "Generally the period between injury and examination was a long one, and in only 5 of these cases was operation considered advisable. Of the 5 patients operated on, only one obtained a reattachment. In the hands of all ophthalmologic surgeons in this vicinity, the results of reattachment operations have been so poor that the trustees of the Boxers and Wrestlers Benefit Fund have been consistently hesitant to authorize such surgical therapy and its attendant expense. They have been willing to have operation attempted only when the prognosis appeared unusually favorable."

"Nearly all eyes showed disinsertion of the retina, with or without other holes. In all of them there was profound disturbance of the vitreous, as evidenced by many opacities, both large and small, present for a long time after the initial injury.... Statistically, at least, boxers who sustain eye injuries make a poor showing for successful medical rehabilitation. Furthermore, the follow-up is embarrassingly poor.... As a class, boxers seem to be quite blind to the fact that their career must of necessity end after a pitifully few years..."

Three years later, [43] wrote specifically describing his great experience with eye injuries resulting from boxing.

According to this author [43], "derangement of the visual apparatus from boxing may conveniently be divided into: (1) Ocular damage; (2) injuries to neighboring structures, including the ocular adnexa, and (3) lesions of the visual pathways and other parts of the brain.

(1) Ocular Damage

One important asset to a boxer is a pair of well-formed orbital margins, but his eyes are nevertheless liable to be damaged by blows falling tangentially upon the cornea from a downward and outward direction, where the orbital cavity is at its shallowest. Moreover, the thumb of a boxing glove can easily impinge upon the eyes even if they be deeply set; hence boxing is particularly dangerous for myopes, because their eyes are not only more prominent but more vulnerable than those of the average emmetrope.

a) *Lesions of the Outer Eye*: Conjunctival hemorrhages are not in themselves of much importance, but they may, of course, be accompanied by damage to other structures. Any or all of the corneal layers may be injured. Small abrasions may heal uneventfully, but larger ones are liable to infection; and the resulting ulcers will sometimes leave dense opacity in their train. Edema and striate opacity of the substantia propria have been repeatedly observed, and Descemet's membrane may be folded or ruptured. Scleral rupture is another serious possibility to be borne in mind, because it can at first be masked by conjuctival hemorrhage, and will commonly be associated with damage to the inner eye.

(b) *Lesions of the Inner Eye:* These occur in bewildering variety. Hyphema often arises from iris hemorrhage and will at first preclude detailed inspection of the fundus. The iris itself may display single or multiple ruptures of the pupillary margin, with or without implication of the sphincter muscle; or its ciliary margin may be partly torn across to produce an iridodialysis. Occasionally the whole peripheral attachment of the iris gives way, and the retracted ball of uveal tissue is later seen lying free in the anterior chamber. Interference with the ciliary body is presumably the explanation for that persistent hypotony which has been detected in some boxers, and sometimes an insidious iridocyclitis supervenes. The worst cases advance relentlessly to a state of phthisis bulbi. Occasionally a lesion of the ciliary body is limited to its muscle; whence follows paralysis of accommodation. The lens may be subluxated or totally dislocated, and cataract is not uncommon. In this connection, it must be remembered that the full effect of lens concussion may be delayed for months or years. Thus, eyes apparently undamaged may in fact have sustained stresses which will betray themselves after a lag. *Cataract* may also emerge as a complication of cyclitis in an eye damaged by boxing.

Hemorrhage into the vitreous may be derived from the anterior or the posterior segment of the globe or from both. In all except very severe cases, absorption tends at first to be complete, but repeated hemorrhages encourage the deposition of those fibrous strands which perhaps herald retinitis proliferans.

Retinal detachment is one of the most dreaded consequences of boxing, and a number of bilateral cases are recorded in the literature. Here it must be emphasized that the chances of permanent reposition by surgical treatment are much less than they are in other types of juvenile detachment. Among those who have testified to this effect is [44]. Operation was considered feasible in only 5 out of his series of 29 retinal detachments due to boxing, and even among these 5 relatively favorable cases, only one retina was successfully reattached. Cystic and pigmentary changes at the macula are another tragic outcome of blows upon the eyes, and retinal hemorrhages are commoner than many people realize.

Choroidal hemorrhages are even more destructive, and almost certainly originate those irregularly shaped, mottled, raised areas of degeneration which are so ophthalmoscopically conspicuous in the seasoned pugilist. Whenever we see a bruiser with a pair of cauliflower ears, let us be on the lookout for cauliflower choroids. These multiple fundus lesions account for many a boxer's defective visual acuity. Then again, a choroidal rupture may involve the macula. Optic atrophy is another possible fundus finding. Avulsion of the optic nerve can produce complete atrophy, and so can hemorrhage into the nerve sheaths. *Partial consecutive atrophy* is a sequel of repeated traumatic hemorrhage, especially from the choroid.

Recurrent congestive glaucoma is another potential danger for a man exposed to repeated blows upon the eyes, and this condition may produce a blind, painful eye; but it is abundantly clear that, for every troublesome eye which has to be removed, several remain as nonfunctioning, though painless, vestiges, and in many others vision is permanently curtailed.

(2) Injuries to Neighboring Structures, Including the Ocular Adnexa

Diffuse thickening of the bone along the orbital margins is not uncommonly evident in ring veterans. *Localized hyperostoses* have also been found encroaching upon the orbital cavity. Any of the bones that form the orbit may be fractured, especially the ethmoid, maxilla, malar, and lacrimal bones. *Orbital emphysema* is apt to arise when the accessory air cells, especially those of the ethmoid, are involved in a fracture; and *obstruction of the nasolacrimal duct* is one of the complications of a broken nose. The lacrimal gland itself may suffer damage, and another possible source of orbit may be fractured, especially the ethmoid, maxilla, malar, and lacrimal bones. Orbital emphysema is apt to arise when the accessory air cells, specially those of the ethmoid, are involved in a fracture; and obstruction of the nasolacrimal duct is one of the complications of a broken nose. The lacrimal gland insert suffer damage, and another possible source of deranged lacrimal function is injury to a canaliculus.

Hearing Impairments

While there exists a vast body of literature concerning the results of single head injuries, only a few papers have been published on the effects of repeated head injuries on the hearing organ. While head injuries usually occur as isolated accidents in the average person's life, boxers are subjected to numerous repeated head injuries over a number of years. The damage to the hearing apparatus is of particular interest to the otologist, since the hearing losses in these cases are caused by repeated injuries to the head.

Disturbances of hearing were first reported by De KLEYN (1941) [59]. The majority of the boxers whom he examined revealed disturbances of hearing at the 4000 Hz frequency.

Impaired hearing after blunt injuries of the head without skull fractures was first demonstrated using audiometric curves after the Second World War.

PAULSEN and HUNDHAUSEN (1971) [60] presented a classic study, they examined 43 men audiometrically; 35 were amateur, the remaining 8 professional, boxers. Twenty-five of them were between 20 and 30 years of age, 11 were under 20 years, and 7 over 30 years. Apart from the question of the frequency and extent of these hearing losses, their reversibility and any typical features of the characteristic audiometric curves of the hearing pattern, the injuries to the hearing function are of particular interest to the otologist because the hearing losses involved in these cases are caused by repeated injuries to the head.

The boxers in this study were grouped by weight into the following classes: (1) Feather-lightweight (up to 61 kg); (2) half welter-welterweight (from 62 to 67 kg); (3) light middleweight-middleweight (68 to 72 kg); (4) light heavyweight (73 to 80 kg); and (5) heavyweight (above 80 kg).

The number of bouts ranged from one to 400. Thirteen boxers were involved in between one and 8 bouts, 12 boxers between 10 and 20 bouts, 9 boxers between 30 and 90 bouts, 6 boxers between 100 and 200 bouts, and 3 boxers between 300 and 400 bouts.

Threshold audiometric recordings were taken of all the boxers, as well as "above threshold" audiometric curves.

The greatest difficulty existed, according to Paulsen et al., in convincing the boxers - amateurs and professionals - to subject themselves to an audiometric examination. More than the boxers, however, it was the trainers and the representatives of the *Amateur Boxing Association of the State of Schleswig-Holstein, Germany*, who rejected the audiometric examination, with the argument that the yearly medical routine examination should be sufficient, and that medical publications concerning the sport of boxing were considered detrimental, especially in regard to young recruits.

It was only with great difficulty that, finally, 43 boxers could be examined. Only those boxers whose hearing impairments could be related only to boxing were examined.

The audiometric findings were evaluated using the following criteria:

(1) The extent of the hearing impairment in the different weight classes.

Due to the greater body weight the striking force of a heavyweight is higher than that of a flyweight. Since in boxing fights two boxers of the same weight class always fight each other, the striking force which connects with the head of the opponent will increase with the increasing weight class.

(2) The extent of the hearing impairment in relation to the total number of bouts.

The longer a boxer is active, the more frequently he is hit by his opponent against the head. It has to be taken into consideration that the boxer is not only subjected to blows against his head in matches and meets, but also during training and while involved in sparring bouts. Each boxer is subjected to repeated blows against his head in every week of his career, since boxers normally train at least twice a week.

Audiometric Findings in the Different Weight Classes

1) *Feather-lightweight* (up to 61 kg - 8 boxers)
Two boxers in this class revealed no hearing losses; the remaining 6 exhibited hearing losses in the frequencies between 1000 and 8000 Hz.

(2) *Half-welter-welterweight* (62 to 67 kg - 13 boxers)
Six audiograms were normal, but the remaining 7 showed hearing losses in the high frequencies. In the mean curves a slight hearing impairment occurred in the higher frequencies.

(3) *Light middle-middleweight* (68 to 72 kg - 10 boxers)
One boxer had a normal audiogram; in two cases there was a bilateral, continuous decrease in the high frequencies. The curve of a boxer with 300 amateur and 98 professional bouts dipped on the left side at 1000 Hz, and on the right side at 1500 Hz to 70 dB hearing impairment and revealed a dip at c^5 with 50 dB hearing loss. The remaining 7 boxers revealed hearing impairments in the middle and high frequencies. In the mean curve, slight hearing impairments can be seen in the middle and higher frequencies.

(4) *Light heavyweight* (73 to 80 kg - 6 boxers)
This group also revealed hearing losses in the middle and higher frequencies. In 3 cases the left ear was more involved than the right. The mean curve revealed a trough-shaped hearing loss above 2000 Hz with accentuation of the frequencies between 3000 and 4000 Hz.

(5) *Heavyweight* (above 80 kg - 6 boxers)
The curves of the 6 boxers in this class revealed, in two cases, depressions between 3000 and 6000 Hz. The remaining 4 audiograms showed a continuous hearing impairment above 1000 or 1500 Hz. This is shown in the mean curve as well.

Threshold Audiometric Findings of Boxers Related to the Total Number of Bouts

(1) *1 to 9 bouts - 13 boxers*
This group was composed of 4 boxers in weight class one (WC 1), 6 in WC 2, two in WC 3, and one in WC 4. The audiogram of 7 boxers revealed no hearing impairments with more than 10 dB. The remaining boxers showed in their audiograms only a slight hearing loss in the higher frequencies. This can be seen in the mean curve as a flat trough between 1500 and 8000 Hz.

(2) *10 to 29 bouts - 12 boxers*
This group was made up of two boxers of WC 1, 4 of WC 2, two of WC 3, two of WC 4, and two of WC 5. Two boxers revealed practically no hearing loss. The audiogram of the remaining boxers revealed a very slight hearing loss in the lower frequencies, on the right side more than on the left, and slight but definite hearing impairments in the form of troughs between 1500 and 12000 Hz. In single cases isolated dips can be seen. The mean curve revealed a slight but definite hearing loss

ın trough form between 1500 and 12000 Hz, mainly in the higher
frequencies.

(3) *30 'to 99 bouts - 9 boxers*

In this group were two boxers of WC 1, two of WC 2, 3 of WC 3,
and two in WC 5. In every case there was a hearing impairment of more
than 10 dB. All together the hearing loss is more pronounced. In one
case there was a continuous dip in the high frequencies, in another case
a steep dip at 1500 Hz with 75 dB hearing loss at 3000 Hz. Single
audiograms had dips in other flat troughs. The mean curve is
characterized by slight to medium hearing losses in the middle but
mainly in the higher frequencies. Bilaterally a slight trough at c^5 is
visible. The hearing impairment on the left side is more pronounced
than on the right.

(4) *100 to 200 bouts - 6 boxers*

This group consisted of one boxer in WC 2, two in WC 3, two in WC
4, and one in WC 5. All audiograms revealed hearing losses, which have
to be considered light to medium. With the exception of one boxer the
left side was more severely damaged than the right side. One boxer who
participated as an amateur for 11 years, with one hundred 41 bouts,
revealed (on the right side) a deep, trough-shaped hearing loss at c^5,
on the left side at fis^4. The mean curves showed on the right side a
flat trough-shaped hearing loss in the middle and especially in the
higher frequencies, with slight c^5 dip, and on the left side a
continuous hearing loss with accentuation in the higher frequencies and
slight fis^5 dip.

5) *300 to 400 bouts - 3 boxers*

All the boxers of this group revealed a marked hearing loss; each
of these boxers is a professional, who has boxed for many years. In two
cases the hearing impairment was bilateral. In the third case the left
side was slightly more damaged than the right side. In each of these
cases there is a continuous hearing loss, extending from the middle to
the higher frequencies. In every case there are dips and troughs, which
are most pronounced at c^5. The mean curve revealed bilaterally a marked
hearing loss in the middle and especially in the higher frequencies.
The hearing loss has already begun at 500 Hz. Bilaterally there was a
slight c^5 dip, wich is more pronounced on the left side than on the
right.

The findings demonstrate that 76.6% of the boxers have a
pathological audiogram.

Two of 8 boxers in the first weight class have normal hearing. In
the second class, there is a hearing loss of less than 10 dB in 7 out of
13 cases. In the third class (light middle - middleweight), only one out
of 10 boxers has no hearing loss. In the fourth and fifth weight classes
(light heavyweight and heavyweight) all boxers revealed hearing losses.

In the lighter weight classes up to 67 kg, no boxers show a steep
decline (dip) in the high frequencies. Troughs exist normally between
2000 and 6000 Hz, with a maximum of 4000 Hz.

Two boxers in the third class showed high tone dips in their
audiograms, with slight c^5 dips. The remaining classes revealed
depressions and troughs between 2000 and 6000 Hz. It is evident that
the troughs in 4 out of 7 cases are wider than in the lower weight
classes.

Depressions and troughs in the middle and higher frequencies also
occur in the light heavyweights. In two cases, depressions in the higher
frequencies are visible along with the troughs at 3000 and 2000 Hz.

In 4 out of 6 audiograms of heavyweights, there were both trough-shaped hearing losses in the middle and higher frequencies and depressions in the higher frequencies.

Extent of the Hearing Loss in Regard to the Number of Bouts

The hearing impairment grows with the increasing number of bouts. Boxers with less than 10 fights have practically normal hearing, with only minimal hearing losses in the high frequencies. In boxers with up to 30 fights hearing impairments can be recognized by depressions and troughs in the middle and especially in the higher frequencies. These hearing losses can be interpreted as minimal, despite the fact that they are more severe than in boxers with a lower number of fights.

Boxers with 30 to 99 fights reveal, usually in the middle and high frequencies, trough-shaped and sometimes continuous hearing losses. The mean curve reveals bilaterally flat troughs. The hearing impairments in boxers with one 100 to 200 bouts are more severe. Here also, in the middle and higher frequencies, are trough-shaped or continuous hearing losses. The mean curve shows bilaterally a slight c^5 dip. The most severe hearing impairment appears in boxers with more than 300 bouts. The hearing deficit is especially severe in the middle frequencies, and hearing is severely impaired.

In summary, it can be said that with an increasing number of bouts, the hearing impairment increases (but it should be mentioned that in single cases the hearing losses can be minimal).

The extent of the hearing impairment after blunt impacts to the head is in general related to two factors, namely the intensity and number of impacts. There authors [60] took both factors into consideration, by evaluating the audiograms as they related on the one side to the weight classes of the boxers, and on the other side to the number of fights. The results show convincingly that with an increasing intensity of impacts (higher weight class) and an increasing number of impacts (number of fights), there is an increase in hearing impairment. The number of fights seems to be of greater importance.

Despite the small number of cases examined the audiograms can be classified into 3 types of curves:

Curve type A - shows slight hearing impairments in the high frequency of the type of a dip at c^5. This dip can appear at higher or lower frequencies. In this area flat trough-shaped hearing impairments can be seen, which do not appear in excessive noise trauma. This type of curve may possibly be interpreted as specific for a status after repeated head impacts.

Curve type B - reveals a wider trough-shaped hearing deficit with a maximum of around 3000 - 4000 Hz. In single cases this trough-shaped hearing deficiency may appear in higher frequencies.

Curve type C - is characterized by a continuous hearing loss beginning in the lower part of the middle frequency with severe damage in higher frequencies combined with a slight c^5 dip.

If one compares these three curve types with the corresponding curves of hearing impairment due to sound and noise trauma, it is impossible then to decide, using the audiogram, whether the cause for the hearing impairments is a mechanical trauma, a noise trauma, or chronic exposure to excessive noise. The ear reacts in the same way to different types of the same noxious event; slight injury leads as a rule to alterations and hearing loss in the high frequencies especially around 4000 Hz; more serious injuries produce more severe and more marked alterations in the form of trough-shaped hearing losses, which can extend into the middle frequencies; and severe injuries, or injuries resulting from repeated impacts over a longer period, lead to a high-tone loss which finally covers large parts of the middle frequencies as well.

In general, the classification of the types of hearing impairment due to boxing is not as simple as the classification due to noise or explosion trauma.

The Relationship of Hearing Impairments to the Localization of the Impact

PAULSEN and HUNDHAUSEN (1971) [60] quoted the literature and came to the conclusion that the nearer the impact occurs to the ear, the heavier is the hearing loss.

The boxer is hit mainly against the frontal parts of his face and on the forehead, but also against lateral parts of the temple and the ear. Blows against the occiput are against the rules, but they are dished out from time to time.

The results of PAULSEN and HUNDHAUSEN [60]reveal a very interesting finding. In 12 cases, the left ear showed a more severe hearing deficit than the right one. The explanation should be that the vast majority of all boxers are right- handed - the left hand leads, and the right hand hits. The most severe blows will be delivered by the right hand against the left side of the head of the opponent.

Above-threshold audiometry: The localization of the hearing impairment due to the results of above-threshold audiometry.

Twenty boxers out of 23 had an above-threshold audiometry. In 17 cases this demonstrated an above-threshold disturbance, and in 3 there was a retro-labyrinthine lesion. All 3 cases were professional boxers who had been involved in a large number of fights, and all had severe hearing losses.

Injuries to the Hand and the Wrist

To understand the injuries of boxer's hands, one must first analyze the position of the fist inside a boxing glove. Boxers in their gloves with fists clenched as tight as possible were x-rayed [61]. It could be shown, that the metacarpophalangeal joints were only flexed to about 50 to 60 o, with the fingers slightly open and the thumb almost straight and abducted from the side. This is largely due to the fact that the hand has to grip the palm of the glove and is therefore more open. Due to the splinting effect of the thumb encasement and the fact that the passing on the side causes the thumb to be a little on one side, the thumb, if not held close into the side of the glove, is placed in a position fo maximum vulnerability and is most liable for injury. The distortion of the metacarpophalangeal joint of the thumb is the more common hand injury of boxers than the metacarpals, followed by distortion of the hand joints and fractures of the navicular bone [62]. It has been suggested that the use of the thumbless boxing glove might not only minimize eye injuries but also protect the thumb from injury.

Only 5o% of boxers end their careers without any trace of injury on their hands [63,64].

Cardiac Injuries

The *heart* and *pericardium,* lying close behind the anterior chest wall, are very vulnerable to blows in the region of the pericardium. Traumatic injuries of the heart in boxers are more frequent than realized. Professional boxers found that the effects of well-placed hooks to the heart usually last for the rest of the fight (Jokl 1941). Fatal injuries were reported by [65-67].

Acute Renal Damage

The changes that occur in a man's urine after he has engaged in a boxing match have been studied by Amelar and Solomon (1954) and Kleiman (1958).

Urine samples in 139 professionals before and after a bout were examined by [68]. The authors found that in 46% of the fighter's urine specimens changed from clear before the fight to turbid immediately afterwards, and the specific gravity increased in 80% of the cases. Traces of aceton were manifest in 14%. The urinary pH decreased in 30%. Sugar was spilled in the urine in 9% of the boxers. Albuminuria, which was not present before the bout, was present in 68% of the boxers after the fight. Microscopically, red blood cells were found in significant pathological amounts in 73% of the boxers after fighting, and 26% were found to have casts of granular or hyaline variety in their urine.

In summarizing their findings, they concluded that they had proved the obvious, namely, that in addition to an effect of exercise, there is also an effect of acute trauma observed in the urine of boxers immediately after the fight and its obvious bearing on the amount of renal trauma.

Significant hematuria in 27% of 764 professional boxers in the postbout specimens of urine were found by [69[. Roentgenographic studies revealed structural abnormatities of the kidneys in many cases of hematuria and suggested that such defects render the kidneys more susceptible to the trauma of boxing (as demonstrated by the high incidence of recurrent postbout hematuria).

DAMAGE TO THE CENTRAL NERVOUS SYSTEM

Different Knock-down and Knock-out Mechanisms

Clinically, boxing injuries can be grouped into *acute* and *chronic types*. The most notable example of the acute group is the knock-down or the knock-out. In a knock-out the boxers is so disabled by a boxing blow or a series of blows that he is unable to stand on his feet after 10 seconds to continue the fight. A technical knock-out is declared when the fight is stopped by the referee or a ring physician due to an apparent injury or the defenselessness of one participant. A distinction must be made between a *cerebral knock-out* and a *body knock-out*.

Cerebral Knock-out

A *cerebral concussion* or *commotio cerebri* with immediate unconsciousness with loss of muscle tone may be the result of a heavy blow with acceleration of the head. The intensity of the impacting glove has, in such a case, been high enough to accelerate the head to a threshold which leads to the concussive syndrome. The unconsciousness and the loss of posture occur instantly, within a fraction of a second after the impact, and the boxer collapses on the spot; he may land on his back, in a prone position, or even draped over the ropes.

Not in every knock-out occurs a cerebral concussion or commotio cerebri. A hard blow may lead to a loss of muscle tone without loss of

consciousness, or the boxer is not able to get up due to severe pain or
vertigo.

Anemia of the brain cannot be used to explain a commotio cerebri,
since the effects of such a process would require at least 8 to 10
seconds. A delayed loss of posture with unconsciousness due to anemia
of the brain is an event in which at least several seconds elapse before
all symptoms become evident. It occurs in boxing, when a boxer goes down
some seconds after being hit.

Oculocardiac Reflex Mechanismen (Aschner-Dagnini-Reflex)

Bernhard Aschner in Vienna [70] and Guiseppe Dagnini in Bologna
[71] reported independently of each other 1908 slowing of cardiac
actions as the result of a pressure on the eye bulb. This phenomenon
received much interest in the medical literature; the phenomenon was
termed a oculocardiac or Aschner-Dagnini reflex. A severe blow or
pressure at the eye can result in bradycardia, decrease in the
respiratory rate and vomiting [72-75].

Several authors have developed theories about a knock-out
mechanism, which cannot be discussed here in detail [76-79].

Body Knock-out

Boxing blows are allowed against all parts of the body above the
waistline.

"Groggy States" and "Pummeling Knock-out" (Verhämmerungs Knock-out)

Occasionally a boxer is *groggy* after a series of blows to the
head. His movements are then slower than normal, less certain, and his
sensorium is impaired. The muscle tone, most obviously that of the neck,
is reduced, and the head moves like a pendulum under the blows. It
therefore sustains higher accelerations and, consequently, more severe
effects. Unless a sensible referee stops the bout it will end with the
boxer hammered into a knock-out state (*"hammering knock-out'* or
"Verhämmerungs-knock-out"), a terminus which speaks for itself, or with
his no longer being able to instigate voluntary motor activity. States
of "grogginess", in which consciousness is reduced, are not rare,
according to the testimony of boxers and descriptions in the medical
literature. The boxer is *"out on his feet"* and is unable to defend
himself. His arms hang loosely down at his sides, and he runs a very
high risk of being subsequently hit and severely injured by a series of
blows to the head and neck.

Boxing Blows Against the Lateral Region of the Neck

The range of boxing blows against the lateral region of the neck
embraces still another possibility of acute damage, namely mechanical
irritation of the carotid sinus and compression of the carotid artery.
Both knock-downs and knock-outs are possible.

The Carotissinus-Syndrome and the so-called Hyperactive Carotissinus-Reflex

Hering [80] called attention to a network of receptor nerves at
the bifurcation of the internal and external carotid artery; he called
these structures "carotid sinus". This author had already alluded to

the possibility that boxers could be knocked-out by blows against the carotid sinus.

Application of mechanical pressure to the carotid artery may result in bradycardia and an asystolia. It may provoke one of the 3 forms of the carotid sinus syndrome; the resulting unconsciousness is the result of a depressive, cardiac, or central type of the syndrome [81]. In the first 2 mentioned forms, the drop in blood pressure, the bradycardia or asystolia lead, respectively, to an hypoxemia or anoxemia of the brain, after which unconsciousness may occur in a few seconds. In the third, disputed form, the immediate unconsciousness with loss of posture occurs reflectively.

Ruptures of internal layers of the carotid artery with lamellar hemorrhages (dissecting aneurysms) and thromboses have been described, which can lead to reduced cerebral blood supply and eventually, due to softening and necrosis of brain tissue in their supporting area, especially that of the middle cerebral artery, to a hemiparesis. Cases were described by [82-84].

Blunt blows against frontal parts of the neck can produce injuries of the larynx and glottis [85]. A boxer hit on the throat may stagger and gasp for air. Press photographs and descriptions of boxers hit against the throat record that these injuries can easily incapacitate.

Blows against the precordial region may produce alterations in cardiac actions which can result in a knock-out.

Blunt flat blows to the thorax and abdomen which cause a marked stimulation of the vagovagal reflex) [6].

Blows against the abdomen may lead to additional extensive reactions. The celiac plexus (solar plexus), which contains many ganglia, is the largest of the vegetative nervous system. It rests upon the abdominal aorta and extends into the area of the branches of the celiac artery, superior mesenteric artery, and renal artery; cranially it connects with the thoracic aortic plexus and caudally with the abdominal aortic plexus.

Chronic Clinical Findings

The chronic clinical pictures of exboxers reveal a considerable variation from case to case, but the one consistent feature is the evidence of many diffuse lesions in the brain. The progressive clinical symptoms become noticeable after a number of years. The occurrence frequently coincides with the end of a boxer's active career, but it may occur a little later. Clinically the boxer exhibits a combination of pyramidal and extrapyramidal disturbances and cerebellar signs, such as disturbed gait and coordination, tremor of the hands and body, slurred dysarthric speech, and psychopathological findings.

It is a shocking experience to read reports of the mental deterioration in boxer's case histories. Typical features of the picture are a lack of reaction, uncritical attitude, illusion about one's capabilities, inadequate euphoric and some times dysphoric tempers, depravation, general deterioration of mental performance and considerable dementia. Many of these exboxers had to be transferred to psychopathic hospitals or asylums.

The pathologist Martland (1928)[87] called attention to the fact that for some time fight fans and promoters had recognized a peculiar condition among prize fighters which in ring parlance, they call "punch-drunk". He noted those most often affected are fighters of the slugging type. They are usually poor boxers and take considerable head punishment, seeking only to land a knock-out blow. It is also common in second rate fighters used for training purposes, who may be knocked-down several times a day. The author would add to this group those boxers with a long career behind them.

This condition known by several names, *dementia pugilistica* [88]. and *chronic progressive traumatic encephalopathy of the boxer* [89] among others. Courville [90] coined the phrase "*psychopathic deterioration of pugilists*". However, it is the slang expressions - *goofy, slug nutty, cuckoo, stumblebum, slap happy, cutting paper dolls* - which illustrate better than medical terms the exboxer's mental deterioration and depravation.

The early symptoms of punch drunkness usually appear in the extremities. There may only be an occasional and very slight flopping of one foot or leg in walking, noticeably only at intervals, or a slight unsteadiness in gait or uncertainty in equilibrium. These may seriously interfere with fighting. In some cases periods of slight mental confusion may occur, as well as distinct slowing of muscular actions. These early symptoms of punch drunkness are well known to fight fans and promotors [87].

Martland [87] stated that many cases remain mild and do not progress beyond these first symptoms. In other a very distinct dragging of the leg may develop, and with this there is a general slowing down in muscular movements, a peculiar mental attitude characterized by hesitancy in speech (dysarthria), tremor of the hands, and nodding movement of the head, necessitating withdrawal from the ring. Later on, in severe cases, there may develop a peculiar tilting of the head, a marked dragging of one or both legs, a staggering propulsive gait with the facial characteristics of the Parkinsonian syndrome, or a backward swaying of the body with tremors, vertigo, and deafness. Eventually a marked mental deterioration may set in, necessitating commitment to an asylum.

The author fully agrees with Martland on the classical clinical findings in punch drunk boxers, but does not agree with his interpretation of the pathomorphology of this syndrome. There is no doubt that this syndrome is the result of repeated blows to the head, but the "multiple concussion hemorrhages" that he mentions as being in the deeper portions of the cerebrum do not exist in this syndrome.

In medical literature it is frequently stated that this condition is due to "multiple petechial hemorrhages" in the deeper portions of the brain, followed by degenerative processes and a reparative gliosis. This view is incorrect. The pathomorphological findings as the result of the numerous repetitive blows against the head of boxers are of the hypoxic type; the neurons are destroyed and replaced by a reactive gliosis. Extensive histological examination of the brains of boxers resulted in the description and quantification of the boxer's encephalopathy [91-95]. These pathomorphological findings are similar, in some cases identical, to those lesions which were described by the author in different species of animals which were subjected to repeated subconcussive impacts, imitating the situation of the boxer in the ring who suffers multiple and repeated blows to the head. The resulting lesions are of the hypoxic type [96-98].

The above mentioned multiple petechial hemorrhages do in fact occur in the deeper portions of the cerebrum in boxers. They are frequently observed as hemorrhagic necroses of the brain and brain stem, which occur as acute findings in boxers who die as the results of complications of head injuries sustained in the ring. *They are the results of complications of head injuries after hemorrhages and hematomas of the enveloping structures of the brain*, of intracerebral hemorrhages, marked brain edema, thrombotic occlusion of extra- and intracranial vessels, etc. These hemorrhagic necroses of the brain develop minutes, hours or days after injuries in the ring and are considered very serious complications, which normally lead to the death of the boxer due mostly to a secondary traumatic midbrain syndrome. *These hemorrhagic necroses are not the substrata of the so-called "punch drunk" syndrome.* This confusion is partly the result of an inadequate nomenclature used by Courville [99], who termed these traumatic alterations "diffuse contusions of the brain"; they are not contusions but hemorrhagic necroses. The multiple petechial hemorrhages of the boxer brain as the morphological substrate of progressive boxer's encephalopathy do not exist, although the two seem inextricably entwined in the pertinent literature.

Beside the usual type of progressive postraumatic encephalopathies of the boxer, forms with hyperkinesias have been described [100-102].

Mawdsley and Ferguson [103] and Spillane [104] stated that the pneumencephalograms of 90% of 11 and 40% of 5 boxers, respectively, with severe clinical symptoms showed a tremendously enlarged cavum septi pellucidi communicating broadly with the ventricular system, as compared with a normal rate of 0,2 to 1,25% of the total number of pneumencephalogram [105-107].

A clinical study was published by Roberts in 1969 [108]. He based his work on a report by a Committee of the Royal College of Physicians in London on the medical aspects of boxing, in 1962. Two hundred and fifty exprofessional boxers from the 16 781 boxers registered between 1929 and 1955 were examined clinically and electroencephalographically in this investigation. The entire sample of boxers was traced, and with the exception of 9 who had emigrated, and 16 who had died, and 1 who had refused, all those traced (224) were examined. Electroencephalograms were available in 168 cases and independent accounts in over half of the sample. Roberts found in 37 cases (17%), there were clinically demonstrable lesions of the central nervous sytem which bore a close resemblance to the syndrome previously described in boxers. "The study has shown the relationship to occupational exposure of an easily recognizable and relatively stereotyped syndrome of disturbed neurological function."

Sixty amateur boxers with a record of more than 100 bouts, who had been observed over a period of 4 years were examined by [109].. Neurological abnormalities were found in 50% of the subjects; 18.3% exhibited mental disorders, and 40% electroencephalographic changes. In 5 cases (8.4%) frank clinical syndromes requiring hospitalization developed.

Computed tomography (CT) has lately been used as a further diagnostic tool in cases of boxers' encephalopathy. Using CT [110] studied 6 professional and 8 amateur boxers, who had been national champion of Finland; they found evidence of brain atrophy in 4 of the 6 professional and one of the amateur boxers. Also, 2 of the professionals and 8 of the amateur boxer had EEG abnormalities. The authors conclude their studies with: "The most predictable and permanent reward... is chronic brain damage... The only way to prevent brain injuries is to disqualify blows to the head."

Ross et al.[111] published their findings on 40 exboxers, of whom 38 had a CT scan of the brain and 24 a complete neurological examination, including an EEG. The results demonstrate a significant relationship between the number of bouts fought and CT changes indicating cerebral atrophy. Electroencephalographic abnormalities were significantly correlated with the number of bouts fought. These authors conclude their studies with the statement that "computed tomography and EEG of the brain should be considered as part of a regular neurological examination for active boxers, and if possible, before and after each

match, to detect not only the effects of acute life threatening brain
trauma such as subdural hematomas, but the more subtle and debilitating
long-term changes of cerebral atrophy."

Pathomorphology - Acute Injuries

All types of *intracranial hemorrhage* as caused by blows to the
head have been found in boxers.

Epidural Hemorrhages

Epidural hemorrhages do not occur often, but a fatal case has been
published [112]. A ruptured tentorium cerebelli at the connection of the
falx cerebri and rupture of the longitudinal sinus in an amateur boxer
[113] were caused by a punch to the chin that must have been strong
enough to produce considerable skull deformation and therefore
overstraining of the dural duplicature.

Subdural Hemorrhages

Subdural hemorrhages are a frequent injury, making up more than
75% of all acute brain injuries combined, and occupy first place among
boxing fatalities. Numerous observations of subdural hemorrhage, mostly
involving amateur boxers, have been published [114-135].

Pathomorphology - Late and Permanent Brain Damage

Morphological studies on late and permanent brain damage in boxers
were carried out by [91-95].

REFERENCES:

[1] Jokl, E., The Medical Aspect of Boxing, van Schaik, Pretoria, 1941.
{2] Pöschl, M. and Krieger, G., "Todesfälle beim Sport und medizinische
Fragen ihrer Prophylaxe", Münchener Medizinische Wochenschrift, Vol.
105, 1963, pp. 2205-2216.
[3] Critchley, M., "Medical aspects of boxing", British Medical Journal,
Vol. I, 1957, pp.357-362.
[4] Winterstein, C.E., "Head injuries attributable to boxers", Lancet,
Vol. II, 1937, pp. 719-720.
[5] Bass, A.L., Blonstein, J.L., James, R.D., and Williams, J.G.P.,
Medical Aspects of Boxing, Pergamon Press, Oxford London New York, 1965.
[6] Sercl, M., and Jaros O., "Boxing and the Damage to the Nervous
System, Sbor Med Praci Hradec Kralov, Supplement to Collection of
Scientific Works of the Faculty of Medicine, Charles University of
Hradec Kralov, 1968.
[7] Unterharnscheidt, F., "About boxing: Review of historical and
medical aspects, Texas Reports on Biology and Medicine, Vol. 28, 1970,
pp. 421-495.
[8] Unterharnscheidt, F., "Traumatische Schäden des Zentralnervensystems
bei Boxern", In: Stucke, K. (ed) Verhandlungen Deutscher Sportärztebund,
24. Tagung, Würzburg, October 14-17, 1971, Demeter, Gräfelfing, 1971,
pp. 116-121.
[9] Unterharnscheidt, F., "Traumatische Hirnschäden bei Boxern. Eine
Übersicht", Schweizerische Zeitschrift für Sportmedizin, Vol. 20, 1972,
pp. 131-175.

[10] Unterharnscheidt, F., Injuries due to boxing and other sports. In: Braakman R. (ed) Injuries of the Brain and Skull, Part I, Vol. 23. In: Vinken, P.J. and Bruyn, G.W. (ed) Handbook of Clinical Neurology, North-Holland Publ. Corp., Amsterdam, 1975, pp. 527-593.

[11} Unterharnscheidt, F., Boxing injuries, Chapter 25. In: Schneider, R.C., Kennedy, J.C., and Plant, M.L. (eds) Sports Injuries. Mechanisms, Prevention, and Treatment, Williams & Wilkins, Baltimore, 1985, pp. 462-495.

[12] Roberts, A.H., Brain Damage in Boxers. A Study of the Prevalence of Traumatic Encephalopathy among Ex-professional Boxers, Pitman Medical Science Publ. Corp., London, 1969

[13] Unterharnscheidt, F, and Sellier, K. "Vom Boxen: Mechanik, Pathomorphologie und Klinik der traumatischen Schäden des ZNS bei Boxern" Fortschritte der Neurologie und Psychiatrie, Vol. 39, 1971, pp.109-151.

[14] Homer, The Iliad, translated by Richard Lattimore, University of Chicago Press, Chicago, 1951.

[15] Pausanias, Description of Greec, books I and II, with an English transaltion by W.H.S. Jones, The Loeb Classical Library,No. 93, Harvard University Press, Cambridge, MA, 1969.

[16] Pausanias, Description of Greece,Books III, IV, and V, with an English tarnsaltion by W.H.S Jones and H.A. Ormerod, The Loeb Classical Library, No.188, Harvard University Press, Cambridge, MA, 1966.

[17] Jüthner J. Über antike Turngeräte. Abhandlungen des epigraphischen Seminars der Universität Wien, Hölder, Wien, 1886.

[18] Brein,F. (ed) Jüthner, Julius, Die athletischen Leibesübungen der Griechen, I. Geschichte der Leibesübungen. Böhlaus Nachfolger, Graz Wien Köln, 1965.

[19] Rudolph, W. Olympischer Kampfsport in der Antike. Faustkampf, Ringkampf und Pankaration in den griechischen Nationalfestspielen. Schriften aus der Sektion für Altertumskunde, Heft 47, Akademie Verlag, Berlin, 1965.

[20] Krause, J.H., Die Gymnastik und Agonistik der Hellenen, 2 Bd., Leipzig, 1841, Reprint, Sändig, Wiesbaden, 1971.

[21] Plato, The Laws, The Loeb Classical Library, Vol. X, books I-IV, No. 187, Harvard University Press, Cambridge, MA, 1926.

[22] Gardiner, E.N., Greek Athletic Sports and Festivals. Mac Millan, London, 1910, Reprint, Brown, Dubuque, IA, 1970.

[23] Philostratos, Gymnastik.

[24]Schröder, B., Der Sport im Altertum, Schoetz, Berlin, 1927.

[25] Mezö, F., Geschichte der olympischen Spiele, München, 1930.

[26] Homer, Odyssey, The Loeb Classical Library, 2 vol., translated by A.T. Murray, No.104 & No. 105, Harvard University Press, Cambridge, MA, 1919.

[27] Antyllus, Oribasius.

[28] Gardiner, E.N., Athletics of the Ancient World, Clarendon Press, Oxford, 1930, Reprint, Ares, Chicago, 1980.

[29] Aristophanes, The Birds, Peace, translated into verse by Benjamin Bickley Rogers, The Loeb Classical Library. No. 79, Harvard University Press, Cambridge, MA, 1924.

[30] Sellier, K. and Unterharnscheidt, F. Mechanik und Pathomorphologie der Hirnschäden nach stumpfer Gewalteinwirkung auf den Schädel, Hefte zur Unfallheilkunde, Heft 76, Springer, Berlin Göttingen Heidelberg, 1963.

[31] Unterharnscheidt, F. and Sellier, K. Mechanics and pathomorphology of closed brain injuries, Chapt. 26, In: Caveness, W.F.and Walker, A.E.

(eds) Head Injury, Conference Proceedings, Lippincott. Philadelphia Toronto, 1966, pp. 321-341.

[32] Unterharnscheidt, F. and Ripperger, E.A. Mechanics and pathomorphology of impact-related brain injuries. In: Perrone, N.(ed) Dynamic Response of Biomechanical Systems, The American Society of Mechanical Engineers, New York, 1970, pp. 46-83.

[33]Unterharnscheidt, F. Translational versus rotational acceleration - Animal experiments with measured input, Proceedings 15th Stapp Car Crash Conference, November 17-19, 1971, Coronado, CA, Society of Automotive Engineers, New York, 1972, pp. 767-770.

[34] Unterharnscheidt, F. and Sellier, K. "Vom Boxen. 1. Mitteilung. Mechanik der traumatischen Schäden des ZNS bei Boxern," Medizin und Sport, Vol.10, 1970, pp. 35-45.

[35] Unterharnscheidt, F. and Sellier, K. "Vom Boxen. 2. Mitteilung. Pathomorphologie und Klinik der traumatischen Schäden des ZNS bei Boxern, Medizin und Sport, Vol. 10. 1970, pp. 111-117.

[36] Palazzi, S. "Cranio-faziale Traumen bei Boxern und Kieferschutzapparat," Zeitschrift für Stomatologie, Vol. 23, 1925, pp. 873-882.

[37] Rolauf, 1937, quoted by Jokl, E., 1941.

[38] Millard, R.D. "Closure of boxing lacerations between rounds," Archives of Surgery, Vol. 86, 1963, pp. 295-298.

[39] Mandl, F. Chirurgie der Sportunfälle, Boxen, Kap. 9, Urban & Schwarzenberg, Wien, 1925, pp. 195-215.

[40] Gottlieb, I. and Gottlieb, O. "Fractura mandibulae opstaet ved Boxning," (Danish with English summary), Ugeskrift for Laeger, Vol. 113. 1951, pp. 1268-1270.

[41] Ellis, M. "Maxillo-facial injuries". In: Bass, A.L., Blonstein, J.L., James, R.R., and Williams, J.G.P. (eds) Medical Aspects of Boxing, Pergamon Press, Oxford London New York, 1965, pp. 23-28.

[42] Seltzer, A.P. "Surgery of the pugilists nose," Annals of Otology, Rhinology, and Laryngology, Vol. 59, 1950, pp. 924-930.

[43] Doggart, J.H. Eye injuries. In: Bass, A.L., Blonstein, J.L., James, R.D., and Wi;lliams, J.G.P. (eds) Medical Aspects of Boxing, Pergamon Press, Oxford London New York, 1965, pp. 3-7.

[44] Albaugh, C.M. "Eye problems in boxing," Journal of the International College of Surgeons, Vol. 17, 1952, pp. 191-194.

[45] Favory, A."Les lésions oculaires dues à la boxe de combat," Presse Medicale, Vol. 45, 1937, pp. 254-257.

[46]Boshoff, P.H. and Jokl, E "Boxing injuries of the eyes," Archives of Ophthalmology, Vol. 39, 1948, pp. 643-644.

[47] Doggard, J.H. "Fisticuffs and the visual organ," Transactions of the Ophthalmological Society (United Kingdom), Vol. 71, 1951, pp. 53-59.

[48] Doggart, J.H. "Blessures à la vision par la boxe," Bolletino d' Oculista, Vol. 44, 1954, pp. 273-284.

[49] Doggart, J.H. "The impact of boxing upon the visual apparatus" Archives of Ophthalmology, Vol. 54, 1955, pp. 161-169.

[50] Faviry, A, and Sedan, J. "Traumatologie oculaire du boxeur," Archives d' Ophthalmologie, Vol. 11, 1952, pp. 429-456.

[51] Glees, M. "Über Boxverletzungen der Augen," Klinische Monatsblätter für Augenheilkunde, Vol. 124, 1954, pp. 101-103.

[52] Löhlein, W. "Zur Prognose der Boxverletzungen der Augen," Klinische Monatsblätter für Augenheilkunde, Vol. 124, 1954, pp. 570-573.

[53] Graham, J.W. Medical care of the boxer. In: Bass, A.L., Blonstein, J.L., James, R.D., and Williams, J.G.P. (eds) Medical Aspects of Boxing, Pergamon Press, Oxford London New York, 1965, pp. 85-91.

[54] Wolff, S.M. and Zimmerman, L.E. "Chronic secondary glaucoma associated with retrodisplacement of iris root and deepening of the anterior angle secondary to contusion," American Journal of Ophthalmology, Vol. 54, 1962, pp. 547-563.

[55]Palmer, E. Lieberman, T.W, and Burns, A. "Contusion angle deformity in prize fighters, Archives of Ophthalmology, Vol. 94, 1976, pp. 225-228.

[56] Hruby, K. "Netzhautablösung beim Boxsport," Klinische Monatsblätter für Augenheilkunde, Vol. 174, 1979, pp. 314-316.

[57] Maguire, J.I. and Benson, W.E. "Retinal injury and detachment in boxers," Journal of the American Medical Association, Vol. 255, 1986, pp. 2451-2453.

[58]Enzenauer, R.W. and Mauldin, W.M. "Boxing-related ocular injuries in the United States Army, 1980 top 1985, Southern Medical Journal, Vol. 82, 1989, pp. 547-549.

[59] De Kleyn, A. Proceedings Koninglijke Nederlande Akademie van Wedenschappen, Vol. 44, 1941, p. 787.

[60] Paulsen, K, and Hundhausen T. "Hörschäden durch Boxen", Zeitschrift für Rhinologie Otologie und Grenzgebiete, Vol. 50, 1971, pp. 297-324.

[61] Farrow, R, Hand injuries. In: Bass, A.L., Blonstein, J.L., James, R.D., and Williams, J.G.D. (eds) Medical Aspects of Boxing, Pergamon Press, Oxford London New York, 1965, pp. 43-50.

[62] Gladden: J.R. "Boxer's knuckle: A preliminary report," American Journal of Surgery, Vol. 93, 1957, pp. 388-397.

[63] Ducroquet, quoted by Schmid, L., 1970.

[64] Schmidt, L. "Die Bedeutung des Boxhandschuhs für die Prophylaxe von Verletzungen," Medizin und Sport, Vol. 10, 1970, pp. 117-119.

[65]Bramann C. von "Lebensgefahr im Kampfsport," Münchener Medizinische Wochenschrift, Vol. 7, 1927, pp. 634-636.

[66] Deutsch, F. "Sekundenherztod im Boxkampf durch Commotio cordis," Wiener Archiv für Innere Medizin, Vol. 20, 1928, pp. 279-286.

[67] Jankovitch, L. "Suites mortelles d'un combat de boxe," Annals de Medecine Legale, Vol. 15, 1935, pp. 795-799.

[68] Amelar, R.D. and SDolomon, C. "Acute renal trauma in boxers," Journal of Urology, Vol. 72, 1954, pp. 145-148.

[69] Kleiman, A.H. "Hematuria in boxers," Journal of the American Medical Association, Vol. 168, 1958, pp. 1633-1640.

[70] Aschner, B. Ueber einen bishrer noch nicht bveschriebenen Reflex vom Auge auf Kreislauf und Atmung: Verschwinden des Radialispulses bei Druck auf das Auge," Wiener klinische Wochenschrift, Vol. 21, 1908, pp. 1529-1530.

[71] Dagnini, G. "Intorno ad un riflesso provocato in alcuni emiplegici collo stimulo dell cornea e colla pressione sub bulbo oculare," Bolletino Sciencia Medicale, Vol. 8, 1908, pp. 380-381.

[72] Bernards, J.A. "The orbitocirculatory reflex. I. Effects of pressure on the eyes on the circulation in the dog, Archives Internationales de Physiologie, Vol. 68, 1960, pp. 761-773.

[73] Hollwich, F., Brandt, H.P. and Zintl,F. "Der okulo-kardiale Reflex in augenärztlicher Sicht," Medizinische Klinik, Vol. 60, 1972, pp. 170-172.

[74] Pruche, A. "Le réflexe oculo-cardiaque; etude electroencephalographique, Archives des Maladies du Coeur, Vol. 26, 1933, pp. 724-751.

[75] Jimenez Espinosa, L. and Espinosa Iberra, J. "Knock-out and syncope in professional boxing: An EEG study, Electroencephalography and Clinical Neurophysiology, Vol. 72, 1960, pp. 196-197.

[76] Sherrington, C.S. Integrative Action of the Nervous System, London, 1906.

[77] Somen, H. "Le mécanisme physiologique du knock-out," Paris Medecine, Vol. 13, 1913/1914, pp. 54-57.

[78] Flint, A. Pugilism, Vol. 2, Chap 44. In: Collected Essays and Articles on Physiology and Medicine, Appleton, New York, 1903, pp. 319-329.

[79] Govons, S.R. "Brain concussion and posture. The knock-down blow of the boxing ring, Confinia Neurologica, Vol. 30, 1968, pp. 77-84.

[80] Hering, H.E. Die Karotissinus-Reflexe auf Herz und Gefäße, vom normal-physiologischen, pathologisch-physiologischen und klinischen Standpunkt. Steinkopff, Leipzig, 1927.

[81] Franke, H. Über das Karotissinus-Syndrom und den sogenannten hyperaktiven Karotissinusreflex, Schattauer, Stuttgart, 1963.

[82] Starassmann, G. and Helpern, M. "Tödliche Hirnverletzungen im Boxkampf," Deutsche Zeitschrift für die gesamte gerichtliche Medizin, Vol. 63, 1968, pp. 70-83.

[83] Hockaday, T.D.R. "Traumatic thrombosis of the internal carotid artery, Journal of Neurology, Neurosurgery and Psychiatry, Vol. 22, 1959, pp. 229-231.

[84] Murphy, F. and Miller, D.H. "Carotid insufficiency - diagnosis and surgical treatment. A report of twenty-one cases," Journal of Neurosurgery, Vol. 16, 195 ,pp. 1-23.

[85] Sury K. von "Boxtodesfall infolge akutem Larynxödems, Deutsche Zeitschrift für die gesamte gerichtliche Medizin, Vol. 1, 1922, pp. 695-696.

[86] Goltz, F. "Vagus und Herz, Archiv für pathologische Anatomie, Vol. 26, 1863, pp. 1-33.

[87] Martland, H.S. "Punch drunk," Journal of the American Medical Association, Vol. 91, 1928, pp. 1103-1107.

[88] Millspaugh, J.A. "Dementia pugilistica (punch drunk)", US Naval Medical Bulletin, Vol. 35, 1937, pp. 297-303.

[89] Critchley, M. "Medical aspects of boxing. Particularly from a neurological standpoint," British Medical Journal, Vol.I, 1957, pp. 357-362.

[90] Courville, C.B. "Punch drunk: Its pathogenesis and pathology on the basis of a verified case, Bulletin of the Los Angeles Neurological Society, Vol. 27, 1962, pp. 160-168.

[91] Brandenburg, W. and Hallervorden, J. "Dementia pugilistica mit anatomischem Befund," Virchows Archiv für pathologische Anatomie, Vol. 325, 1954, pp. 680-709.

[92] Grahmann, H, and Ule,G. "Beitrag zur Kenntnis der chronischen cerebralen Krankheitsbilder bei Boxern (Dementia pugilistica und traumatische Boxerencephalopathie)," Psychiatria et Neurologica,, Vol. 134, 1957, pp. 261-283.

[93] Neubërger, K.T., Sinton, D.W. and Denst, J. "Cerebral atrophy associated with boxing," Archives of Neurology and Psychiatry, Vol. 81, 1959, pp. 403-408.

[94] Payne, E.E. "Brains of boxers," Neurochirurgia, Vol. 11, 1968, pp. 173-188.

[95] Corsellis, J.A.N., Bruton, C.J. and Freeman-Brown, D. "The aftermath of boxing, Psychological Medicine, Vol. 3, 1973, pp. 270-303.

[96] Unterharnscheidt, F. "Experimentelle Untersuchungen über die Schädigungen des ZNS durch gehäufte stumpfe Schädeltraumen," Zentralblatt für die gesamte Neurologie und Psychiatrie, Vo. 147, 1958, p. 14.

[97] Unterharnscheidt, F. Die gedeckten Schäden des Gehirns. Experimentele Untersuchungen mir einmaliger, wiederhiolter und gehäufter Gewalteinwirkung auf den Schädel, Monographien aus dem Gesamtgebiet der Neurologie und Psychiatrie, Heft 103, Springer, Berlin Göttingen Heidelberg, 1963.

[98] Unterharnscheidt, F. Neuropathology of rhesus monkeys undergoing - Gx impact vector acceleration. In: Ewing, C.L., Thomas, D,J., Sances, A., and Larson, S.J. (eds) Impact Injury of the Head and Spine, Thomas, Springfield, 1983, pp. 94-176.

[99] Courville, C.B. "The mechanism of boxing fatalities: Report of an unusual case with severe brain lesions incident to impact of boxer's head against the ropes," Bulletin of the Los Angeles Neurological Society, Vol. 29, 1964, pp. 59-69.

[100] Grewel, F. "Encephalopathia traumatica bij boksers, Nederlands Tijdschrift voor Geneeskunde, Vol. 85, 1941, pp. 154-160.

[101] Huszar, I, and Környey, E. "Über neuropsychiatrische Aspekte des Boxens," Psychiatrie, Neurologie und medizinische Psychologie, Vol. 17. 1965, pp. 335-338.

[102] Parker, H.L. "Traumatic encephalopathy ("punch-drunk") of professional pugilists," Journal of Neurology and Psychopathology, Vol. 15, 1934, pp. 20-28.

[103] Mawdsley, C. and Ferguson, F.R. "Neurological disease in boxers," Lancet, Vol. II, 1963, pp. 795-801.

[104] Spillane, J.D. "Five boxers," British Medical Journal, Vol.II, 1962, pp. 1205-1210.

[105] Bergleiter, R. and Frekas, L. "Das Cavum septi pellucidi und Cavum Vergae im Röntgenbild," Fortschritte der Neurologie und Psychiatrie, Vol. 32, 1964, pp. 361-399.

[106] Grahmann, H, and Peters, U.H. "Das erweiterte Cavum septi pellucidi und das Cavum Vergae, Nervenarzt, Vol. 35, 1964, pp. 343-349.

[107] Unterharnscheidt, F, Jachnik, D, and Gött, H, Der Balkenmangel. Monographien aus dem Gesamtgebiet der Neurologie und Psychiatrie, Heft 128, Springer, Berlin Heidelberg New York, 1968.

[108] Roberts, A.H. Brain Damage in Boxers. A Study of the Prevalence of Traumatic Encephalopathy among Ex-professional Boxers, Pitman, London, 1969.

[109] Jedlinski, J., Gatarski, J. and Szymusik, A. "Encephalopathia pugilistica," Acta Medica Polona, Vol. 12, 1971, pp. 443-451.

[110] Kaste, M., Vikki, L. Sainio, K, Kuurne, T,, Kata Vuo, K. and Meurala, H. "Is chronic brain damage in boxing a hazard of the past?" Lancet, II, 1982, pp. 486-488.

[111] Ross, R.J., Cole, M,, Thompson, J.S., and Kim, K.H. "Boxers - computed tomography and neurologic evaluation," Journal of the American Medical Association," Vol. 249, 1983, pp. 211-213.

[112] Krefft, F. "Über Todesfälle beim Boxen," Deutsches Gesundheitswesen, Vol. 7, 1952, pp. 1559-1564.

[113] Werkgartner, A. "Gezelteriß durch Boxhieb," Zeitschrift für gerichtliche Medizin, Vol. 25, 1936, pp. 41-44.

[114] Benes, V. "Death as a result of boxing, (Czech with English summary), Czechoslovak Neurologie, Vol. 19, 1956, pp. 167-170.

[115] Bergleiter, R, and Jokl, E. "Hirnschädigungen durch Boxsport," Zentralblatt für Neurologie, Vol. 116, 1956, pp. 28-43.

[116] Cruikshank, J.K., Higgens, C.S. and Gray, J.R. "Two cases of acute intracranial hemorrhage in young amateur boxers," Lancet, Vol. I, 1980, pp. 626-627.
[117] Felc, W. "Zwei neue Todesfålle beim Boxkampf, (Polish), Ref. Zentralblatt für Neurologie, Vol. 94, 1939, p. 595.
[118] Foerster, A. "Plötzlicher Tod beim Boxkampf," Monatsschrift für Unfallheilkunde, Vol. 39, 1932, pp. 441-445.
[119] Fraenkel, P. "Tod im Boxkampf," Deutsche Zeitschrift für die gesamte gerichtliche Medizin, Vol. 1, 1922, pp. 481-486.
[120] Gurdjian, E.S., and Webster, J.E. Head Injuries: Mechanisms, Diagnosis and Management, Little Brown, Boston, 1958.
[121] Horowitz, D. "Verletzungs und Todesfälle beim Boxen und die gerichtsärztliche Begutachtung, Pam Wilenskiego Tow Lek, Vo. 9, 1933, pp. 1-20, Ref. Deutsche Zeitschrift für die gesamte gerichtliche Medizin, Vol. 22, 1933, p. 82.
[122] Kappis, M. "Über die t¨dlichen verletzungen beim Boxkampf," Zentralblatt für Chirurgie, Vol. 65, 1938, pp. 934-938.
[123] Kohlrausch, W. "Boxunfälle mir tödlichem Ausgang," Archiv für klinische Chirurgie, Vol.118, 1921, pp. 902-907.
[124] Krauland, W. Über die Quellen des akuten und chronischen subduralen Hämatoms, Thieme, Stuttgart, 1961.
[125] La Cava, G. "La cranio-encephalopahie traumatique des boxeurs," Bruxelles Medical, Vol. 29, 1949, pp. 3233-3245.
[126] Marenholtz, von "Tod im Boxkampf," Medizinische Welt, Vol. 6, 1932, pp. 556-557.
[127] Munck, W. "Tilfelde of Dodsfald ved Boksning," (Danish), Ugeskrift for Laeger, Vol. 85, 1923, pp. 848-850.
[128]Pampus, F. and Müller, N. "Über einen Todesfall nach Boxkampf," Deutsche Zeitschrift für Nervenheilkunde, Vol. 174, 1956, pp. 177-180.
[129] Paul, M. "A fatal injury at boxing (traumatic decerebrate rigidity), British Medical Journal, Vol. I, 1957, pp. 364-366.
[130] Popielski, B. "Todesfälle beim Boxen," (Polish), Polska Gaz Lek, Vol. 13, 1934, pp. 293-295, Ref. Deutsche Zeitschrift für die gesamte gerichtliche Medizin, Vol. 5, 1935, p. 448.
[131] Rozmaric, A. "Tod beim Boxen," (Czeck), Casopis Lekaru Ceskych, Vol. 63, 1924. pp. 1693-1696., Ref. Deutsche Zeitschrift für die gesamte gerichtliche Medizin, Vol. 5, 1925, p. 448.
[132] Stille, G. "Todesfälle durch Boxschlag," Medizinische Dissertation, Universität Hamburg, 1938.
[133] Weimann, W. "Zum Tod im Boxkampf," Deutsche Zeitschrift für die gesamte gerichtliche Medizin, Vol. 16, 1931, pp. 341-344.
[134] Wolff, K. Boxsport und Boxverletzungen. Eine kritische Studie unter Mitteilung eigener Beobachtungen," Deutsche Zeitschrift für Chirurgie, Vol 208, 1928, pp.341-344.
[135] Wolff, K. "Todesfälle durch Boxkampf," Deutsche Zeitschrift für die gesamte gerichtliche Medizin, Vol. 12, 1928, pp. 392-401.

Ayub K. Ommaya[1], Lawrence E. Thibault[2], Robert J. Boock[2], and David F. Meaney[2]

HEAD INJURED PATIENTS WHO TALK BEFORE DETERIORATION OR DEATH: THE TADD SYNDROME

REFERENCE: Ayub K. Ommaya, Lawrence E. Thibault, Robert J. Boock, and David F. Meaney. "Head Injured Patients Who Talk Before Deterioration Or Death: The TADD Syndrome.", Head and Neck Injuries in Sports, ASTM STP 1229, Earl F. Hoerner, Ed., American Society for Testing and Materials, Philadelphia, 1994.

Abstract: A review of a class of head injured patients who display a lucid interval before onset of coma which defines an important category of brain trauma. A hypothesis explaining the mechanism of this syndrome (T.A.D.D.) is developed on the basis of in-vitro testing of venous and arterial responses to tensile strains and the relevant clinico-pathologic data are reviewed. Venospasm is proposed as the cause of secondary ischemic hypoxia associated with a high incidence of acute subdural hematomas and brain swelling. Suggestions for further testing of this hypothesis and implications for preventive management are discussed.

Keywords: Venospasm, lucid interval, brain injury mechanisms, acute subdural hematoma, tensile strain, blood vessels, brain swelling

INTRODUCTION AND NATURE OF THE PROBLEM.

Mechanisms of head injury caused by direct or indirect impacts have been extensively studied and are relatively better understood when

[1]Professor of Neurosurgery, The George Washington University Medical Center, President, Center for Interdisciplinary Brain Research (C.I.B.R.), 8006 Glenbrook Road, Bethesda, MD 20814, o. (301)654-0801, fax. (301) 654-2563.
[2]Professor of Bioengineering, Assistant Professor of Bioengineering, and Assistant Professor of Bioengineering respectively, University of Pennsylvania, Dept. of Bioengineering, Room 120/Hayden Hall, 240 So. 33rd Street, Philadelphia, PA 19104-6392

immediate loss of consciousness is produced and maintained for variable times prior to subsequent recovery, deterioration or death [1],[2]. Neuropathologically, the hallmark of such cases is the presence of diffuse damage to axons in the white matter as first described by Sabina Strich [3],[4]. This appears to be true for varying levels of injury severity, from the mild to the severe and fatal [5],[6]. Biomechanically, the mechanism is related to the intensity of strains in the brain distributed as predicted by the centripetal theory for traumatic unconsciousness, with diffuse axonal injuries (DAI) caused by impact-induced head motions with significant rotational components [1],[2],[7]. A significant clinical category of initially mild to moderate but ultimately severe head injuries, however, does contain a majority of cases which do not exhibit DAI as the ubiquitous neuropathologic marker of injury severity. These patients have been described as the head injured who "talk and die or deteriorate" (TADD). They are of particular interest in sports injuries, and may constitute up to one third of all severely head injured patients. Autopsies in fatal cases with the TADD syndrome generally fail to reveal evidence of DAI in the majority of brains examined [8]. The cause of death or disability in this category of severe head injuries is currently attributed to abnormally high intracranial pressure (ICP) caused by focal lesions, e.g., intracranial hematomas and contusions or non-DAI diffuse damage, e.g. brain swelling with ischemic hypoxia, a condition more often seen in younger brains [9],[10]. The mechanism for some of these cases is indeed obviously explicable by the effect of focal lesions causing brain herniation in some of the patients, e.g., with extradural hematomas and relatively chronic subdural hematomas, but these lesions are found in a minority of such patients with the TADD syndrome. In the majority, however, and particularly in all cases with acute subdural hematoma (ASDH) of relatively small volume and brain swelling not attributable to large contusions as well as in cases with no focal lesions, the mechanism for the period of lucidity prior to onset of coma is unclear. As in all biologic categories, there is an overlap of clinico-pathologic correlation between the two categories described above, i.e., those who do and those who do not talk and die or deteriorate after suffering a head injury. As will be shown, this overlap is related to how we define primary and secondary damage to the brain after head injury. Graham, et. al. have recently summarized the neuropathology of head injury and define secondary injuries to the brain as follows, "complicating processes that are initiated at the moment of injury but do not become clinically evident for a period of time after the injury" [6]. This definition is of particular relevance to our problem and also illustrates the difficulty in segregating primary from secondary injuries. A better understanding of the biomechanics will probably clarify this and other aspects of our problem to the extent that a reasonable hypothesis may be tested with available data. The following review of some of the clinical and pathological data will bring out some of the facts that require a better explanation embodied in the development of such a new hypothesis for the mechanism of the specific "complicating process" initiated at the moment of injury which determines the course for patients with the TADD syndrome. Our hypothesis is developed on the basis of the clinico-pathologic data reviewed as well as a series of in-vitro experiments on the responses of venous and arterial segments subjected to tensile strains.

CLINICO-PATHOLOGIC PHENOMENOLOGY.

In a previous publication on the biomechanical aspects of head injuries in sports, an attempt was made to hypothesize why falls and blows to the head in athletes and other persons would generate more non-DAI type of cases as compared to head injuries caused by motor vehicle crashes. This report also sought to emphasize that DAI-type cases form a minority of head injuries. We did not, however, bring out the key dimension of the TADD syndrome [11]. Based on a review of clinical data, Gennarelli and Langfitt suggested that immediate onset of prolonged coma without intracranial mass lesions, i.e., diffuse brain damage, occurred in about half of all severe head injuries and that this diffuse injury, mainly DAI, was the cause of death in about 35% of all head injury deaths [12]. These clinical data should be considered in the context of the pathological evidence. Adams and his colleagues have reported an extensive histopathologic study of 434 fatal head injury cases in which 122 cases with DAI were identified (28%), with a significant association of focal lesions, such as gliding contusions and basal ganglia hematomas. Based on experimental grading of DAI severity, the majority of these brains showed Grade 3 DAI severity, i.e., with focal lesions in the dorsolateral quadrants of the brain stem [13]. Thus it would appear that the majority (72%) of fatal head injuries died of causes not simply related to DAI. It is of particular interest that 17 of these 122 DAI cases had a period of talking lucidity clearly showing the overlap between the various histologic markers of head injury severity [13].

The first report describing the clinical syndrome of "talk and die" patients after head injury was by Reilly, Adams, Graham & Jennet from Glasgow [8]. A consecutive series of autopsied cases (N = 151) were examined and 58 (38%) were identified as having had a lucid interval specified by the ability to talk. A second consecutive series of non-fatal head injuries (N = 163) were also examined and lucidity was found in 50 (31%), i.e., there was a relatively similar incidence of lucidity in "talk and die" and "talk and deteriorate but survive" patients with severe head injuries. Of the 58 patients with lucidity, 44 had hematomas, the majority of which were ASDH (93%). An additional 8 patients without hematomas from an earlier data set were added to bring the total to 66 patients. Thus 75% of the patients had intracranial hematomas and 25% (22 cases) had no hematomas. The cause of death in these latter cases was attributed to brain swelling with contusions and hypoxic ischemic injury as the cause of brain shift and herniation associated with elevated intracranial pressure. When the clinical features of patients with and without hematomas were compared, there were more similarities than differences. The only significant difference was that patients with hematomas were more often found to have initial disturbance of consciousness persisting for more than 1 hour, i.e., not having the clinical features of the TADD syndrome. Both groups had an equivalent percentage without any initial loss of consciousness (23 and 25% respectively). In the initial series of patients who were autopsied, no pathologic evidence of DAI was found as compared to the 17 cases (14%) of severe head injury patients with lucidity and DAI discussed in the later series of 122 cases with DAI as the main focus of the investigation [8],[13]. It would appear therefore that DAI plays a relatively insignificant role in the mechanism of the TADD syndrome. (Table I)

More recent reports of what may be called essentially "Non-DAI" cases of severe head injury with the TADD syndrome have reported incidences ranging from a low of 10-12% to a high of 25-32% [14],[8],[9]. Marshall, et. al. reported on the first 325 patients entered into the National Traumatic Coma Data Bank and found 35 cases with the TADD syndrome [14]. Primary differences between such patients who talked and survived versus those who talked and died were mean age (32 versus 50) and midline shift on CT (< 15 mm in survivors), i.e., nothing that would appear to be specific to the phenomenon of lucidity. ASDH were significantly more common in the TADD cases, particularly in those who died and more than 90% also had midline shift. Two cases with no shift had bifrontal contusions with compression of basilar cisterns [14]. The largest series of TADD patients was reported by Lobato, et. al. in 1991 consisting of 838 consecutive cases of severe head injury with 211 (25.1%) cases with this syndrome (TADDS) [9]. Significant differences were found between the cases with and without lucidity for the presence of multiple trauma, hypotension and hypoxia at an early stage and increased vulnerability with age for the non-TADDS group and for presence of focal lesions for the TADDS group. No significant difference was found for the occurence of seizures as a prodomal factor between the two groups [9]. The types of lesions found were classified into four groups, epidural, ASDH alone, cerebral contusions and hematomas and "no focal lesions". The majority (42%) had brain contusions associated with cerebral hematomas while the other 3 groups had relatively equal distributions, i.e., about 20% each. It should be noted that the "no focal lesion" group had a 75% incidence of brain swelling and a 30% incidence of subarachnoid hemorrhage found either as small parenchymal or interventricular locations. This combination of abnormalities in the "no focal lesion" group, coupled with the fact that patients with ASDH usually did not have hematoma volumes large enough to explain the post-lucidity deterioration and the highest mortality rate on the basis of a straight forward space occupying lesion effect, are of great interest to us in arriving at a mechanistic explanation of the TADD syndrome.

Lobato, et al also calculated the statistical significance of various factors as predictors of the outcome in their patients. The duration and quality of the lucid interval (the latter measured by the verbal Glasgow coma score) and the cause of injury (e.g. falls, motor vehicle crashes, assaults, etc.) were not significant. The most significant factors were the GCS after deterioration and the highest mean ICP measurement. A lesser degree of significance was found for age, presence of midline shift and the type of lesion (Table II). Onset of epileptic siezures were not noted as a contributing factor.9 Lobato's finding of no statistical correlation of type of injury causation in TADD patients, e.g., falls vs. motor vehicle crashes, contrasts with the finding that 72% of the patients with ASDH are found to have been injured in falls or assaults and only 24% (6) in motor vehicle crashes overall. This would suggest that other unique factors, e.g. age and specific anatomical variations, also play a role in causation for the TADD syndrome. (Table II)

TADD SYNDROME IN SPORTS HEAD INJURIES.

Head injuries in Sports are usually not severe and are generally classified as mild or moderate [15]. The incidence for mild concussions in secondary school football is given as 19 per 100 per year

constituting 24% of all football injuries   [16]. Alves & Barth examined
data on 2350 college football players at 10 Universities who had
undergone neuropsychological testing prior to and serially after a head
injury sustained while playing. They found decrements in cognitive
function and information processing which usually recovered within 5 to
10 days [16],[17]. The reported numbers of such minor head injuries
are probably underestimated because a subconcussive "ding" with
reversible amnesia and no loss of consciousness may be ignored. The
potential for such minor head injuries evolving into the TADD syndrome
has not been specifically addressed by any report analyzing significant
numbers of head injury cases in specific sports although Dacey, et. al
assessed the risk of complications in a series of 610 "minor" head
injuries [18]. Anecdotal case reports for football induced head
injuries collected by Schneider illustrate the type of clinical and
pathological phenomena which must be explained by any worthwhile
hypothesis for the mechanism of TADDS [19] The actual potential for
the evolution of TADDS and other potentially serious complications after
apparently minor head injuries has been evaluated without separating
TADD patients as a separate category by Mendelow, et. al., in a series
of 1442 consecutive head injuries of all degrees of severity [20].
About 4% had intracranial hematomas and of 865 patients initially alert
and oriented 1.3% developed such lesions. Discharge diagnosis was
cerebral concussion in 87% of these patients. In a second report on
36,637 admissions for all head injuries in non-neurosurgical units in
Scotland there were 545 cases with intracranial hematomas, an incidence
of 1.5% [21]. A prospective study at the University of Virginia looked
at the risk of serious complications in minor head injuries. Of 610
consecutive cases selected for transient impairment of consciousness,
vision, memory or speech with 13 - 15 GCS scores in the emergency room
18 (3%) required neurosurgical treatment of which 3 had subdural
hematomas and 7 had ICP monitors placed. Eight of these 18 cases had an
initial GCS of 15. The most common lesion in this prospective study was
also the ASDH and in one case, prompt removal failed to save the patient
who died of tentorial herniation [18]. Reilly, et. al. had previously
pointed out the high incidence of this type of lesion in the TADD cases.
It should be emphasized that the true incidence for all TADD cases is
not yet established because the majority are classified as severe head
injuries and not as complications of mild to moderate cases. The
reported variations in incidence of TADD reflect the type of selection
bias made in the studies discussed above.

One of the most puzzling features of the TADD syndrome is the
apparently trivial nature of the causal impact which is often noted to
be compatible with a full lucidity or only brief disturbance of cerebral
functions. This has been reported following single impact events in
children and young adults as well as following sequential minor impacts
occurring in contact sports [10],[22],[23],[24].   The catastrophic
deterioration that follows often within the space of minutes thus seems
difficult to explain. This severe effect of minor impacts has been
described in contact sports and particularly in football. Prior to the
clear recognition of the TADD syndrome by Reilly et. al., R. C.
Schneider had published an excellent monograph on "Head and neck
Injuries in Football" in 1973 [8],[19]. In a series of 69 cases with
subdural hematomas, Schneider found 28 fatalities and 41 survivors from
the head injuries for the period from 1931 to 1970. The number of
people playing football during this period was estimated at 2.5 million
annually. Incidence of direct fatalities (mainly due to head and neck
injuries) for 1970 was 2 out of 100,000 participants for high schools

and colleges combined as reported by Blyth and Arnold in the 36th Annual
Survey of Football fatalities (1931 - 1970). In the 1990 survey of
football fatalities by Mueller & Schindler, the incidence per 100,000
players for 1990 was 0. They discuss the significant increase in total
deaths between 1964 and 1972 with subsequent decrease beginning in 1973
and further significant decrease after 1976 when rule changes were
introduced aimed at preventing use of the head for blocking and tackling
[25]. Schneider's comment on his unique survey of the data on head
injuries in football players is notable for what seems to be an indirect
description of the TADD syndrome. "Many of these players sustained
their injury and shortly thereafter, within 30 - 60 minutes became
deeply comatose and arrived at a hospital in an agonal state with the
pupils dilated and fixed [19]. A summary of six of these case reports
can serve to illustrate clinico-pathologic correlations which can shed
further light on our understanding of the TADD syndrome. Three
additional personally reviewed cases are also described. The first
series (A) consists of football related head injuries, whereas the
second series (B) consists of one football injury, one motorcycle crash
and one boxing injury.

SELECTED CASE REPORTS.

A. R.C. Schneider (1973) Series (Case numbers are as given in this
   reference) [19].
   I. Three TADD patients with Acute Subdural Hematoma (ASDH).
      1. (Case no. 4.) A 17 year old blocked a charging opponent,
         staggered, complained of dizziness, walked to the side line and
         complained of headache and within a few minutes became comatose
         with decerebrate rigidity and fixed dilated pupils. Initially
         hypertensive and as blood pressure fell, stopped breathing.
         Surgery after intubation revealed ASDH with two large torn
         bridging veins. No improvement and died 9 hours after head
         injury. Past history: Exactly similar episode 1 year earlier up
         to stage of decerebrate rigidity and then rapid recovery without
         surgery. EEG done 1 week prior to fatal impact was normal and was
         released to play football exactly one year after first impact.
      2. (Case No. 9.) A 17 year old had a helmeted head to head impact,
         stood up and walked 30 feet before collapsing with coma, Cheyne
         Stokes respiration, fixed dilated pupils. Surgery for ASDH of no
         avail and death ensued 3 days later. Autopsy revealed brain edema
         with hemorrhages in brain stem and between dural leaves of
         tentorium on the right side plus wide spread areas of degenerative
         changes in cerebral hemispheres bilaterally (infarcts).
         Past history: No previous head injuries or neurological problems.
      3. (Case No. 46) A 14 year old suffered a hit on his helmeted head
         in a scrimmage at 5:30 pm. Left game complaining of dizziness and
         talking; about three minutes later collapsed with dilated right
         pupil and taken to hospital (6:05 pm). Hypertonic glucose (100
         cc, 50%) given in E.R. and burr holes done by 6:30 pm. Large (125
         cc) ASDH removed with complete neurological recovery by 3rd week
         post-trauma.
         Past history: No previous head injuries or neurological problems.

   II. Three TADD patients without ASDH.
      1. (Case No. 8) A College football player was observed to be
         walking the wrong way from the line, apparently confused but
         continuing to play for a few plays before collapse into coma. No

head strike observed. Death followed within 24 hours. Autopsy revealed hemorrhagic infarcts of cerebral hemisphere and brain stem.

Past history was positive for a mild head injury recently with full recovery.

2.   (Case No. 10) A 17 year old tackled with his head and hit opponent who was running away from him. No loss of consciousness and complained of severe headache, but continued to play until collapse in huddle about 5 minutes later. Able to walk with assistance to side line where he collapsed again with loss of consciousness, unequal pupils, decerebrate rigidity and Cheyne-Stokes respiration. Steroids were given intravenously and within 2 to 3 hours he began to improve, talking but with residual diplopia and confusion. Within 3 weeks full recovery noted with normal neurological and radiological findings.

Past history indicates he had complained of headaches for the past 1 week.

3.   (Case No. 28) A 17 year old tackled with left side of head to opponent's helmet, got up immediately and shortly thereafter vomited x2, fell down and was briefly unconscious and then semicomatose, but talking slowly. No evidence of external injury to scalp or skull, but had bilateral pyramidal signs with "blindness", disorientation and incontinence. Radiological studies included angiography and no lesions noted. Spinal tap revealed normal CSF pressure after completion of angiography (many hours post-impact). CSF protein 103 mgm. and EEG showed gross bilateral diffuse abnormalities only.

Final outcome: Visual agnosia with minimal to no visual evoked responses. Marked memory deficits with Parkinsonian masking of face and slow movements with long term survival.

Past history: No previous head injuries or neurological problems.

Comment: These six cases illustrate the common role of brain swelling causing ischemic hypoxia with the ASDH adding its own contribution to the cerebral circulation and abnormal intracranial pressures. Both are related to strains in the venous elements.

B. Personally reviewed cases.

1. A 15 year old linebacker on the third day of practice was tackled by his opponent and struck on the face mask of his helmet and thrown down during a practice session. Standing up immediately, he congratulated his attacker with the words, "Good hit!" Leaving the practice, he went to the side lines and began complaining of headache as he sat down next to one of his teammates. Within the next 5 minutes he laid back on the ground and continued talking and complaining of headache and quite suddenly stopped talking and was found to be comatose with a right fixed dilated pupil. Rushed to a hospital, CT scans revealed a right holoconvexity ASDH, which was surgically removed. No significant contusions seen, but some adhesions to the temporal lobe were described. Post-operative CT showed persisting shift and elevated ICP with GCS at 7 (Verbal). Due to persistent elevated ICP he was put into pentobarbital coma which diminished the ICP and after a stormy 3 weeks, his GCS was 10 - 11 rising to 13 over the next few days Talking was resumed one month post trauma and a residual left hemianopia and 3rd nerve palsy were noted at the time of transfer to rehabilitation. MRI scans confirmed an ischemic infarct in the right parieto-occipital region.

Past History. He had complained repeatedly over the past months about headaches and had fallen, spraining his ankle a few weeks earlier.

Comment: The trauma in this case was apparently quite minor and the history of earlier headaches with temporal lobe adhesions suggests the role of previous trauma as a tethering factor for cortical veins.

2. A 22 year old male motorcyclist lost control of his vehicle on a rainy night directly in front of a community hospital with a level I Trauma Center. His helmet was removed in the ER and showed no evidence of damage and there was no evidence of scalp damage. The patient was combative, talking coherently at times and confused at other times, oriented to person but not to place or time. Level of consciousness deteriorated rapidly in about 15 minutes after admission and CT scanning showed an intact skull, no focal lesions in the brain, but evidence of mild diffuse brain swelling with bilaterally narrowed frontal horns without shift and mildly compressed basal cisterns. Level of consciousness decreased significantly over the next 24 hours without any significant change in CT scans in spite of intubation and controlled ventilation. Intracranial pressures fluctuated between 10-12 and 15-18 mm Hg under treatment with steroids, Mannitol and Pentobarbital. Over the next 5 days, the level of consciousness did not improve in spite of relatively low intracranial pressures with pCO_2 between 28 and 30 and pO_2 at normal levels. Daily CT scans showed improvement of the brain swelling with normal ventricles and cisternal CSF spaces without development of any delayed mass lesions. Patient expired on the 6th day without regaining consciousness. Autopsy was refused.

Past History. No previous head injuries or neurological problems.

Comment. This TADD patient had diffuse swelling of the brain as the only observable abnormality on CT scan which improved over the next 5 days according to serial CT scans, but with no improvement in his clinical deterioration to death in 6 days. Ischemic hypoxia as the causation factor was proposed secondary to diffuse brain swelling.

3. A 25 year old boxer was in an amateur boxing match when he sustained a blow to the head toward the end of a round. He was able to walk back to the corner, sit and talk briefly. Within a brief period after this, he rapidly became unconscious and was taken to the Emergency Room of a nearby hospital. He was unresponsive and then began to have a series of seizures. After rapid infusion of Manitol (25 grams) Decadron (25 mgm) and Lasix (40 mgm), he underwent C.T. Scanning. A large right parieto-temporal acute subdural hematoma was identified and the patient was immediately taken to surgery and the clot removed. Post-operative, he began to show decerebrate movements of his extremities but remained in a comatose state with decorticate posturing and responsive only by withdrawal to deep pain. He was subsequently transfered to a long term care facility with the diagnosis of persistent vegetative state.

Comment: All three of these cases indicate the dual role of brain swelling occurring early after the lucidity with and without ASDH.

A HYPOTHESIS FOR THE MECHANISM OF TADD.

A common factor for patients with the TADD syndrome is a significant degree of initial brain swelling with or without focal lesions, particularly ASDH. The brain swelling occurs rapidly and is found at time durations too short to invoke cerebral edema of the post-traumatic vasogenic type as being the causative factor for the swelling seen, particularly in the absence of contusions and lacerations. Thus ischemic hypoxia due to vasospasm is a reasonable etiologic factor for the common mechanism to which is added the deleterious effect of space occupying focal lesions such as the fairly ubiquitous ASDH seen in the majority of TADD patients. Arterial vasospasm has been described as a biphasic phenomenon in 2 conditions; rupture of cerebral aneurysms, particularly those related to the circle of Willis and its nearby branches, and in head injuries [26]. Many investigations aimed at uncovering the causation of such arterial vasospasm have failed to reveal its pathogenesis. A study of angiograms in 33 patients suffering from fatal head injury revealed a 57.5% of incidence of arterial vasospasm [21]. However, the relatively slow time course of the appearance of clinically significant arterial vasospasm with subarachnoid hemorrhage after aneurysmal rupture and the lack of correlation between the amount of blood in either aneurysmal or head injury cases and the extent of arterial vasoconstriction would argue against this mechanism as the primary event in the causation of ischemic hypoxia or brain swelling in the TADD syndrome. Arterial vasoconstriction secondary to some delayed release of vasoactive compounds, e.g., secondary to a degree of mechanical damage to the hypothalamic region is certainly possible as a secondary complication. Finally, even the early phase of arterial vasoconstriction occurs over a time course of hours, not minutes. By exclusion, therefore, one is left with the role of the venous structures on the surfaces of the brain, which are also subject to significant deformation during impacts. Until the recent work of Thibault and his colleagues in the Department of Bioengineering at the University of Pennsylvania, the role of venous obstruction as a cause of ischemic hypoxia was usually considered secondary to mass effects in the brain analogous to the hypothesized occlusion of posterior cerebral arteries on the edge of the tentorium secondary to cerebral edema and brain shifts caused by space occupying lesions. As described below, direct testing of the response of blood vessels (arterial and venous) subjected to axial deformation suggest that venous vasospasm may well be a key element in the evolution of the TADD syndrome. An immediate and prolonged venous vasoconstriction with a varying extent of involvement of the surface and basal draining veins of the brain would explain the varying durations of the lucid interval, acting in concert with other lesions, e.g. the well described association with ASDH as the result of a higher level of strain tearing bridging veins. The increased susceptibility of the brain to what has been described as the "Second impact in catastrophic contact sports head trauma" could well be initiated by this proposed mechanism as follows:" [22].

1. Head impacts below the threshold for traumatic disturbance of consciousness would trigger a degree of venous constriction resulting in mild to moderate brain swellingdue to increased blood volume sufficient to decrease the CSF space over the cerebral hemispheres. If strains are greater in bridging veins some can also be torn leading to presentation as the TADD syndrome with or without the ASDH. If the swelling is enough to decrease CSF space and no veins are torn and the patient survives the mild swelling, she becomes vulnerable to a second hazard.

2. The normal relative weight of the brain (1/5 of the brain weight when it is "floating" in the normal CSF space) is increased by approximately five times due to the obliteration of the CSF space as a result of the brain swelling. If the degree of swelling is

not enough to lead to ischemic hypoxia, prolonged contact pressures between brain and dura could lead to adhesions.
3. A second blow now can produce greater injurious effects on the brain due to this relative increase in weight as well as amplifying the existing extent of venoconstriction in the pre-stressed venous structures.

EXPERIMENTAL DATA ON BLOOD VESSELS.

Recent work at the University of Pennsylvania has focused upon the development of a system to test isolated blood vessels undergoing dynamic elongation. The emphasis is placed upon the functional response of the blood vessels (vasoreactivity) when subjected to high strain rate extension. Although the structural failure of neurovascular elements is of obvious importance, we believe that strain induced changes in vascular resistance will effect cerebral blood flow and therefore can affect regional brain injury severity.

METHODS

Albino male Wistar rats weighing from 300 to 750 g were anesthetized with intramuscular injections of Ketamine/Xylaxaine cocktail (87 mg/kg ketamine, 13 mg/kg Xylaxaine). All procedures were performed using protocols approved by the University of Pennsylvania Institutional Animal Care and Use Committee. Using sterile microsurgical technique, approximately 1 cm segments of both femoral artery and vein were exposed. These vessels were tied off distally for arteries and proximally for veins. Any side branches were tied off and then cut. This ensures full inflation of the vessel while cannulation procedures are accomplished. The vessels were cannulated using specially prepared needle tips. These needle tips (27 or 30 gauge) were blunted and notched, and then sterilized using alcohol. The needle tips prior to surgery were filled with heparin allowing several drops to remain in the tip. When cannulating, the heparin was drawn into the vessel by capillary action. This heparin ensured a minimum of clotting within the vessel. The vessel was then nicked and the cannula was placed within. The vessel was then sutured closed around the cannula. The notch provided purchase for the suture to ensure that no vessel slippage occurred during any one of the procedures. It should be noted that blood continued to perfuse these vessels until the second cannulation was made. The vessels were then removed after their in situ length is measured and transported to the small scale materials testing machine. The entire procedure from first cannulation to mounting took no more than 25 minutes. The experimental procedure used a dynamic square wave function to trigger the solenoid at a fixed strain rate of 24 sec-1. A spring return system returns the specimen to its pre-stretch length. Viable perfused blood vessels thus obtained from the rat were stretched using our custom small scale material testing platform. Force and displacement were measured in real time in response to these impulsive loading conditions at several levels of ultimate strain and at a constant strain rate. Post-injury developed force and luminal cross-sectional area changes were continuously measured immediately following mechanical insult. In addition, photographic measurements have been taken on the vessel at various times post stretch.

RESULTS

The average vessel length was 1.04 cm for the veins and 1.07 cm for the arteries. The average diameter of the veins was 0.0458 cm and 0.0535 cm for the arteries. Estimated average wall thickness was 0.00071 cm for the veins and 0.00226 for the arteries.

Venous Response

Sixteen veins were loaded to different levels of ultimate strain of physiologic importance [Margulies et al., 1990]. These experiments have been divided into four groups based on post injury developed force and ultimate strain delivered as the mechanical stimulus for the experiment. Several variables from these experiments have been correlated. Figure 1 shows the maximum post injury developed force versus maximum strain delivered for the entire data set. A curve fit through these points indicates a linear relationship between these variables with a correlation coefficient of 0.96. The isometric developed force post injury ranges from 1.7 grams to 13.4 grams for the experiments ranging from 6 to 22 percent strain. In addition, maximum strain has also been correlated to the percentage diameter decrease measured in the video analysis of these experiments. This is shown in Figure 2. This shows a luminal decrease ranging from 8 percent to 28 percent for the experiments with strains of 6 to 22 percent.

Arterial Response

The only vessels to react to the lower levels of strain have been the veins, although greater numbers of arteries were tested. Arterial response occurs at extremely high levels of strain. These levels would be large enough to produce structural failure in the veins. We hypothesize that equivalent loads applied to the arteries result in lower stress in the walls and thus lower strains in the cells that will react to this stimulus (vascular smooth muscle).

Chemical controls

Six vessels were tested using a bolus of saturated KCL solution injected in the perfusate. This testing involves 3 artery-vein pairs. The isometric developed force post perfusion for the veins range from 17.9 grams to 24.3 grams. The isometric developed force post perfusion for the arteries range from 25.6 grams to 32.6 grams. These developed forces, on average, start immediately post perfusion, peaking at 127 seconds, and returns to baseline by 250 seconds. Several vessels were also tested post stretch, upon return to baseline, with this KCL solution and showed the same magnitude response as those tested with only this KCL solution.

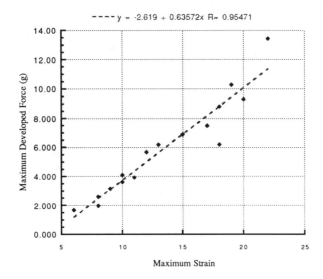

FIG. 1.

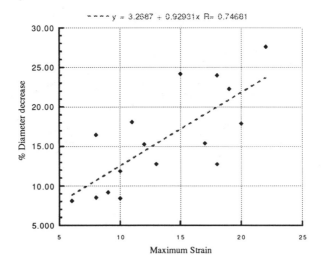

FIG. 2.

DISCUSSION

In vitro experiments confirm the vasoreactive response of isolated blood vessels to a single uniaxial high strain rate load. We have now developed a dose-response relationship for the blood vessels in response to an impulse load and can compare these values to those measured in the physical models of the brain undergoing inertial loading [27],[28].

During our experiments we have noticed a difference in time course between two of the measured functional changes. The first and nearly immediate change is the luminal dimension decrease. This must be compared to the developed force that has a delay of tens of seconds before any significant tension is developed. This can reasonably be explained if we notice the methods in our protocol. Since we do not allow the vessel length to shorten there must be a significant reduction in radial dimension before enough tension is developed in the axial direction. Conversely, if we allowed the vessel to shorten and not develop an isometric axial tension one would predict an increased radial constriction. Lastly, if we assume simple Hagen-Pouiselle flow as a model for associated hemodynamic events, then the radial constriction causes a change in pressure related to the fourth power of this response. From these calculations it can be shown that for even small changes in radius, significant flow changes at constant pressure drop can be developed. These experimental data provide adequate support for our hypothesis for the role of venous vasoconstriction in the genesis of the TADD syndrome after head impact. The result would be a marked obstruction to blood flow out of the brain resulting in cerebral engorgement with a realative stagnation of blood flow. Strains in bridging veins exceeding their tensile strength could result in rupture and ASDH [29]. In a recent paper by Wilberger, et. al., clinical data on 101 patients with ASDH were reviewed. Their findings supported the pathophysiological evidence that the extent of primary brain injury "is more important than the subdural hematoma clot itself in dictating outcome; therefore the ability to control intracranial pressure is more critical to outcome than the absolute timing of subdural blood removal [30]. When the injury mechanism leads to immediate loss of consciousness, i.e., a DAI type of case, the primary brain damage (with or without focal lesions) is well described in the existing neuropathological literature [4],[6],[7],[13]. In the case of the TADD syndrome, however, this is not the case and an important distinction has to be made. This distinction relates to the point raised earlier on primary vs. secondary lesions. Thus causation has to be explained in a 2 step manner; first, the cause of the patient's initial clinical presentation and secondarily, his later clinical status in terms of the biomechanics and physiopathologic changes induced. In this sense, the biomechanical mechanism is always primary and secondary together, whereas the secondary clinical and neuropathologic manifestations are always secondary to the "complicating processes initiated at the moment of injury" [6]. In this report, we have sought to make a distinction between the TADD and DAI "types" of head injury. However, we would also emphasize that while only a few TADD cases have DAI lesions, such lesions may not play a significant role in 72% of all fatal cases [13]. The proposed mechanism of TADD, i.e., venous vasoconstriction is, however, most probably also present in the majority of severe and fatal head injuries and in combination with the DAI mechanism could well explain the majority of head injury cases with the worst outcome. The ASDH is thus a key focal lesion signifying a severe head injury in which the level of venous element strains are more than sufficient to add the

deleterious effects of venous vasoconstriction to the space occupying
role of the ASDH itself. This would hold for both DAI and non-DAI cases
with ASDH as well as those TADD and non-TADD cases without ASDH.

Two suggestions for further research emerge from a consideration of
the facts and concepts reviewed above. Firstly, we propose to look for
clinical data to test our hypothesis. MRI scans can now visualize
venous channels within and near the dura with significant precision.
Thus in a patient with spontaneous intracranial hypotension due to a CSF
leak, marked distortion of the pons, displacement of the optic chiasm
and downward cerebellar herniation were seen on the MRI scan along with
marked dural enhancement of the tentorial, supratentorial,
intrahemispheric and infratentorial dura [31]. This enhancement
resulted from the venous dilatation resulting from the venous blood
replacing the decreased CSF volume following the Monroe-Kellie rule that
CSF volume fluctuates reciprocally with changes in intracranial blood
volume when the skull is intact [32],[33]. The dural enhancement seen
on the MRI scan in the patient reported by Fishman and Dillon provided
confirmation of the patients severe postural headache and other clinical
deficits, all of which were reversed when the CSF leak was closed. A
repeat MRI scan showed reversal of the abnormal findings seen including
marked reduction of the dural enhancement [31]. Quantification of
dural venous flows with early MRI scans would be a practical method to
test our hypothesis for the TADD syndrome mechanism.

A second line of inquiry results from the availability of a
standardized system for testing isolated blood vessels which enables a
systematic exploration of the chemical changes associated with the
venous (and arterial) vasospasm undergoing dynamic elongation. Coupled
with this methodology one could also test putative vasospasm reversing
chemical substances, e.g., nitrous oxide. We look forward to
investigating these questions further.

REFERENCES

[1] Ommaya, A.K. and Gennarelli, T.A., "Cerebral Concussion and Traumatic Unconsciousness." Brain. Vol. 97, 1974, pp 633-654.

[2] Ommaya, A.K., "Mechanisms of Cerebral Concussion, Contusions and Other Effects of Head Injury." Neurological Surgery. Ed. Youmans, J. Vol. 4, pp 1877-1895. W. B. Saunders, 1982.

[3] Strich, S.J., "Shearing of Nerve Fibres as a Cause of Brain Damage Due to Head Injury. A Pathological Study of Twenty Cases." Lancet, Vol. 2, pp 443-448.

[4] Strich, S.J., "Cerebral Trauma", Greenfield's Neuropathology. Ed. W. Blackwood and J.A.N. Corsellis. Year Book Publishers, 3rd. Edition, 1976.

[5] Oppenheimer, D.R., "Microscopic Lesions in the Brain Following Head Injury." Journal of Neurology, Neurosurgury and Psychiatry, Vol. 31, 1968, pp 299 - 306.

[6] Graham, D.I., Adams, J.H., Gennarelli, T., "Pathology of Brain Damage in Head Injury", Head Injury, 3rd Edition. Ed. Cooper, P.R. Williams & Wilkins, 1993.

[7] Gennarelli, T.A., Thibault, L.E., Adams, J.H., et. al., "Diffuse Axonal Injury and Traumatic Coma in the Primate." Annals of Neurology, Vol. 12, 1982, pp 564-574.

[8] Reilly, P.L., Graham, D.I., Adams, J.H., et. al., "Patients with Head Injury who Talk and Die.", Lancet, Aug. 30, 1975, pp 375 - 377.

[9] Lobato, R.D., Rivas, J.J., Gomez, P.A., et. al., "Head Injured Patients Who Talk & Deteriorate into Coma: Analysis of 211 Cases Studied with Computerized Tomography. Journal of Neurosurgery, Vol. 75, 1991, pp 256-261.

[10] Bruce, D.A., Alavi, Al, Bilanink, L., et. al., "Diffuse Cerebral Swelling Following Head Injuries in Children: The Syndrome of 'Malignant Brain Edema'", Journal of Neurosurgery, Vol. 54, 1983, pp 285-288.

[11] Ommaya, A.K., "Biomechanical Aspects of Head Injuries in Sports." Chapter 8. In Sports Neurology, Ed. Jordan, B.D., Tsairis, P. & Warren, R.F. Aspen Publishers, Maryland, 1989.

[12] Gennarelli, T.A., Spielman, G.A., Langfitt, T.W., et. al., "Influence of the Type of Intracranial Lesion on Outcome from Severe Head Injury", Journal of Neurosurgery, Vol.56, 1982, pp 26-36.

[13] Adams, J.H., Doyle, D., Ford, I., et. al, "Diffuse Axonal Injury in Head Injury: Definition, Diagnosis & Grading", Histopathology, Vol. 15, 1989, pp 49-59.

[14] Marshall, L.F., Toole, B.M., Bowers, S.A, "The National Traumatic Coma Data Bank, Part 2. Patients who Talk & Deteriorate: Implications for Treatment", Journal of Neurosurgery, Vol. 59, 1983, pp 285-288.

[15] Gerberich, S.G., Priest, J.D., Boen, J.R., "Conscussions, Incidence and Severity in Secondary School Varsity Football Players", American Journal of Public Health, Vol. 73, 1983, pp 1370.

[16] Barth, J.T., Alves, W.M., Ryan, T.V., et. al., "Mild Head Injury in Sports: Neuropsychological Sequelae and Recovery of Function."

[17] Levin, H.S., Eisenberg, H.M., Benton, A.L.(eds), Mild Head Injury, Oxford University Press, New York, 1989.

[18] Dacey, R.G., Alves, W.M., Jane, J.A., et. al., "Neurosurgical Complications after Apparently Minor Head Injury: Assessment of Risk in a Series of 610 Patients", Journal of Neurosurgery, 1986, pp 203 - 210.

[19] Schnieder, R.C., "Head and Neck Injuries in Football: Mechanisms, Treatment and Prevention", Williams & Wilkins, Baltimore, MD, 1973.

[20] Mendelow, A.D., Teasdale, G., Jennet, B., et. al., "Risk of Intracranial Hematoma in Head Injured Adults", British Medical Journal, Vol. 287, 1983, pp 1173 - 1176.

[21] Mendelow, A.D., Campbell, D.A., Jeffrey, R.R., et. al., "Admission after Mild Head Injury: Benefits and Costs", British Medical Journal, Vol. 285, 1982, pp 1530-1532.

[22] Saunders, R.L, & Harbaugh, R.E., "The Second Impact in Catastrophic Contact Sports Head Trauma", JAMA, Vol. 252(4), 1984, pp 538 - 539.

[23] McQuillen, J.B., McQuillen, E.N., Morrow, P., "Trauma, Sport & Malignant Cerebral Edema", American Journal of Forensic Medical Pathology, Vol. 9(1), 1988, pp 12 - 15.

[24] Kelley, J.P., Nichold, J.S., Filley, M., et. al., "Concussion in Sports. Guidelines for the Prevention of Catastrophic Outcome", JAMA, Vol. 266(20), 1991, pp 2867 - 2869.

[25] Mueller, F.O., Schindler, R.D., "Annual Survey of Football Injury Research, 1931 - 1990", American Football Coaches Association.

[26] Mcpherson, P., Graham, D.I., "Arterial Spasm and Slowing of the Cerebral Circulation in the Ischemia of Head Injury", Journal of Neurology, Neurosurgery & Pshiciatry, Vol. 36, 1973, pp 1069 - 1072.

[27] Margulies, S.S., Tibault, L.E., Gennarelli, T.A., "Physical Model Simulations of Brain Injury in the Primate", Journal of Biomechanics, Vol. 23(8), 1990, pp 823-836.

28 Boock, J.R., Thibault, L.E., "An Experimental and Analytical Approach to the Development of a Range of Neruovascular Trauma Indicies", Proceedings of IRCOBI, Lyon, France, 1990.

29 Lowenhielm, P., "Dynamic Properties of Parasaggital Bridging Veins", Z. Rechsmedizin, Vol. 74, 1974, pp 55 - 62.

30 Wilberger, J.E., Harris, M., Diamond, D.L. Acute Subdural Hematoma: Morbidity, Mortality and Operative Timing", Journal of Neurosurgery, Vol. 74, 1991, pp 212-218.

31 Fishman, R.A., Dillon, W.P., "Dural Enhancement and Cerebral Displacement Secondary to Intracranial Hypotension", Neurology, Vol. 43, 1993, pp 609-611.

32 Kellie, G., "An Account of the Appearances Observed in the Dissection of 2 or 3 Individuals Presumed to have Perished in the Storm of the 3rd and Whose Bodies were Recovered in the Vicinity of Leith with Some Reflections on the Pathology of the Brain", Trans. Edinburgh Medical Chirological Society, Vol. 1, 1824, pp 84-169.

33 Ommaya, A.K., O'Tuama, L.A., Lorenzo, A.V., "CSF Dynamics, Hydrocephalus and Leaks", in Principles of Nuclear Medicine, 2nd Ed. Wagner, H.N. (Ed.), 1993.

Christopher D. Ingersoll[1]

MEASUREMENT OF SENSORY FUNCTIONING AND INTEGRATION
FOLLOWING CLOSED HEAD INJURY

REFERENCE: Ingersoll, C. D., **"Measurement of Sensory
Functioning and Integration Following Closed Head Injury,"**
Head and Neck Injuries in Sports, ASTM STP 1229, Earl F.
Hoerner, Ed., American Society for Testing and Materials,
Philadelphia, 1994.

ABSTRACT: A protocol for measuring sensory functioning and
integration is discussed along with different approaches
for examining the information collected. This protocol
involves performing six variations of the Romberg test on a
force platform. The six test conditions either eliminate
sensory input or produce inaccurate visual and/or surface
orientation inputs. Total, anterior-posterior, and medial-
lateral sway are calculated from force platform center of
pressure data. Five Romberg coefficients were formulated to
determine the relative destabilizing effects of the last
five test conditions. Center of pressure data were also
subjected to a Fast Fourier Transform to examine the
frequency spectrum associated with postural sway. Five
frequency bands representing visual input, semicircular
canal function, otolith function, and somatosensory input
are evaluated. The results of studies examining each of
these methods of evaluating sensory function and
integration are presented.

KEYWORDS: closed head injury, fast fourier transform,
motor control, postural control, postural sway,
somatosensory input, vestibular input, visual input

Establishing externally valid criteria for returning
athletes to athletic competition following head injury is
essential for safe participation. Numerous diagnostic
techniques are described in the literature with this
purpose, but do not have functional applicability. For
example, MRI findings correlate poorly with other
neurological signs in boxers [21]. The purpose of this

[1]Assistant Professor, Sports Injury Research
Laboratory, Athletic Training Department, Indiana State
University, Terre Haute, IN 47809

review is to describe the use of stabilometry as a
diagnostic tool for identifying subtle functional deficits
following closed head injury. Several methods of measuring
postural control are described and preliminary data using
each are presented.

POSTURE AS A DIAGNOSTIC TOOL

Identifying sensorimotor deficits following closed
head injury is important because integrated and coordinated
movement is essential for optimal athletic performance.
Posture is a good method of identifying sensorimotor
deficits because it provides a simple model to test the
many elements of the nervous system that interact to
produce motor control. Standing posture has been used for
this purpose, particularly in otolaryngology, for some
time.
Posture is maintained by three systems: vision,
vestibular input, and somatosensory input [10,25,40]. Each
system has a different role in maintaining posture,
although there is interaction and cooperation among them.
Contributions of visual input to dynamic movements
include, but are not limited to: timed leg extensor
activity prior to landing from a jump [34], descending
stairs [16], and controlling arm extensor activity in
self-initiated forward falls [14].
The vestibular apparatus of the inner ear consists of
the three semicircular canals, the utricle, and the
saccule. The semicircular canals are thought to respond
only to angular accelerations, although they may respond to
linear forces as well [18]. The utricular otoliths and
saccule are thought to sense linear accelerations [52].
However, the involvement of the otoliths during balance has
been questioned [42].
The somatosensory system also assists in the
maintenance of posture. Afferent inputs from
mechanoreceptors in the ankles or the soles of the feet,
spindles in the leg muscles, or possibly some other source
help maintain posture. Which input source(s) are important
contributors to posture has not been resolved [15].
Several interactions between the sensory modalities
have been described. Lestienne et al. [29] explained the
visual-vestibular interaction as follows: "...the otoliths
detect no acceleration, the discrepancy between the visual
system, which detects motion, and the vestibular system,
which does not, is solved in the following manner: it is
assumed by the CNS that a backwards pitch has induced a
component of gravity on the utriculus which cancels the
effects of linear acceleration. The body is then felt as
being inclined (backwards) with respect to a new
'subjective' position of gravity ('subjective vertical').

This, in turn, induces a postural readjustment (forward) in order to realign the body with the supposed direction of gravity."

There is also interaction between the proprioceptive system and the vestibular system. Dietz et al. [13] stated that after reducing the proprioceptive input of the lower leg muscles, the vestibular system becomes the dominant regulating factor for maintaining posture. They contend that the vestibular system operates with longer delays and compensates the body shift mainly by trunk and head movements.

METHODS OF MEASURING POSTURAL CONTROL

Test Conditions

The Romberg test can be modified to systematically remove or conflict one or more of the three sensory modalities that control posture [45] (Figures 1-6). This allows evaluation of individual sensory modalities as well as interaction between them.

Three visual and two surface conditions are used. Vision can be allowed, disallowed, or confused with a visual conflict dome. The standing surface can be the hard surface of the force platform or a square of foam placed over the force platform. Vestibular input cannot be directly manipulated, but its interaction with the other two modalities can be evaluated.

Sway Variables

Postural control has been measured since the middle of the nineteenth century. The evolution of these measurement techniques has paralleled the technological development of man. It all began with an observation made by German neurologist M.H. Romberg [44].

Romberg [44] first described a method of determining the presence and/or extent of neurological disease using a simple balancing task. He explained his test as follows: "If he (the patient) is ordered to close his eyes while in the erect posture, he at once commences to totter and swing from side to side; the insecurity of his gait also exhibits itself in the dark. It is now ten years since I pointed out this pathognomic sign, and it is a symptom which I have observed in other paralyses. . . Since then I have found it in a considerable number of patients, from far and near, who have applied for my advice; in no case have I found it wanting." Since then, attempts have been made to quantify the amount of sway present in Romberg's test.

The development of modern electronic equipment improved not only the accuracy of measurement of posture,

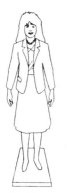

Figure 1. Test condition #1 - eyes open, normal surface condition.

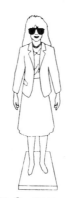

Figure 2. Test condition #2 - eyes closed, normal surface condition.

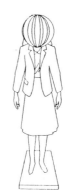

Figure 3. Test condition #3 - visual conflict dome, normal surface condition.

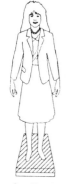

Figure 4. Test condition #4 - eyes open, standing on foam.

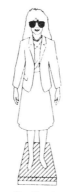

Figure 5. Test condition #5 - eyes closed, standing on foam.

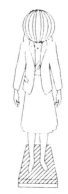

Figure 6. Test condition #6 - visual conflict dome, standing on foam.

but the ability to diagnose the mechanism of the postural instability. Posture has been measured using various types of force plates [6,37], variable resistance balance boards [35], foot-ground pressure pattern devices [3,4], acceleration registrography [26], pedascope [20], cinematography [20,47], seesaw boards [36], and sway magnetometry [9].

The variables measured by such devices include anterior-posterior (AP) sway, medial-lateral (ML) sway, total sway, sway velocity, and frequency spectrum analyses.

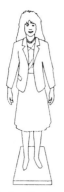

Figure 1. Test condition #1 - eyes open, normal surface condition.

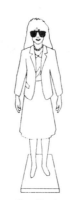

Figure 2. Test condition #2 - eyes closed, normal surface condition.

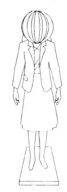

Figure 3. Test condition #3 - visual conflict dome, normal surface condition.

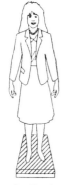

Figure 4. Test condition #4 - eyes open, standing on foam.

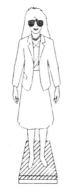

Figure 5. Test condition #5 - eyes closed, standing on foam.

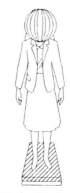

Figure 6. Test condition #6 - visual conflict dome, standing on foam.

but the ability to diagnose the mechanism of the postural instability. Posture has been measured using various types of force plates [6,37], variable resistance balance boards [35], foot-ground pressure pattern devices [3,4], acceleration registrography [26], pedascope [20], cinematography [20,47], seesaw boards [36], and sway magnetometry [9].

The variables measured by such devices include anterior-posterior (AP) sway, medial-lateral (ML) sway, total sway, sway velocity, and frequency spectrum analyses.

These measurements have also been combined mathematically to form normalized measurements, such as Romberg's coefficient [51]. Electromyographical (EMG) measurements of various postural muscles [5,8,42] and cinematographical analyses [27] have also been investigated.

AP sway is the average amount of forward and backwards sway, usually considered as the y axis in a stabilograph. AP sway is generally larger than medial-lateral sway, which is limited by the anatomical structure of the ankle joint.

ML sway is the average amount of sway to the left and right. ML sway is usually considered as the x axis in a stabilograph.

Total sway or sway path is the total distance the center of pressure travels during a specified period of time (e.g., 30 seconds). Total sway takes into account both AP and ML sway (i.e., has an x and y coordinate), but is not a mean (average) position.

Romberg's coefficient, expressed as an eyes closed sway variable divided by an eyes open sway variable times 100, is a very useful measurement of sway because it reduces variation between subjects [9] providing a normal distribution. Romberg coefficients have also been used to express the relative destabilizing effects of the last five test conditions described by Shumway-Cook & Horak [45] as compared to the test condition with all sensory modalities available (test condition #1, refer to Figures 1-6) [22].

The frequency spectrum analysis takes the time-domain function of postural sway and converts it to its equivalent frequency-domain representation by the use of a Fourier transform. Since the Fourier transform is very time consuming, the Fast Fourier Transform (FFT) is often used to perform the frequency spectrum analysis. The FFT presents displacement amplitude on the ordinate and frequency on the abscissa. The FFT shows the frequency of oscillations during static equilibrium. This information allows interpretation of the contribution of the sensory modalities during stance. Changes in frequency bands reflect the interplay of the various diffuse neural control mechanisms involved in posture maintenance [46].

Nashner [38,43] stated that each of the three sensory modalities operate in specific frequency ranges, with some overlap, demonstrating that they are not redundant but function together to maintain postural equilibrium. Changes in specific frequency bands have been observed in studies involving disease states affecting the three sensory modalities that control posture.

There are a number of frequency bands that are either normal or caused by normal functioning that should to be considered when interpreting spectral analyses. The mean frequency while standing quietly has been described as approximately 0.7 Hz [15], while the body's natural frequency, when treated as a one-link system, without

elastic couplings, should be 0.45 Hz [2]. Respiratory
rhythm occurs between 0.3 and 0.4 Hz [29]. Brauer & Siedel
[7] made reference to center of gravity changes reflected
in the spectral analysis. They claim that center of gravity
displacements are represented by increases in the 0.025 to
0.2 Hz frequency band and center of gravity displacement
accelerations are measurable in frequencies greater than 1
Hz.

Spectral changes brought about by loss of
somatosensory input usually involve an increased amplitude
in the 0.7 to 1.2 Hz frequency band [1], with a peak at
approximately 1 Hz [30,32]. The increased amplitude around
1 Hz has been observed in patients with Tabes Dorsalis
[31], Friedreich's ataxia [12], chronic muscle afferent
disturbance [1], and in normals with blockage of muscle
afferents [1,30,32]. Anterior lobe atrophy results in
increased AP sway between 2 and 4 Hz., mainly 3 Hz., with
eyes closed [12].

Increased amplitude at 1 Hz is thought to be due to
vestibularly-induced trunk movements [32]. This vestibular
oscillation occurs at 1 Hz due to the long latency and high
threshold of the vestibulospinal reflexes [31,39]. Changes
in 1 Hz range are also observed in conditions with lesions
of certain structures of the CNS [19], but the exact nature
of changes in the 1 Hz area are not fully understood [17].

Visual stabilization posture has been described in the
frequency ranges of 0.5 to 1.0 Hz [50] and 0.03 to 0.3 Hz
[12]. Studies exposing subjects to large moving visual
scenes in order to induce visual disturbance of posture
indicate that visual stabilization of posture occurs
largely in low frequency ranges [10,29,33]. The optical
righting reflex via the cerebral cortex is thought to
increase ML sway at approximately 0.3 Hz [49].

The working frequency range of the vestibular system
can only be estimated [11]. Nashner [41] stated that the
semicircular canals function in frequencies above 0.1 Hz
and that the otoliths sense sway below 0.1 Hz. Brauer &
Seidel [7] further refined the frequency range of otolithic
function, stating that the otoliths sense sway in the 0.025
to 0.1 Hz. range.

**THE EFFECTS OF CLOSED HEAD INJURY ON SENSORY FUNCTION AND
INTEGRATION**

Postural Sway

Ingersoll & Armstrong [24] demonstrated differences in
postural stability for different levels of head injury.
Severely head-injured subjects (unconscious for > 6h)
evidenced greater AP and ML sway than mildly head-injured
or normal subjects, but there was no difference in total

sway between the groups. We concluded that head-injured subjects do not sway more, but maintain their center of pressure at a greater distance from the center of their base of support and make fewer postural corrections. This was particularly evident when one or more of the sensory modalities were conflicted or eliminated.

Lehmann et al. [28] demonstrated similar results using different test conditions. They felt that sway measures accurately reflected subjects performance and could be used to evaluate the success of treatment programs.

Romberg Coefficients

Ingersoll [22] demonstrated differences between severely head-injured subjects and moderate, mild and non-head-injured subjects for RQ41, RQ51 and RQ61 in AP, ML and total sway. RQ41 represents sway for test condition #4 divided by sway for test condition #1 times 100. RQ51 and RQ61 are calculated in the same manner. All differences involved test conditions with altered surface support (i.e., standing on foam), suggesting proprioceptive deficits.

Spectral Changes

Spectral changes have been identified in numerous disease states. Patients with a bilateral loss of labyrinthine excitability show a peak of 0.4 Hz in AP sway with eyes open [48,49]. Increases at 0.4 Hz have also been demonstrated in patients with Foville syndrome and cervical myelopathia [49]. Unilateral disturbance of the labyrinthine or stimulation of the vestibular system results in increases around 0.2 Hz [25,49]. Patients with Meniere's disease demonstrate increased AP sway in frequencies below 0.1 and between 0.6 and 0.7 Hz with eyes closed, decreased sway between 1.4 and 2.0 Hz, as do subjects with paroxysmal positional vertigo and vestibular neuritis [53].

Tokita et al. [49] also noted changes in the frequency spectrum for a number of other neurological disorders. Cerebellar disturbance was reported to increase sway in the 0.1 to 0.2 Hz. range, Parkinson's disease in the 0.25 to 0.6 Hz. range, cervical cord disturbance at 0.4 Hz., and disturbance of spinal reflexes in the 0.04 to 0.8 Hz. range.

Ingersoll & Armstrong [23] detected differences for frequency bands representing semicircular canal functioning, visual input and somatosensory input. Severely head-injured subjects differed from moderate, mild and non-head injured subjects. Semicircular canal functioning was different under test condition 4. Visual input was different for all test conditions except test condition 1.

We concluded that severely head-injured subjects relied heavily on vision to maintain standing posture, even though somatosensory input was unaltered. Faulty processing of somatosensory information was offered as a possible explanation.

CONCLUSION

Postural control testing demonstrates promise as a diagnostic tool for identifying subtle functional changes following closed head injury in athletes. Further research is necessary to determine the criterion-based validity of the sensory function and integration variables and the clinical feasibility of each.

REFERENCES

[1]   Aggashyan, R.V., Gurfinkel, V.S., Mamasakhlisov, G.V., and Elner, A.M. "Changes in Spectral and Correlation Characteristics of Human Stabilograms at Muscle Afferentation Disturbance," Agressologie, Vol. 14D, 1973, pp 5-9.

[2]   Aggashyan, R.V. "On Spectral and Correlation Characteristics of Human Stabilograms," Agressologie, Vol. 13D, 1972, pp 63-69.

[3]   Arcan, M., Brull, M.A., Najenson, T., and Solzi, P. "FGP Assessment of Postural Disorders During Process of Rehabilitation," Scandinavian Journal of Rehabilitation Medicine, Vol. 9, 1977, pp 165-168.

[4]   Arcan, M., and Brull, M.A. "A Fundamental Characteristic of the Human Body and Foot, the Foot-Ground Pressure Pattern," Journal of Biomechanics, Vol. 9, 1976, pp 453-457.

[5]   Basmajian, J.V., and Bentzon, J.W. "An Electromyographic Study of Certain Muscles of the Leg and Foot in Standing Posture," Surgery, Gynecology & Obstetrics, Vol. 98, 1954, pp 662-666.

[6]   Bourassa, P., and Therrien, R. "A Force Platform for the Evaluation of Human Locomotion and Posture," Biomechanics VIII-A. Matsui, H., and Kobayashi, K., Eds., Human Kinetic Publishers, Champaign, 1983, pp. 582-588.

[7] Brauer, D., and Seidel, H. "Time Series Analysis of Postural Sway," *Agressologie*, Vol. 20B, 1979, pp 111-112.

[8] Burke, D., and Eklund, G. "Muscle Spindle Activity in Man During Standing," *Acta Physiologica Scandinavica*, Vol. 100, 1977, pp 187-199.

[9] Dean, E.M., Griffiths, C.J., and Murray, A. "Stability of the Human Body Investigated by Sway Magnetometry," *Journal of Medical Engineering & Technology*, Vol. 10, 1986, pp 126-130.

[10] Dichgans, J., Mauritz, K.H., Allum, J.H.J., and Brandt, T.H. "Postural Sway in Normals and Atactic Patients: Analysis of the Stabilizing Effects of Vision," *Agressologie*, Vol. 17C, 1976, pp 15-24.

[11] Diener, H.C., Dichgans, J., Guschlbauer, B., and Bacher, M. "Role of Visual and Static Vestibular Influences on Dynamic Posture Control," *Human Neurobiology*, Vol. 5, 1986, pp 105-113.

[12] Diener, H.C., Dichgans, J., Bacher, M., and Gompf, B. "Quantification of Postural Sway in Normals and Patients with Cerebellar Diseases," *Electro-encephalography and Clinical Neurophysiology*, Vol. 57, 1984, pp 134-142.

[13] Dietz, V., Mauritz, K.H., and Haller, M. "Regulation of Human Posture During Balancing," (Abstract) *Pflugers Archives*, Vol. 379, 1979, pp R43.

[14] Dietz, V., and Noth, J. "Pre-Innervation and Stretch Responses of Triceps Brachii in Man Falling With and Without Visual Control," *Brain Research*, Vol. 142, 1978, pp 576-579.

[15] Era, P., and Heikkinen, E. "Postural Sway During Standing and Unexpected Disturbance of Balance in Random Samples of Men of Different Ages," *Journal of Gerontology*, Vol. 40, 1985, pp 287-295.

[16] Freedman, W., Wannestadt, G., and Herman, R. "EMG Patterns and Forces Developed During Step Down," *American Journal of Physical Medicine*, Vol. 55, 1976, pp 275-290.

[17] Gagey, P.M., Bizzo, G., Debruille, O., and Lacroix, D. "The One-Hertz Phenomenon," *Vestibular and Visual Control on Posture and Locomotor Equilibrium. 7th International Symposium of the International Society for Posturography*, Igarashi, T., and Black, F.O., Eds., Karger, Basil, 1983, pp 89-92.

[18] Goldberg, J.M., and Fernandez, C. "Vestibular Mechanisms," *Annual Reviews of Physiology*, Vol. 37, 1975, pp 129-162.

[19] Gurfinkel, V.S., and Elner, A.M. "On Two Types of Postural Disorders in Patients With Local Lesions of the Brain," *Agressologie*, Vol. 14D, 1973, pp 10-14.

[20] Hirasawa, Y. "Study of Human Standing Ability by Multipoint XY-Tracker and Pedoscope," *Agressologie*, Vol. 17B, 1976, pp 21-27.

[21] Holzgraefe, M., Lemme, W., Funke, W., Felix, R., and Felten, R. "The Significance of Diagnostic-Imaging in Acute and Chronic Brain-Damage in Boxing - A Prospective Study in Amateur Boxing Using Magnetic Resonance Imaging. *International Journal of Sports Medicine*, Vol. 13, 1992, pp 616-620.

[22] Ingersoll, C.D. "Stabilometric Analyses of Recovered Brain-Injured and Normal Subjects: A Study Using Romberg Coefficients," Presented at the International Congress and Exposition on Sports Medicine and Human Performance, Vancouver, BC, Canada, April 20, 1991.

[23] Ingersoll, C.D., and Armstrong, C.W. "The Effect of Closed Head Injury on the Frequency Spectrum of Postural Sway," *Medicine and Science in Sports and Exercise*, (Abstract), Vol. 23, 1991, pp S3.

[24] Ingersoll, C.D., and Armstrong, C.W. "The Effects of Closed-Head Injury on Postural Sway," *Medicine and Science in Sports and Exercise*, Vol. 24, 1992, pp 739-743.

[25] Kapteyn, T.S., and DeWit, G. "Posturography as an Auxilliary in Vestibular Investigation," *Acta Otolaryngologica*, Vol. 73, 1972, pp 104-111.

[26] Kitahara, M. "Acceleration registography: A New Method of Examination Concerned With the Labyrinthine Righting Reflex," *Annals of Otology*, Vol. 74, 1965, pp 203.

[27] Koozekanani, S.H., Stockwell, C.W., McGhee, R.B., and Firoozmand, F. "On the Role of Dynamic Models in Quantitative Posturography," IEEE Transactions on Biomedical Engineering, Vol. 27, 1980, pp 605-609.

[28] Lehmann, J.F., Boswell, S., Price, R., Burleigh, A., deLateur, B.J., Jaffe, K.M., and Hertling, D. "Quantitative Evaluation of Sway as an Indicator of Functional Balance in Post-Traumatic Brain Injury," Archives of Physical Medicine and Rehabilitation, Vol. 71, 1990, pp 955-962.

[29] Lestienne, F., Soechting, J., and Berthoz, A. "Postural Readjustments Induced by Linear Motion of Visual Scenes," Experimental Brain Research, Vol. 28, 1977, pp 363-384.

[30] Mamasakhlisov, G.V., Elner, A.M., and Gurfinkel, V.S. "Participation of Various Types of Afferentation in Control of the Orthograde Posture in Man," Agressologie, Vol. 14A, 1973, pp 37-41.

[31] Mauritz, K.H., and Dietz, V. "Characteristics of Postural Instability Induced by Ischemic Blocking of Leg Afferents," Experimental Brain Research, Vol. 38, 1980, pp 117-119.

[32] Maurtiz, K.H., Dietz, V., and Haller, M. "Balancing as a Clinical Test in the Differential Diagnosis of Sensory-Motor Disorders," Journal of Neurology, Neurosurgery & Psychiatry, Vol. 43, 1980, pp 407-412.

[33] Mauritz, K.H., Dichgans, J., and Hufschmidt, A. "The Angle of Visual Roll Motion Determines the Displacement of Subjective Vertical," Perception & Psychophysics, Vol. 22, 1977, pp 557-562.

[34] McKinley, P.A., and Smith, J.L. "Visual and Vestibular Contributions to Prelanding EMG During Jump Downs in Cats," Experimental Brain Research, Vol. 52, 1983, pp 439-448.

[35] Mechling, R.W. "Objective Assessment of Postural Balance Through Use of the Variable Resistance Balance Board," Physical Therapy, Vol. 66, 1986, pp 685-688.

[36] Mizuno, Y., Hayashi, R., Miyake, A., and Watanabe, S. "Analysis of Body Sway on Seesaw Board," Biomechanics VIII-A, Matsui, H. and Kobayashi, K., Eds, Human Kinetic Publishers, Champaign, 1983, pp 597-603.

[37] Murray, J.F. "Construction of a Stabilometer Capable of Indicating the Variability of Non-Level Performance," Perceptual & Motor Skills, Vol. 55, 1982, pp 1211-1215.

[38] Nashner, L.M. "Analysis of Stance Posture in Humans," Handbook of Behavioral Neurobiology, Vol. 5. Motor Coordination, Towe, A.L., and Luschei, E.S., Eds., Plenum Press, New York, 1981, pp 527-561.

[39] Nashner, L.M. "Adapting Reflexes Controlling the Human Posture," Experimental Brain Research, Vol. 26, 1976, pp 59-72.

[40] Nashner, L.M. "Vestibular and Reflex Control of Normal Standing," Control of Posture and Locomotion, Stein, R.B., Pearson, K.G., Smith, R.S., and Redford, J.B., Eds., Plenum Press, New York, 1973, pp 291-203.

[41] Nashner, L.M. "Vestibular Postural Control Model," Kybernetic, Vol. 10, 1972, pp 106-110.

[42] Nashner, L.M. "A Model Describing Vestibular Detection of Body Sway Motion," Acta Otolaryngologica, Vol. 72, 1971, pp 429-436.

[43] Nashner, L.M. "Sensory Feedback in Human Posture Control," Massachusetts Institute of Technology Report, Vol. MVT 70-3, 1970.

[44] Romberg, M.H. Lehrbuch der Nervenkrankheiten des Menschen, 2nd Ed., A. Hirschwald, Berlin, 1851.

[45] Shumway-Cook, A., and Horak, F.B. "Assessing the Influence of Sensory Interaction on Balance: Suggestion From the Field," Physical Therapy, Vol. 66, 1986, pp 1548-1550.

[46] Soames, R.W., Atha, J., and Harding, R.H. "Temporal Changes in the Pattern of Sway as Reflected in Power Spectral Density Analysis," Agressologie, Vol. 17B, 1976, pp 15-20.

[47] Spaepen, A.J., Peeraer, L., and Willems, E.J. "Center of Gravity and Center of Pressure in Stabilometric Studies: A Comparison With Film Analysis," Agressologie, Vol. 20B, 1979, pp 117-118.

[48] Tokita, T., Maeda, M., and Miyata, H. "The Role of the Labyrinth in Standing Posture Regulation," Acta Otolaryngologica, Vol. 91, 1981, pp 521-527.

[49] Tokita, T., Miyata, H., Matuoka, T., Taguchi, T., and Shimada, R. "Correlation Analysis of the Body Sway in Standing Posture," *Agressologie*, Vol. 17B, 1976, pp 7-14.

[50] Tokumasu, K., Ikegami, A., Tashiro, N., Bre, M., and Yoneda, S. "Frequency Analysis of the Body Sway in Different Standing Postures," *Agressologie*, Vol. 24B, 1983, pp 89-90.

[51] Van Parys, J.A.P., and Njiokiktjien, C.J. "Romberg's Sign Expressed as a Quotient," *Agressologie*, Vol. 17B, 1976, pp 95-100.

[52] Van De Graaf, K.M., and Fox, S.I. *Concepts of Human Anatomy and Physiology*, Wm. C. Brown Publishers, Dubuque, 1986, pp 569-570.

[53] Yoneda, S., and Tokumasu, K. "Frequency Analysis of Body Sway in the Upright Posture. Statistical Study in Cases of Peripheral Vestibular Disease," *Acta Otolaryngologica*, Vol. 102, 1986, pp 87-92.

Protective Equipment Applications

Hugh H. Hurt, Jr.[1] and David R. Thom[2]

ACCIDENT PERFORMANCE OF MOTORCYCLE AND BICYCLE SAFETY HELMETS

REFERENCE: Hurt, H. H., Jr. and Thom, D. R., "Accident Performance of Motocycle and Bicycle Safety Helmets," Head and Neck Injuries in Sports, ASTM STP 1229, Earl F. Hoerner, Ed., American Society for Testing and Materials, Philadelphia, 1994.

ABSTRACT: Motorcycle and bicycle safety helmets must adhere to specific technical requirements in order to provide protection. Various helmet configurations illustrate success with the application of these principles as well as failure by the neglect of these technical principles. The most critical feature of truly protective headgear is the use of a significant amount of energy absorbing material for the liner of the safety helmet. The most successful safety helmets have been built to standards that incorporate these technical requirements as basic performance in the areas of retention systems and impact attenuation. The qualification of the safety helmet to the basic technical requirements insures protection to the covered integument as well as prevention of a class of "contact" injuries including skull fractures and intracranial injuries. In addition, the qualified safety helmet is shown to prevent or reduce most of a class of "inertial" injuries, but with certain limitations of specific rotational injuries which can not be excluded by any protective device.

KEYWORDS: Helmets, helmet effectiveness, motorcycles, bicycles, head injuries, contact injuries, inertial injuries, impact attenuation

INTRODUCTION

The development of protective headgear has relied upon very simple, basic science to provide effective protection from typical accident threats. The applications in aviation, motor vehicles and sports have proved the real value of modern safety helmets. Similar situations exist for traffic accidents involving motorcycles and bicycles, where contemporary safety helmets have been shown to give significant reductions in injury. However, the voluntary use of safety helmets by motorcyclists and bicyclists is low, and the mandatory use of safety helmets is always debated and challenged in the arena of politics, but never in the arena of science. While there are certain limitations to the protection provided by safety helmets, the overall value of their use is well documented in research.

[1]Professor of Safety Science, Head Protection Research Laboratory, University of Southern California, Los Angeles, CA 90089-0021

[2]Director, Head Protection Research Laboratory, University of Southern California, Los Angeles, CA 90089-0021

The application of the Lombard principles[1] to helmet design and construction has produced a wide variety of highly effective head protection for aviation, motor vehicle racing, motorcycling and bicycling. The application of the various standards of the American National Standards Institute (ANSI), American Society for Testing and Materials (ASTM), British Standards Institute (BSI), Canadian Standards Association (CSA), Department of Transportation (DOT), Snell Memorial Foundation (Snell), etc., have insured a high level of basic qualification to safety helmets. However, there are notable problems in qualified head protection: industrial safety helmets provide protection only for falling objects of low energy and are extremely vulnerable to side impact; fire hats must accommodate a variety of life support equipment and are vulnerable to ejection; unqualified helmets used in many equestrian events give the illusion of protection but actually offer very little protection; and bogus motorcycle helmets intended to circumvent mandatory helmet use laws provide no real protection.

Finally, a major factor affecting the availability of protective headgear has been the last fifteen years of product litigation. Any safety helmet will be associated with injury events in an accident, simply because of its intended function. Because of this, safety helmets have been the target of litigation to the extreme, with both adverse and proverse effect. Many manufacturers have not been able to withstand the litigation, and the cost of product insurance has been severely increased to those remaining in the market. On the other hand, the many qualified safety helmets now availables represent the very best in head protection.

PRINCIPLES OF HEAD PROTECTION

Safety helmet design experienced a significant change in the middle 1950's with the development of truly protective headgear for aviation. The principles established by Lombard[1] were confirmed by detailed investigations of the performance by these helmets in many aircraft accidents. The patents of this configuration were acquired then applied to the design and development of the motor racing helmets produced by Bell Helmets, and the following years established the reputation for protection performance for these helmets.

The basic requirements for the truly protective headgear were established by Lombard and follow traditional thoughts on crashworthiness: the protection system must remain in place during the accident events, the system must furnish a barrier to prevent penetration and distribute impact force, and the impact energy must be absorbed to prevent transmission of energy to the brain. This requirement for an energy absorbing liner was the critical ingredient missing in most previous designs of helmets and was the most unique feature of the Lombard, Toptex and Bell helmets. As various designs of helmets evolved, various materials for energy absorption were applied, including nitrile-vinyl rubber, polyurethane foam, expanded polystyrene bead foam, e.g. EPS or "styrofoam", and polypropylene. Most modern designs of safety helmets employ various bead configurations of EPS because of the suitability for impact attenuation and convenience of foam molding. Exceptions are rare and usually limited to sports helmets where low energy impacts are repeated or applications where the EPS is vulnerable to handling damage and environment, e.g., fire hats.

Figure 1 shows the construction of a typical safety helmet, with the principal parts of the hard shell, the retention system and the energy absorbing liner. An impact to the outer surface of the shell is distributed to a wide area of the liner, depending on the stiffness of the shell and the geometry of the impacting object. The objective is to prevent penetration by sharp impacts and provide a wide area of loading to the liner beneath that impact site. In that way, a large volume of

the liner is available to crush and absorb the energy of impact thus
attenuating the impact and reducing the shock transmitted to the head
and brain. The shell and liner do not act independently in some simple
way but interact in very complicated ways depending upon the type of
impact threat. When the impact involves a sharp edge or point, the
demands for shell strength and stiffness are severe; when the impact
involves a flat or compliant surface, high shell strength and stiffness
will distribute the force too widely and will not allow yielding
deformation of the liner. In that instance of flat or compliant surface
impact, it is desirable to have a flexible shell, or even no shell at
all, as found in many modern bicycle helmets.

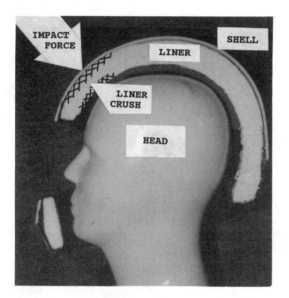

Figure 1
Safety Helmet Construction

The configurations of safety helmets which can incorporate the basic
requirements are numerous and varied, and the most familiar are the
three types of motorcycle safety helmets. Figure 2 shows the partial
coverage, full coverage and full facial configurations of safety
helmets. It is important to note that helmet design followed the Bell-
Toptex design of the 1960's for a very good reason: it was very
difficult to improve upon the early Bell design and many competitors
simply bought Bell helmets and copied them outrightly. The development
of the full facial configuration by Bell Helmets was a major improvement
to add facial protection, and this too was copied by many other
manufacturers with success. There were some very original designs which
evolved in the 1970's some of which offered important advances in
protection. The Shoei S-20 and S-27 were a major improvement in the
incorporation of an extremely large volume of EPS liner, far beyond
other helmets with styrofoam well below test requirements and also
beneath the chin bar. These helmets illustrated an extension of the
Lombard principles: energy absorbing foam liner is good, and more liner-
giving more coverage is better. Currently, the helmets made by Shoei,
Bell, Arai, Kiwi, Bieffe, etc., demonstrate superior protection

performance because those designs incorporate large volumes of energy absorbing foam in their liners, e.g., four plus litres of foam volume.

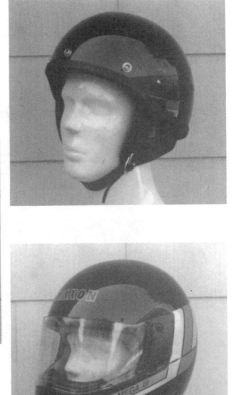

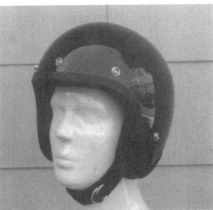

Full

Full Facial

Figure 2
Safety Helmet Coverage

It is very important to distinguish the inherent simplicity of truly protective headgear. The load spreading shell, the retention system and the energy absorbing liner combine to produce the protection required, and an acceptable design can take a variety of forms as long as the principal ingredients are included. In this way, the truly appropriate standards for safety helmets must be requirements of performance only, with specific elements of construction and materials left to the ingenuity of the designer. Accident research[2] has shown that a great variety of safety helmet configurations can provide spectacular reduction in injury, as long as the helmet has the "right stuff." On the other hand, if the helmet does not have the critical ingredients, especially the energy absorbing liner, that helmet is sure to fail in protection of the head. In recent time, there is no better example than the contradictions in bicycle safety helmets. Before the introduction of the ANSI Z-90.4 bicycle helmet standard, there was a great variety of bicycle helmets, some designs having the proper ingredients but many not having the "right stuff." A similar situation existed for equestrian helmets. Prior to the introduction of the ASTM F1163-90 standard, most of the equestrian helmets available were not capable of adequate head protection. Comparison of laboratory and accident performance of contrasting designs[3] has completely confirmed that those helmets without the energy absorbing liner give only the illusion of protection and offer nothing to protect the wearer in an accident. Figure 3 shows a bicycle helmet which violates all three parts of the Lombard principles: there is no substantial outer shell, there is no energy absorbing liner but there is a resilient padding which actually increases impact response, and the retention system is feeble and fragile. Incredibly, such a helmet has many advocates and users, but also several severely injured former users who now appreciate the illusion of protection as result of their accident and accompanying head injury.

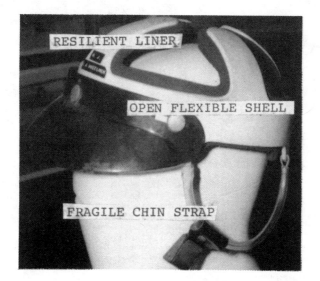

Figure 3
Unqualified Bicycle Helmet

Completely elastic, resilient materials cannot serve as effective liners because the impact energy is stored then rebounded rather than absorbed. Consequently, elastic foam materials do not absorb impact but have the prospect of amplifying impact dynamics. The suitable liner material must demonstrate the energy absorbing characteristic, by deforming permanently when impact occurs. It is this characteristic that allows an accident-involved safety helmet to be disassembled and examined for its accident performance[4]. Figure 4 shows an accident-involved motorcycle safety helmet disassembled to expose the severe impact damage to the exterior and the corresponding damage to the EPS liner underneath that impact location. There is damage to the exterior of the shell at the impact site marked "A", and the styrofoam liner beneath that impact "A"

shows a large area of permanent compression and bead damage, which is
outlined by the arrows. The area of liner compression carries many
features of functional damage such as noticeable reduction of thickness
due to crush, interbead cracking on both inner and outer surfaces and
palpable softening due to the crushing.

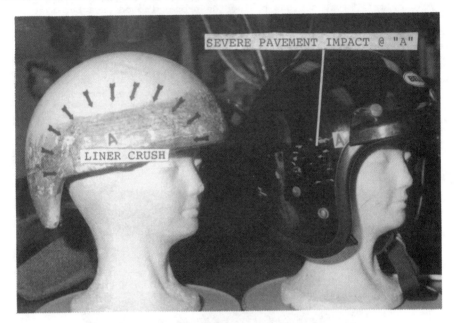

Figure 4
Disassembled Accident Involved Motorcycle Helmet

Sports helmets used in football and hockey have different impact
requirements when compared with safety helmets for motorcycles or
bicycles. The football or hockey helmet must have the ability to
recover from one low energy impact then sustain other similar impacts.
Proper protection from repeated low energy impacts requires a suitable
viscoelastic material (Kelvin solid) with rapid recovery. Typically,
such viscoelastic materials do not have the high energy absorption
characteristics needed for motor sports helmets.

DESIGN REQUIREMENTS AND STANDARDS

The situations which require head protection are not simple and
predictable but typically involve a variety of impact agents such as
pavement, curbs, Botts Dots, roll bars, A-pillars, roof rails, bumpers,
undercarriage, foot pegs, roll bars, rocks, falling objects, guard
rails, trees, power poles, windshields, fenders, tires, soil,
vegetation, mud, snow, ice, animals, including other humans, and
environments of fire and heat, cold and wet, electric and toxic, etc.
When the designer of a safety helmet is faced with such a variety of
potential impact surfaces, special attention to one type of impact
condition can result in a vulnerability for some other impact condition.
For example, if a safety helmet were designed to contend with multiple
high energy impacts from an automobile roll bar at a given location,
that same helmet may have unfavorable response to a single impact into a
very compliant surface such as sand or mud. Obviously, this sort of
complication can occur often in the design of safety helmets and thus

the need for suitable standards is apparent. Proper standards will have established priorities for potential accident threats and thereby specify particular performance of the safety helmet rather than particular constructional features. ANSI, ASTM, BSI, CSA, DOT, Snell, etc., standards allow the manufacturer to focus on more traditional design factors of comfort, convenience, graphics, reliability, maintainability, and cost. This is an example of the traditional reliance upon standards by small industry which does not usually possess the capability for in-depth scientific analysis of design requirements.

The development of the original standards for protective headgear properly focused upon three areas of requirements: (1)retention system strength and stiffness, (2)penetration resistance, and (3)impact attenuation. In each area, there were requirements for a specific minimum performance to satisfy the standard, and test procedures which have improved with time. The most durable of the standards for motor vehicle helmet applications is the ANSI Z-90.1 or Snell 68, which has evolved to the DOT FMVSS 218 without major change. The application and enforcement of this DOT standard has been shown by Liu[5] to produce major improvements in the protection quality of motorcycle helmets available to the public. The DOT motorcycle helmet standard requires the following performance: the retention test requires sustaining a central downward pull of 1335N (300 lb.), while limiting deflection to 25mm (1.0 in.). The penetration test requires impact of a 3 Kg. penetrator dropped from a height of 3 m. without violation of the protected space. The impact attenuation test requires drop tests of two successive impacts onto flat anvils with specific energy[3] of 1.8 m. (6 ft.), or hemispherical anvils with specific energy of 1.4 m. (4.5 ft.). Headform acceleration limit for these tests is 400g, and dwell time limits are 2.0 ms. at 200g and 4.0 ms. at 150g. While some parts of this standard may seem arbitrary, it is sure that an inferior helmet could not survive these tests. In fact, one of the most confounding aspects of the DOT standard is that some helmets qualified to much higher impact energies fail the DOT tests. A common example would be an expensive helmet qualified to the 1985 Snell standard but failing the DOT 200g dwell time limit at the flat anvil cold condition test[6].

Regardless of the completeness and detail of the standard, the designer of a safety helmet must consider typical accident events to account for the expected use of the helmet and insure proper function of the helmet. A typical example of additional consideration is the area of retention system performance of motorcycle safety helmets. The ANSI-DOT type standard for retention system performance requires sustaining a 1335N (300 lb.) central symmetrical pull while limiting deflection to 25mm (1.0 in.) The satisfaction of this simple requirement will provide completely satisfactory retention performance in the great majority of motorcycle accidents, but yet allow helmet ejection if some special requirements are not considered. One of the typical problems is the failure to provide a special geometry for the retention system to prevent forward roll-off when the motorcyclist suffers impact to the anterior chest. Then the helmet develops inertial forces tending to displace the helmet forward on the head. If the geometry of the properly fastened retention system allows such mobility, the retention system will fail to resist such forward roll-off and the helmet will be ejected in the sequence illustrated in Figure 5.

Ejection of the helmet by forward roll-off as shown in Figure 5 is clearly a problem of geometry and kinematics[7], rather than a simple problem of strength. While such problems can be described analytically and easily understood in a practical sense, many makers of safety

---

[3]Specific energy is mechanical energy per unit weight or mass, and has linear dimension.

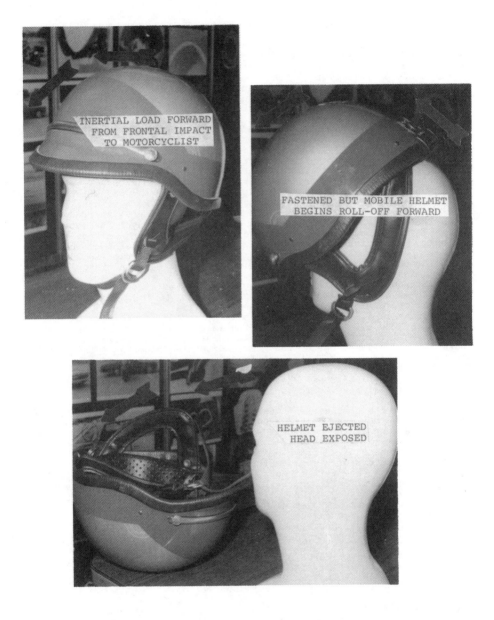

Figure 5
Forward Roll-Off Helmet Ejection

helmets have produced designs which allowed this mobility and potential
for ejection. The mobility for forward roll-off is conveniently limited
by proper location of the retention attachment to the shell so that
roll-off kinematics produce tightening rather than loosening of the chin
strap. Of course, the helmet coverage is a major factor in roll-off
mobility with full facial coverage helmets having the least mobility and

partial coverage helmets having the greatest mobility. In the case of the partial coverage helmet, it is often necessary to limit helmet mobility by the addition of an inconvenient and uncomfortable nape strap, etc. Procedures for testing helmet roll-off characteristics have been developed recently by the ASTM F08 committee.

The retention system design must also consider that the accident events may not apply a simple symmetrical pull to the retention system, so eccentric loads must be considered. Since the attachment of the retention system to the shell is a simple rivet, that rivet system should be capable of withstanding at least 25% of the retention system force in a lateral/medial direction[2]. Also, the cervical spine is not without limits and cervical distraction can occur at approximately 3600N to 4400N (800 to 1000 lbs.), so the retention system should have upper limits of strength which respect this mode of cervical injury. This sort of consideration denies the proposition that "stronger is better," especially for protective headgear. Dynamic crash tests and detailed examination of accident-involved motorcycle safety helmets have shown that the actual loads in a helmet retention system are relatively low, e.g., far less than 900N (200 lbs.) Of course, the exception is that instance when the helmet is snagged on an bumper or undercarriage of an automobile, then higher forces are developed, but retention of the helmet in such circumstances is not necessarily desirable because of potential injury to the neck. Some standards have attempted to include dynamic "jerk" tests on the retention system of motorcycle and bicycle safety helmets, but there is simply no evidence that the complication of such tests will better simulate accident events and produce better retention systems if asymmetrical loads and roll-off are not yet considered.

Helmet ejection in motorcycle accidents is primarily associated with failure to fasten the chin strap securely, or loosely fitted helmets, which increases helmet mobility and enhances forward roll-off in frontal impacts. In very severe frontal impacts involving facial fractures, fracture of the mandible destroys the retention support and allows subsequent ejection of any helmet.

Penetration tests of typical standards employ the impact of a sharp pointed device, attempting to penetrate the shell and liner. The concentration of 54J to 88J (40 to 65 ft-lbs.) of energy onto the penetrating point is severe; the energy density corresponding to that of a small caliber handgun. Such a penetration threat demands a substantial shell and liner, thus such a test would surely penetrate any inferior helmet. While there is little evidence that such tests represent actual accident events, such a test serves very well to eliminate inferior helmets from qualification.

Impact attenuation tests are required to prove the fundamental protection capability of a safety helmet, and such tests are the major part of any helmet standard. The most typical test involves a rigid headform with a sensitive accelerometer mounted inside. The helmet is mounted on the headform then dropped in a guided free fall to impact on an anvil surface, usually a rigid steel flat or hemispherical surface.

Figure 6 shows a conventional test system with a bicycle helmet prepared for testing. Conventional impact test systems of this sort have proved their value over the years because the rigid anvils and headforms provide highly repeatable test procedures, and require the helmet to perform all parts of the impact attenuation process. Some detractors of this rigid headform/anvil combination proffer the use of compliant headforms and more realistic anvil surfaces, but compliant headforms absorb some significant part of the impact energy and fail to determine the limits of helmet performance. The most important requirement of any helmet standard and corresponding test system is repeatability, and

experience has shown that rigid headforms and anvils provide that
quality in safety helmet testing.

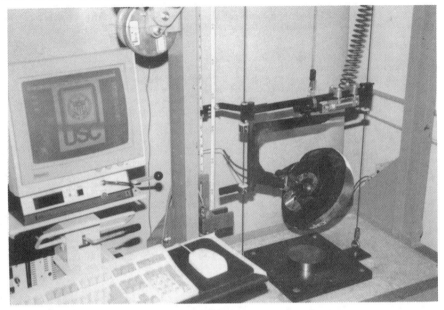

Figure 6
Conventional Helmet Test Equipment

In some fields of safety helmets, there have been no industry consensus
standards and little information available to the designer of a helmet.
For example, before the introduction of the ASTM F1163-90 standard for
equestrian helmets, most helmets available to the public offered great
style and light weight but very few provided real protection from
impact. In the absence of standards, a designer should apply the Lombard
principles and develop basic criteria suitable to the protection
requirements. In most instances, these requirements can be very basic
and without great technical complications. For example, in the middle
1970's, such was the case of Bell Helmet's development of the first
truly protective bicycle helmet, which was reported by Newman[8] and
then available to others interested in those bicycle sport applications.
Few manufacturers took advantage of that information at that time
because of lack of interest in that consumer market, ignorance or
economics.

An alternative for a designer without standards and basic criteria is to
simply select an existing standard with somewhat similar applications.
For example, a good bicycle helmet meeting ANSI Z-90.4 standard is a
suitable roller skating or skateboarding helmet. Also, a good motorcycle
helmet meeting DOT standards is a suitable helmet for hang glider and
ultralight aircraft pilots, at least due to the high level of protection
offered and lack of a requirement for communication equipment. On the
other hand, a good football helmet does not make a suitable aviation
helmet; a good aviation helmet does not make a suitable motorcycle
helmet; a good motorcycle helmet does not make a suitable football
helmet, etc. Regardless of the protection quality of a helmet design,
the suitability for the intended use is a critical factor, especially

where use of protective headgear is voluntary and has important social aspects involved.

In the arena of high energy impact protection, motor vehicle safety helmets have been developed to a high degree. Current motorcycle safety helmets are qualified to either DOT or Snell standards, or both. The compliance with the DOT standard is not optional; compliance with Snell standards is by agreement with the Snell Memorial Foundation. The specific energy for the DOT impact attenuation test is 1.8 m. (6 ft.) for the flat anvil and 1.37 m. (4.5 ft.) for the hemispherical anvil; the specific energy for Snell motorcycle impact attenuation test is 3 m. (10 ft.) for both flat and hemispherical anvils. Both standards require two successive impacts at each test site and the limits for headform acceleration are effectively 300g for Snell and 400g for DOT.

The test zone on the helmet for the DOT standard is illustrated by the lines on the helmet as shown in Figure 7; the test zone for Snell is basically the same except for being slightly lower at the rear of the helmet. This area includes approximately 80% of the most severe impacts which occur in motorcycle accidents[2] but yet excludes the necessary visual space, hence excludes a great part of the face from impact protection. In Figure 7, the adjacent model head has a sectioned full facial coverage helmet to compare the areas of the head actually covered with those required to be qualified by the DOT standard. It is important to respect this basic limitation of such protective headgear; motorcycle riders and all other helmet users must have a clear visual space so impact protection for the face has severe limitations.

The impact attenuation requirements for DOT have an unusual effect in actual performance: the most convenient way to meet the difficult 200g dwell time limit is to simply limit the overall impact response to less than 200g, so that there is no dwell time at 200g level. Most current helmets with only DOT qualification perform in this way, and thus demonstrate a very "soft" impact response in general. A helmet so qualified for DOT can not withstand both of the Snell impacts, especially the hemispherical anvil impacts, but most of these DOT helmets can withstand the first flat anvil Snell impact with lower peak g's than a Snell qualified helmet. In order to withstand the higher specific energy of the Snell tests, a helmet must have greater shell strength and liner density, if the helmet is so equipped. DOT qualification surely does not guarantee Snell qualification and likewise Snell qualification does not guarantee DOT qualification, especially for the 200g dwell time limit. Since the Snell qualified helmet must also qualify to the DOT standard, the Snell qualified helmet does not have the "soft" impact response of the DOT helmet but is capable of withstanding the greater variety of more severe impacts. Finally, whenever various standards for motor vehicle safety helmets are compared it is important to return to reality: DOT specific energy of 1.8 m. (6 ft.) corresponds to 6 m/sec. (13.4 mph) impact; Snell M90 specific energy of 3 m. (10.0 ft.) corresponds to 7.75 m/sec. (17.3 mph) impact; 8.9 m/sec. (20 mph) impact corresponds to 4.1 m. (13.4 ft.); 13.4 m/sec. (30 mph) corresponds to 9.1 m. (30 ft.); 26.8m/sec. (60 mph) corresponds to 36.6 m. (120 ft.)! The fundamental issues of head protection involve relatively LOW SPEED impact conditions and any expectation for a high level of head protection in direct impact at greater than 9 m/sec. (20 mph) is unrealistic.

The basic physics of impact determine the physical requirements of helmet design, as well as the materials suitable for helmet construction. In the presence of current technology, approximately 40mm (1 1/2 in.) of helmet thickness is necessary to meet Snell M90 impact attenuation requirements at specific energy of 3 m. (10.0 ft.). If the same technology were applied to specific energy of 4 m. (13.4 ft.), at least 65mm (2 1/2 in.) of helmet thickness would be required, swelling

overall helmet dimensions considerably beyond expected consumer
acceptance.

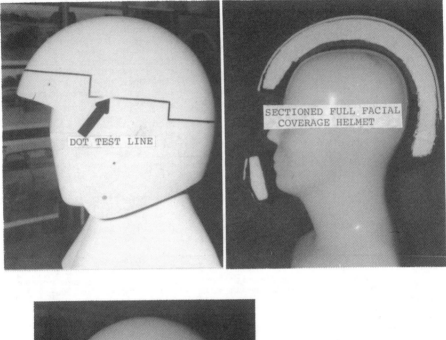

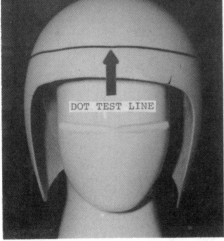

Figure 7
DOT FMVSS 218 Test Zone

Detailed statistics for head impacts are incomplete, and there is little
known about the specific energy associated with various accident impact
conditions. In the case of motorcycle accidents[2], it has been
determined that the DOT flat anvil specific energy corresponds
approximately to the 90th percentile of helmet impacts in motorcycle
traffic accidents. Further estimates find that the Snell M90 corresponds
approximately to the 97th percentile for helmet impacts in motorcycle
traffic accidents. Since both standards require TWO successive impacts
at each test site, it is evident that the Snell standard requires
performance at the extreme of impact energy. Other motorcycle and
bicycle accident data show that the predominating impact surfaces were
flat (87%)[2], (75%)[9] or blunt (8.6%) and pavement (71.6%) or metal
(21.8%). Comparison with U.S. Army Aviation accident data establishes a
significant correlation for SPH-4 helicopter helmet accident impact
surface geometry.

HEAD INJURIES AND PROTECTION PERFORMANCE

The types of head injuries are classified by Ommaya[10] generally
according to anatomic locations, while suggesting some of the
biomechanical origins of the injuries. This description of injuries can
be useful in the evaluation of the accident performance of safety
helmets, and is presented in Table 1.

In order to correlate this typology of head injuries with the typical
safety helmet, Figure 8 shows the sectioned full facial coverage
motorcycle safety helmet in place with head and neck anatomy. In this
way, it is clear that injuries to the integument of the head are easily
prevented by that coverage. Abrasions are possible only where the
integument is exposed to tangential motion of the impacting agent;
lacerations are easily prevented by the immediate presence of the hard
shell and underlying liner. Contusions, bruises and subgaleal hemorrhage
generally require direct contact with severe pressure to injure the
adjacent tissue hence such injuries are easily prevented by the load-

TABLE 1
TYPES OF HEAD INJURIES
(After Ommaya)

I.   Integument, Scalp
      a. abrasion
      b. laceration
      c. contusion, bruise, subgaleal hemorrhage,
         hematoma
      d. avulsion
      e. burn
II.   Skull
      a. suture separation, diastasis, often juvenile
      b. linear fracture
      c. indentation, e.g., ping-pong fracture,
         usually juvenile
      d. depressed fracture
      e. crushing, massive comminution
III. Extracerebral Hemorrhage, Hematoma
      a. subarachnoid hemorrhage
      b. epidural hemorrhage,
         usually associated with skull fracture
      c. subdural hemorrhage
IV.   Brain Tissue Damage
      a. concussion, diffuse axonal injury
      b. brain contusion
      c. intracerebral hemorrhage
      d. cerebral laceration
      e. avulsion, extrusion

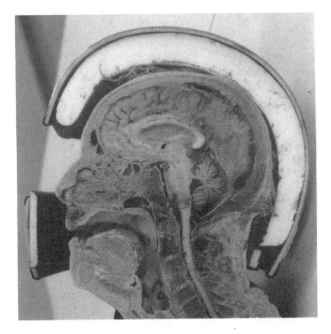

Figure 8
Sectioned Helmet with Head and Neck Anatomy
Photo by P.M. Fuller, Ph.D.

spreading of the shell and energy absorption of the underlying liner. The external ear can suffer severe injury when unprotected and uncovered, and avulsion of the pinna is a typical injury when the unprotected head encounters pavement, sharp metal objects, etc., so that safety helmet coverage easily prevents such injuries. While most safety helmets do not have specific qualifications for thermal protection, any substantial coverage and heat sink will do much to prevent burns from short duration thermal threat.

These capabilities for protection of the integument by various forms of protective headgear deserve special attention because such injuries to the integument are the most common injuries to the unprotected head in all forms of accidents. The injuries to the integument are rarely more than minor or moderate severity but they are the most frequently encountered injuries. Of course, the helmet coverage determines the extent of protection to the integument, and research[2,5,11] shows that more coverage is more protection to the integument, e.g., the full facial coverage helmet is better than the full coverage helmet, which is better than the partial coverage helmet, which is better than no helmet at all.

If the helmet is ejected during accident events, or not in use before the accident, such protection of the integument does not occur and abrasions, laceration, contusions, etc. will result. A stellate laceration plus abrasion of the parietal region of the scalp denies the presence of a safety helmet, unless that helmet has very severe structural damage in that corresponding location. To be sure, every safety helmet will have structural limits determined by design and related standards, and impacts to the exterior which are within those limits typically generate only minor contusion beneath these limiting impacts. Impacts which are beyond those limits will typically cause adjacent subgaleal hematoma, then laceration when the shell and liner capacity are exhausted.

It is necessary to involve certain biomechanical principles to explain the further effects safety helmets in the protecting regions of the head beneath the integument. Head impacts occur in a variety of accident configurations, with the moving head striking a hard surface, with the body free, or sometimes restrained, with a blunt object striking the head, etc. But head injuries can also occur without direct impact to the head, as in severe whiplash from blunt force trauma to the chest[12]. When the head is impacted directly, there is contact with the agent of injury and the possibility of injuries at that location. Also, when the head is not restrained, such an impact will produce motion response according to the laws of dynamics, and inertial forces will be developed within all of the masses of the head. Such inertial forces due to accelerations have the prospect of producing injury because of the relative motions of the parts of the brain and local stresses and strains in those tissues. Gennarelli[13] has provided a biomechanical description and classification of this system of injuries, shown in Table 2.

TABLE 2
MECHANISTIC TYPES OF HEAD INJURY
(After Gennarelli)

CONTACT INJURIES (requiring impact to the head; but head motion is not
                  necessary)

    Integument Injuries

    Skull Deformation Injuries
    Local: a. skull fractures (suture separation,
                    indentation, linear, depressed, crushing,
                    massive comminution)
            b. epidural hemorrhage, hematoma
            c. coup contusions, lacerations, maceration,
               avulsion, extrusion
    Remote: a. vault and basilar fractures

    Stress Wave Injuries
            a. contrecoup contusion
            b. intracerebral hematoma

INERTIAL INJURIES (direct impact to the cranial vault not necessary;
                   head acceleration necessary)

    Surface Strains
            a. subdural hematoma
            b. contrecoup contusion
            c. intermediate coup contusion

    Deep Strains
            a. concussion syndrome
            b. diffuse axonal injury

Because a qualified safety helmet will spread the contact impact force and provide for energy absorption beneath that contact point, the "contact" injuries defined by Gennarelli are those injuries most probably prevented by the helmet. Consider the example of a severe fall with a specific energy on the order of 1.8 m. (6 ft.), as might happen in an industrial slip and fall, a fall from a motorcycle or bicycle, or ejection from an automobile to fall to the roadway. If the unprotected side of the head is impacted on the hard surface, the typical injury system is as follows: an injury of abrasion, laceration, or contusion to the integument at the contact site, severe concussion, an underlying linear fracture of the temporal bone with laceration of the middle meningeal artery, causing a large developing epidural hemorrhage and hematoma, with consequent brain compression and injury. This system of "contact" injuries could be completely excluded by the use of a qualified DOT motorcycle helmet or ANSI Z90.4 bicycle helmet, and the inertial injury of concussion could be reduced to a light concussion which would not be an irreversible injury.

The use of qualified safety helmets allow the damage to be developed in the helmet, not the head. When the safety helmet is subject to impacts within qualification, the integument is protected, the skull is protected from fracture (with some exceptions), the associated epidural hemorrhage and hematoma are prevented, and coup contusions, lacerations, etc., are prevented. When the qualified safety helmet is subject to impacts beyond its qualification, there is increasing probability of contact injuries as the capability of the helmet is exhausted, and the damage to helmet will give evidence that the helmet structure has been overwhelmed. The typical indications are that the liner has suffered limiting deformation and has been crushed severely, or "bottomed-out;" the fiberglass shell will have developed considerable delamination and fracture, and the polycarbonate shell will have evidence of ductile fracture. Since polycarbonate materials are vulnerable to embrittlement in several ways, the possibility of premature brittle fracture requires investigation. Preexisting cracks, fractures originating at obvious stress concentrations, and smooth initial fracture surfaces require further investigation of the material properties. Fiber reinforced plastics using glass, kevlar and carbon fiber usually require no more than an investigation of the proper hardening of the resin, which can be done by BARCOL portable hardness testing.

Actually, within the perspective presented here, fracture of the shell is favorable because that would ordinarily represent additional energy absorption. The effect is adverse when the fracture occurs prematurely, prevents load spreading and the loss of structural integrity allows helmet ejection to expose the head to subsequent injury. Generally, detailed examination of the fracture and inspection of the adjacent liner will determine the chronology of events: if there is a deep localized gouge of the liner beneath the fracture, the fracture was premature or the impact surface was a sharp edge; if the liner shows a wide area of liner deformation, the fracture occurred at the end of the impact events, or the impact surface was flat and the shell had little function in those events. Laboratory tests confirm that shell fracture is favorable within these provisions because of the additional energy absorption.

Because the qualified safety helmet attenuates this impact and reduces the acceleration of the head within the helmet, the probability of contrecoup contusion and intracerebral hematoma is reduced, and when the acceleration is reduced below tolerance levels, the injuries are prevented. Of course, this means that impacts within the design range should not allow such injury, given that the tolerance levels are appropriate. Obviously, individual head impact tolerance levels vary, especially with health, age and ethanol involvement, but the qualified safety helmet will provide benefit nevertheless by reducing the contact injury threat in all cases.

A special exception must be noted in the case of basilar skull fractures, which can be specifically related to head motion as a result of the impact to the helmeted or unhelmeted head. Detailed dissections of the head and neck were conducted on a large number of helmeted and unhelmeted fatally injured motorcyclists[11] and many basilar skull fractures were found to be associated with the extremes of head and neck motions. A consistent system of basilar skull fracture was determined in both helmeted and unhelmeted fatalities: left side head impact produced the extreme of right lateral flexion and left sided basilar skull fractures, right side head impact produced the extreme of left lateral flexion and right sided basilar skull fractures; extremes of hyperextension or hyperflexion produced bilateral basilar skull fractures. In this system, a qualified safety helmet can reduce the probability of extreme head and neck motions hence reduce the probability of basilar skull fractures, but finally no helmet can exclude these severe injuries when severe head and neck motion occur[11,14]. Basilar skull fractures are generally associated with contact injuries but severe chest impact can generate severe head and neck motions and produce basilar skull fractures even without any sort of head contact or impact[11]. Of course, no helmet could alleviate this deadly threat.

The "inertial" injuries outlined in Table 2 are the results of the head being accelerated (most usually by impact) then all distributed and concentrated masses within the cranium develop forces resisting the acceleration, i.e., inertial forces. Just like the jet pilot experiences maneuvering accelerations that wrench his internal organs and drain the blood from the head and brain, the components of the brain are deformed and displaced relative to each other when head accelerations result. As a result of helmet function, an impact is attenuated and the head receives less shock, so the probability of these inertial injuries is reduced, so protective headgear can prevent these inertial injuries when the accelerations are within tolerance. In this way, the helmet cushions the impact and reduces the transmitted head acceleration, which corresponds to injury reduction. When a safety helmet is subjected to an impact beyond its capability, a typical result is an increase in head acceleration to dangerous levels hence injury. Evidence of extreme impact conditions would be wide areas of damage to the shell and large areas of liner crush approaching exhaustion of the crush capability, or "bottoming-out." It should be appreciated that impacts at the edge of the protection zone, such as around the face opening, have obvious limits and less protection than the qualified regions. Well designed helmets will carry the full thickness of liner down to the forehead region, but lesser helmets will have liners tapered to reduce thickness at the forehead to simplify molding and reduce liner costs.

The origins of inertial injuries are the responses to the energy of the accident events, and some accident impact configurations will generate conditions favoring inertial injuries and essentially eliminating contact injuries. Such limits to the function of motorcycle safety helmets have been described by Newman[15] and deal primarily with helmet impacts on compliant surfaces. When a helmeted head is impacted on hard pavement, the shell and liner have specific functions of load spreading and energy absorption; when a helmeted head impacts in soft mud or sand, these functions are severely limited in conventional helmets and the load is spread and the energy is absorbed only in a way which is determined by the compliant surface. The result is that the contact injuries are eliminated by the compliant surface, and the helmet can do very little to limit inertial injuries. When a qualified helmet happens to impact on a compliant surface, the only possible function would be to eliminate trivial integument injuries. If such a compliant surface impact were the ONLY consideration in design, the helmet could be made with more flexible shell and softer liner to contend with that special impact condition, but the helmet would then be vulnerable to unexpected hard object impacts.

A major part of the "surface" and "deep" strains causing inertial injuries is rotation of the head, as a result of direct impact to the head or response from impact to some other part of the body. Clearly there is a kinematic restraint of the head in motion since it is connected to the neck, etc., so impact to the head produces both linear and angular acceleration of the head, and the linear and angular accelerations are kinematically constrained. For example, if the head is impacted to produce 100g's of linear acceleration, an approximate instantaneous radius of rotation of 22cm (8 1/2 in.) corresponds to a rotational acceleration of about 4500 rad/sec^2. In this example, the linear acceleration of 100g's is tolerable by all standards and would not correspond to injury of any sort, but the high angular acceleration would correspond to the threshold of critical head injury, with significant inertial injuries and threat to life. In this way, a qualified safety helmet can reduce inertial injuries but these rotational injuries can not be excluded by any helmet.

An important limitation for any protective headgear is protection for the face. Because of the visual space requirements, all configurations of safety helmets will be vulnerable to facial impacts, and it is well established that facial impacts can have serious consequences. Facial injuries can be severe and difficult to repair; facial impacts can transmit force and acceleration to the brain to cause injury there. Figure 4 shows a disassembled motorcycle helmet which had a severe pavement impact at the right frontal-temporal region, at "A". In addition to the pavement impact on the helmet at "A", there was severe impact to the right zygoma and maxilla, which transmitted additional acceleration to the brain, which could not be reduced by this helmet. The resulting inertial head injury (due primarily to rotation) was a combination of that part of the impact on the helmet at "A" which was attenuated, plus the unattenuated impact transmitted through direct facial impact.

Clinical examination of fatal motorcycle accident cases[11] provided examples where impact to the mandible was transmitted to the base of skull to produce displaced basilar skull fracture and brain laceration, in both helmeted and unhelmeted motorcyclists. In contradiction, nonfatal clinical cases provided examples of severe facial fractures which apparently absorbed a major part of the impact energy and prevented brain injury, in both helmeted and unhelmeted motorcyclists.

The use of full facial coverage contributes additional coverage with the prospect of additional protection. If the chin bar has the proper construction such protection will result. The chin bar must have adequate strength and stiffness, such as would be required by Snell M90, and should have energy absorbing liner beneath that chin bar. Not all full facial helmets provide energy absorbing liner beneath the chin bar and thereby have limits to the protection offered. Some motorcycle full facial helmets have only thin resilient foam and sharp edges around the chin bar, so that impact to that chin bar produces an action similar to a "cookie-cutter" with injury rather than protection.

SUMMARY OF ACCIDENT PERFORMANCE

Contemporary safety helmets show significant reduction of head injury when those helmets have the critical ingredients for protection. Those critical ingredients are the hard shell, effective retention system and (especially) an energy absorbing liner.

The most effective safety helmets are those in motor vehicle applications where effective standards are in use[2,10]. The least effective helmets are those without the critical ingredients, where standards do not exist and industry is inactive in developing criteria.

Qualified safety helmets offer protection related to the coverage of the helmet, with the full facial configuration offering the greatest coverage and protection. Damage to the helmet shell and liner is the expected result of the protection function, and allows evaluation of impact severity and helmet function.

Qualified safety helmets are very effective in preventing or reducing the severity of contact type injuries. Qualified safety helmets are very effective in preventing and reducing the severity of inertial injuries, but many accident configurations create severe rotational acceleration of the head, which can not be excluded by any safety helmet.

REFERENCES

[1]   Lombard, C.F., Advani, S.H., "Impact Protection of the Head and Neck," USAF-Industry Two-Wheel Motor Vehicle Safety Seminar, 1966 (also refer to U.S. Patent No. 2,625,683 of January, 1953).

[2]   Hurt, H.H., Ouellet, J.V. and Thom, D.R., "Final Report-Motorcycle Accident Cause Factors and Identification of Countermeasures," NTIS PB81-206443, U.S. DOT-NHTSA, January, 1981.

[3]   Hurt, H.H., and Thom, D.R., "Laboratory Tests and Accident Performance of Bicycle Safety Helmets," Proceedings, 29th Annual Conference of the Association for the Advancement of Automotive Medicine, 1985.

[4]   Hurt, H.H., Ouellet, J.V., and Wagar I.J., "Analysis of Accident-Involved Motorcycle Safety Helmets," Proceedings, 20th Annual Conference of the Association for the Advancement of Automotive Medicine, 1976.

[5]   Liu, W.J.J., "Analysis of Motorcycle Helmet Test Data for FMVSS 218", Proceedings, International Conference on Motorcycle Safety, Motorcycle Safety Foundation, 1980.

[6]   Thom, D.R. & Hurt, H.H., "Conflicts of Contemporary Motorcycle Helmet Standards," Proceedings, 36th Annual Conference of the Association for the Advancement of Automotive Medicine, 1992.

[7]   Newman, J.A., "Dynamic Retention Characteristics of Motorcycle Helmets," Biokinetics and Associates, Ltd. 2470 Don Reid Dr., Ottawa, Ontario, Canada, 1979.

[8]   Lewicki, L.R., and Newman, J.A., "Head Protection for the Bicyclist", Proceedings, 19th Conference of the Association for the Advancement of Automotive Medicine, 1975.

[9]   Williams, M., "The Protective Performance of Bicyclists' Helmets in Accidents," Accident Analysis and Prevention, Vol. 23, Nos. 2/3, pp.119-131, 1991.

[10]   Ommaya, A.K., "Biomechanics of Head Injuries-Experimental Aspects, Biomechanics of Trauma," A.M. Nahum and J. Melvin, Eds., Appleton-Century-Crofts, 1985.

[11]   Hurt, H.H., Ouellet, J.V., and Rehman, I., "Epidemiology of Head and Neck Injuries in Motorcycle Fatalities," Mechanism of Head and Spine Trauma, A. Sances, D.J. Thomas, C.L. Ewing, S.J. Larson and F. Unterharnscheidt, Eds., Aloray, 1986.

[12]   Ommaya, A.K. and and P. Yarnell, Subdural Hematoma After Whiplash Injury, Lancet 2:237-239, August 1969.

[13]   Gennarelli, T.A., "Biomechanics of Head Injury", Biomechanics of Impact Trauma, International Research Council on the Biomechanics of Impact, 1984.

[14]   Thom, D.R., "Basilar Skull Fractures in Fatal Motorcycle Accidents," M.S. Thesis, University of Southern California, 1993.

[15]   Newman, J.A., "Motorcycle Helmets-Their Limits of Performance", Proceedings, International Conference on Motorcycle Safety, Motorcycle Safety Foundation, 1980.

Robert C. Shiffer[1]

ASTM F-1292 AS A TOOL FOR PLAYGROUND INJURY SEVERITY
REDUCTION

REFERENCE: Shiffer, Robert C., **"ASTM F-1292 as a Tool for
Playground Injury Severity Reduction,"** Head and Neck
Injuries in Sports, ASTM STP 1229, Earl F. Hoerner, Ed.,
American Society for Testing and Materials, Philadelphia,
1994.

ABSTRACT: In 1986 an activity was undertaken by ASTM
Committee F08 to develop a standard specification for
testing playground surfaces impact attenuation. This
activity resulted in the 1991 publication of ASTM F-1292
"Standard Specification for Impact Attenuation of Surface
Systems Under and Around Playground Equipment." This
specification sought to clarify the 1981 United States
Consumer Product Safety Commission (CPSC) guideline
recommendation of instrumented headform deceleration levels
less than 200 G-max when tested at accelerations equal to
play equipment critical heights. As such, it specifies test
methodology to be used for surface testing to be conducted
both in the laboratory and in the field and allows the
determination of the maximum drop height at which G-max does
not exceed 200. In the 1991 CPSC guideline recommendation,
a second criteria of less than 1000 Head Injury Criteria
(HIC) was added to the 200 G-max requirement. Revisions to
ASTM F-1292 are currently being balloted to include this
1000 HIC requirement and attendant acquisition methodology.

KEYWORDS: Playground surfaces, impact attenuation,
instrumented headform, play equipment critical heights, HIC,
ASTM F-1292

This paper will review the contents of ASTM F-1292
including laboratory and in-field surface testing
requirements. Some background will be given on the history
and applicability of instrumented headforms and G-max and
HIC for serious head injury prediction. Finally, an

---

[1]Chief Chemist, Research and Development, Carlisle Tire
& Rubber Company, Carlisle, PA 17013

overview of CPSC comments will be given on the applicability of general surface types that are desirable surfacing under and around playground equipment.

INSTRUMENTED HEADFORM STANDARD DEVELOPMENT

Use of instrumented headform drop testing to compare impact attenuation performance of various surfaces used under and around playground equipment began in the United States with the 1981 publication of the HANDBOOK FOR PUBLIC PLAYGROUND SAFETY by the United Stated Consumer Product Safety Commission (CPSC). This document contained the following:

> **SECTION 12:2, Recommendation** - When tested in accordance with the suggested test method in Paragraph 12.3 a surface shall not impart a peak acceleration in excess of 200 G's to an instrumented ANSI headform dropped on a surface from the maximum estimated fall height (see Reference 32).

This recommendation was based on testing conducted by the National Institute of Standards and Technology (NIST, formerly National Bureau of Standards, NBS) as documented in the "Impact Attenuation Performance of Surfaces Installed Under Playground Equipment," NBSIR 79-1707; February, 1979 (Reference 32 of Section 12.2, above). The researchers selected the ANSI rigid headform due to its use in current headgear standards, reproducibility and the analysis that it gave a more conservative estimate of head response than a resilient headform of the time. Further, they analyzed head injury tolerance data for head-first falls of children that estimated a peak acceleration of 200-250 G's as the tolerance limit and felt that these data were in good agreement with those reported by Hodgson, et al. that the risk of serious head injury due to a head-first fall is minimal when the peak acceleration imparted to the head is 200 G's or less [1]. They, therefore, proposed that a surface should not impart a peak acceleration in excess of 200 G's to the instrumented ANSI headform dropped on the surface from the maximum estimated fall height [2].

In 1986 ASTM Committee F08 on Sports Equipment and Facilities created a Task Group on Playground Surfacing. The initial goal undertaken was to develop test methodology and performance criteria for the impact attenuation properties of surface systems under and around playground equipment. After consideration of a number of alternatives, it was decided to base the standard on the work leading to the issued CPSC guideline recommendation of 200 G's maximum acceleration to an instrumented ANSI headform. This effort

culminated in 1991 with the ratification and issuance of
ASTM F-1292 "Standard Specification for Impact Attenuation
of Surface Systems Under and Around Playground Equipment."

ASTM F-1292 STANDARD SPECIFICATION CONTENT

The stated goal of this specification is to establish a
uniform means for measure to compare characteristics of
materials in order to provide the potential buyer with a
useful yardstick by which to measure available materials as
a surface under and around playground equipment. The
rationale states that government statistics indicate that
approximately 70% of all playground injuries requiring
hospital treatment each year are a direct result of falls
from play equipment to the underlying surface. The
specification establishes a method to determine the maximum
drop height at which G-max does not exceed 200, when tested
in accordance with ASTM F-355 Procedure C. Procedure C
requires the use of the ANSI Size C metal headform. A
warning is also contained in the specification that
compliance does not imply that an injury cannot be incurred.

A number of aspects were included in the specification
to give the user some understanding of the technology on
which the standard was based, and to present surface system
performance versus 200 G-max under a variety of laboratory
conditions. First a terminology section was prepared. This
includes definitions of such applicable terms for
acceleration, G, G-max, impact attenuation, impact velocity,
loose fill, non-loose fill system, and theoretical drop
height. Requirements were added that all surfaces had to be
tested at 30°, 72° and 120°F. (-1°, 23°, and 40°C.). Impact
testing must be performed at heights one foot (.3 meters)
over and under the drop height at which G-max did not exceed
200 at all test temperatures. A recommended test report
form was generated to further aid data analysis and
comprehension. Finally, test procedures were developed so
that testing of installed surfaces could be accomplished.

To assure the technical accuracy and reproducibility of
results, a substantial number of equipment and sample
requirements were specified in addition to those found in
the ASTM F-355 base standard. Accuracy of temperature
measurements, acceleration system recording resolutions, and
the filtering of the accelerometer signal were covered.
Minimum size samples for laboratory testing were specified
to best simulate surface system performance in actual use.
Round robin tests were conducted in order to justify a
precision statement. The round robin was conducted by a
total of six university, independent testing and industrial
laboratories. Sample types included four non-loose fill and
two loose fill types. Results of the round robin led to

method reproducibility being estimated at ± 15% which includes all errors encountered within and between laboratories.

In summary, as it was published in 1991, ASTM F-1292 was in agreement with and further delineated a method for determining the 1981 CPSC guideline recommendation of 200 G-max for the impact attenuation characteristics of surface systems used under playground equipment.

HIC INCLUSION

In late 1991, CPSC revised the HANDBOOK FOR PUBLIC PLAYGROUND SAFETY. In addition to other changes, the new guideline contains a dual criteria for surface impact attenuation to be under both 200 G-max and 1000 HIC when tested in accordance with ASTM F-1292. The guideline authors referenced work by Collantes in explaining this inclusion [3]. Collantes noted that, while G-max measures surface impact attenuation characteristics, it does not take into account the duration of the acceleration. HIC does consider duration and, thus, would be a better predictor of severe head impact injuries.

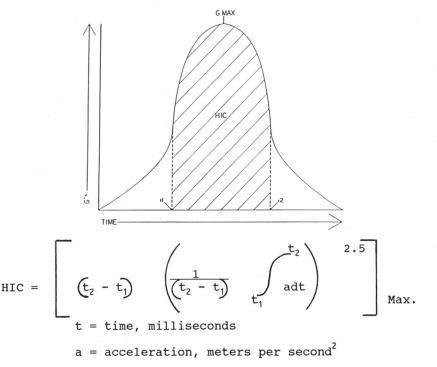

$$HIC = \left[(t_2 - t_1) \left(\frac{1}{(t_2 - t_1)} \int_{t_1}^{t_2} adt \right)^{2.5} \right]_{Max.}$$

t = time, milliseconds

a = acceleration, meters per second^2

Acceleration/time curve and HIC calculation formula

In order to maintain consistency with the new CPSC guideline and to minimize consumer confusion, ASTM F-1292 is currently being revised to include the 200 G-max and 1000 HIC dual criteria. Definition, mathematical formulation, and a computer program for calculating HIC are included. The document is currently in the last balloting stages.

SURFACING TYPE APPLICABILITY

Section 10.4 of the 1991 CPSC HANDBOOK FOR PUBLIC PLAYGROUND SAFETY contains information on a wide variety of surfacing materials. Asphalt and concrete are found to be unsuitable except as a base for a shock absorbing unitary material such as a rubber mat or foam padding. Soils, hard packed dirt, grass and turf surfaces are not recommended because their effectiveness in absorbing shock can be reduced considerably due to compaction, wear and environmental conditions. Unitary materials, such as rubber mats, foams, or bound rubber-like materials, are satisfactory but information on specific properties and installation practices are to be obtained from the manufacturer. Some loose fill materials have acceptable shock absorbing properties when installed and maintained at sufficient depth. Included are results of a number of generally available loose fill materials which were tested in accordance with ASTM F-1292.

SUMMARY

The use of instrumented headforms for the determination of the shock absorbing properties of surface systems under and around playground equipment has become an accepted practice. Further, the relationship of performance levels under 200 G-max and 1000 HIC to the likelihood of substantial reduction of severe head injuries caused by falls from equipment has been outlined. The use of ASTM F-1292 "Standard Specification for Impact Attenuation of Surfaces Under and Around Playground Equipment" has been established as an effective and accepted test protocol and performance requirement.

REFERENCES

[1]   Mohan, D., Snyder, R. G., and Foust, D. R., "A Biomechanical Analysis of Head Impact Injuries to Children," presented at the Ninth Annual Neuroelectric Society Meeting, December 1977.

[2]   "Impact Attenuation Performance of Surfaces Installed Under Playground Equipment," Product Technology Division, National Bureau of Standards, NBSIR 79-1707, February 1979.

[3]   Collantes, Margarita, "Evaluation of the Importance of
       Using Head Injury Criteria (HIC) to Estimate the
       Likelihood of Head Impact Injury as a Result of a Fall
       onto Playground Surface Materials," U.S. Consumer
       Product Safety Commission, Washington, D.C. 20207,
       October 1990.

[1]Edward D. Williams, DMD[1]

Jaw-Joint Disorders in Contact-sports' Athletes . Diagnosis and Prevention

REFERENCE: Williams, E. D., "Jaw-Joint Disorders in Contact-Sports' Athletes: Diagnosis and Prevention," Head and Neck Injuries in Sports, ASTM STP 1229, Earl F. Hoerner, Ed., American Society for Testing and Materials, Philadelphia, 1994.

ABSTRACT: Clinical and radiologic findings in contact-sports' athletes who sustained injury to the Vital Cranial Triad (VCT), a complex of bones consisting of the temporomandibular joint (TMJ), the tympanic temporal bone and the inferior surface of the petrous temporal bone, were studied. Approaches to the diagnosis of temporomandibular disorders focused on findings from patient history, clinical examination and a modified transcranial radiographic examination. Indications for radiography included headache, earache, nausea, vomiting, vertigo, impaired hearing and balance, muscle weakness, occlusal disturbances, TMJ pain and other symptoms associated with neurologic and circulatory deficit secondary to trauma. Radiologic findings included compression fractures, condylar neck fracture, degenerative condylar remodeling, obliteration of the articular eminence, atresia of the ear canal and other damage to the VCT. Structural damage to the VCT is described and the associated symptoms are discussed in the context of 4 exemplary cases. The use of a customized mandibular orthopedic repositioning appliance to prevent injuries to the VCT is discussed. Damage to the VCT leads to painful and tragic sequelae which can and must be prevented in contact sports.

KEYWORDS: vital cranial triad, tempomandibular disorders, modified transcranial radiography, intraoral jaw-joint protection appliance, strength testing, symptomatology, diagnosis, prevention, repetitive impact loading, sequelae, jaw-joint disorders, contact sports

The relationship of trauma to temporomandibular disorders (TMD) has, until recently, been ignored or underestimated by many health-care providers possibly because of difficulties in demonstrating TMJ damage with conventional radiographic techniques and possibly because of inadequate provider training in craniomandibular physiology.

Clinicians agree that TMD arises from several pathologic conditions which affect mandibular opening, deglutition, mastication and other neurologic functions in which pain and discomfort predominate. TMD is one of the health hazards uniquely associated with contact sports such as hockey, football, soccer and boxing, the most frequent cause being repeated subconcussive blows to the head, chin or jaw, directly or via the headgear. In practically all instances, the vital cranial triad (VCT), which includes the TMJ, the tympanic temporal bone and the inferior surface of the petrous temporal bone, is violated. This complex of bones houses and ports important cranial nerve trunks as they exit from the base of the brain; it also houses the blood supply to the brain and the auditory and balance mechanisms, among others. Specifically it performs three important functions: it permits multiplanar motion of the mandible; supports the mandible and a variety of hard and soft tissue structures at the base of the skull; and, most importantly, it serves as a protective conduit for cranial nerve trunks and blood vessels. Thus, it should come as no surprise that athletes with VCT injuries often present with symptoms reflecting neurologic and circulatory deficit. These symptoms include headache, earache, facial pain, bloodshot eyes, photosensitivity, muscle weakness, pain and numbness of extremities, vomiting, vertigo and impaired speech among others (Table 1).

[1]CEO, WIPSS Inc., 1432 E. Washington Lane, Philadelphia, PA 19138

Table I. Symptoms-Athletes Jaw Disorder

EYES
- Sensitivity to light
- Pulsating pain behind eyes
- Bloodshot eyes

MOUTH
- Discomfort when chewing
- Discomfort when at rest
- Pain when opening mouth
- Clicking or popping when opening mouth
- Limited opening of mouth
- Jaw jumps or deviates to one side when opened
- Jaw locks in open position when eating, yelling, or yawning
- Teeth do not seem to fit together properly; can't locate "bite"
- Unconscious grinding of teeth, during times of anxiety or asleep
- "Migraine" type headaches

HEAD
- Radiating headache pain from forehead to eyebrow area
- Pain and pressures similar to sinus problems
- Ache in temple area-above and in front of the ear
- Hair or scalp painful to touch
- Radiating pain in back of head
- "Migraine" type headaches

EARS
- Clogged or itching ear with no infection or foreign body
- Dizziness or vertigo; ringing, hissing, or buzzing sound
- Earache but no infection
- Decrease in hearing capacity

THROAT
- Sore throat but no infection

NECK
- Sore, tired, and stiff neck muscles
- Pain and numbness in arms and fingers
- Rotator cuff-shoulder and neck pain
- Frequent shoulder and neck pain
- Recurring stiff-neck pain

MOTOR FUNCTIONS
- Impaired speech
- Nausea
- Impaired sense of balance
- Decrease in voice volume

There are a few studies which identify trauma as a major cause of TMD in the general population and few, if any, standardized approaches to diagnosis of TMD [1-11]. To our knowledge, there are no studies which link trauma and its sequelae to VCT injuries in male athletes. There are a variety of methods employed for visualizing the TMJ/VCT, each with specific indications, limitations, availability and attendant risks. Arthroscopy, for example, provides excellent visualization of adhesions, perforations and displacements of the articular disc, as well as an indication of the contour of the meniscus and its relationship to the condyle and the articular fossa [12-16]. Its use is complicated by pain, hemorrhage, lacerations, instrument breakage and limited field [12-18]. It is also invasive, expensive, not easily available and requires specialized equipment and training. Panoramic images provide good visualization of hard structures associated with mastication, but show a loss of the true shape of the condyle because of the lateral projection of the beam [19]. Moreover, articular fossa are often obscured if the patient has limited mandibular opening [12-15]. With tomography, bony changes and functional relationships are easily visualized and non-osseous structures can be seen without dye injection. However, its use is limited by cost, availability, high levels of radiation and limited definition [12,15,20]. MRI is used for soft tissue analysis. It is more accurate than arthrography in providing soft-tissue contrast, is virtually free of ionizing radiation and is noninvasive. However, its linear focus has a limited depth of field and poor definition of structures. Like most of the other methods, it is very expensive, not easily available and not adaptable for office use.

The most practical and most affordable alternative to the methods described is a modified transcranial radiographic technique which we have developed. It is also relatively inexpensive, noninvasive, easily adaptable for use in medical, dental and sports facilities, and carries less risk of ionizing radiation than other methods. There is also less distortion due to overlapping structures than with conventional radiography, and sharper definition of bony structures. In addition, the pathologic results of trauma to the VCT are radiologically demonstrable with this technique. In this communication the pathologic results of trauma to the VCT of athletes are described and the symptoms associated with VCT damage are discussed in the context of 4 exemplary cases.

METHODS AND MATERIALS

Bilateral transcranial radiographs of 31 male and 3 female athletes, ages 17-43 years were selected for study of destructive changes of the VCT. The patients, all referrals, had presented with one or more symptoms of pain, dysfunction, clicking, locking, occlusal difficulties, vertigo, tinnitus, crepitus, and hearing impairment, among others (Tables 1 and 2). Headache, stiff neck and shoulder weakness were predominant symptoms. All had described a relationship between onset of symptoms and previously incurred trauma to the jaw.

Usually, symptoms became apparent 2 to 3 months after injury and had lasted for periods varying from 3 months and beyond. In some, symptoms became apparent

CLINICAL SYMPTOMS
Athletes Jaw-Joint Disorders (n=34)

	FOOTBALL (n=12)	BOXING (n=12)	SOCCER (n=10)
Stiff neck	12	12	9
Headache	12	12	10
Ear sounds	10	7	8
Blackout	12	3	1
VCT sounds	8	11	4
Sinus pain	9	5	7
Rotator cuff	12	12	4
Locking jaw	3	2	5

Table 2

immediately. All patients were evaluated by standard methods including a full mouth and trans-cranial radiographic examination, physical examination of the head, neck, jaw and shoulder areas and a medical history. In addition, two simple strength tests were conducted using the Nicholas MMT (Model 01160). Both were used to ascertain loss of strength in athletes with VCT injury. Injury to the VCT results in the loss in strength and physical endurance because of localized neurologic impairment at the nerve trunk. Essentially the condyle was unloaded by moving the lower jaw by mechanical means to an inferior and anterior position away from the injured VCT. Various muscle groups were then tested for strength loss or gain and the results were recorded.

RADIOGRAPHY
Transcranial radiographs were made with a Bennett Head Unit. The patient's head was positioned laterally, with the imaginary ala-tragus line parallel to the floor. The tragus was positioned so that the lateral view of the TMJ/VCT would include the external auditory meatus, the total translatory space of the condyle, and the tympanic temporal bone to exclude unwanted cranial bones from the radiograph. Angulation was also described and standardized for the cassette holder and the radiation source to minimize angulation changes that would adversely affect the radiograph. Semi-axial lateral projections were made with both open-and closed-mouth positions. An 8 x 10 inch or a 24 x 30 mm cassette with screen was placed on the horizontal plane of

Fig. 1   Fig. 2

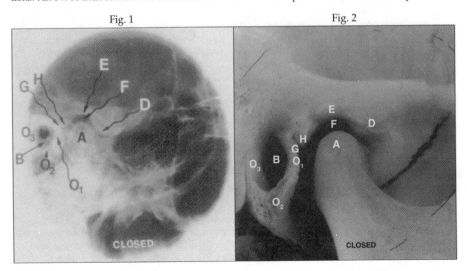

the cassette holder and an adapter was used. The X-ray source was collimated to the aperture of the adaptor to create 2 circular exposures of the same film. An X-ray grid was used to eliminate scatter radiation effects on the film. The mAs (mA x time), was calibrated with the kVp at 70 to 80. The films were exposed, processed, traced, and examined. The volume of joint space and the destructive changes in and around the VCT area were studied and compared with dried skull specimens and the reference transcranial radiographs described as normal.

Radiographs of a 53 year-old male volunteer (Fig.1) which approximated normal VCT findings were used as reference. These were then compared with a series of dried skulls. A representative dried skull was chosen (Fig.2) which showed anatomical markings typical of a so-called "normal" VCT complex. A comparison of Figs. 1 and 2 reveals a relatively normal condyle morphology except for an early change at the antero-superior head of the condyle (Fig. 1). Glenoid fossae are congruent with the condylar heads, the tympanic temporal bone forms two well-formed walls and floor of the external auditory meatus, i.e., the anterior wall (0-1), the inferior portion of the wall (0-2) and part of the posterior wall (0-3). The anterior wall of the tympanic temporal bone was convex facing the condyle; the posterior surface of the condyle is convex facing the temporal tympanic bone; the antero-superior surface of the anterior wall of the tympanic temporal bone is contiguous (G) with the infero-posterior or surface of the postglenoid process (H); the articular eminence (D) is well-defined with rounding slopes, and the assumed disc space (F) suggests adequate disc thickness.

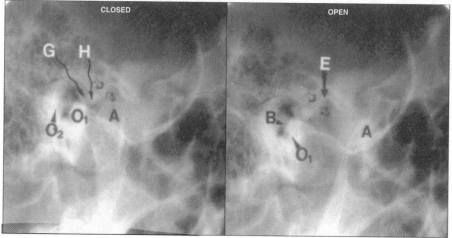

Fig. 3 Right Transcranial

Case Reports

Case 1. A 24-year-old football player complained of shoulder pains, frequent stiff neck, gurgling and raspy voice patterns, headaches of unknown origin, periodic tingling and smarting sensations of the upper extremities and fingertips, and a steady decline in the amount of weight he could lift on bench press. The right transcranial radiograph (Fig.3) reveals an increase in the sclerotic density of the tympanic temporal bone (O-1, O-2); traumatic displaced fracture (G) of the supero-anterior surface of the tympanic temporal bone and the postero- inferior surface of the postglenoid process (H). A change in the condyle/fossa congruence; flattening of the superior surface of the condyle (A); pyramidal reshaping of the of the fossa (E); change in the definition of the external auditory meatus (B) as a result of the green-stick fracture of the anterior wall of the tympanic temporal bone; degenerative changes of the posterior slope of the glenoid fossa (nondisplaced healed fracture)(2 open arrows); and increase in sclerotic density and thickening of the postglenoid process. In some instances such blows can force the condyle into the external ear canal.

The left transcranial study (Fig 4) shows structural damage similar to that seen on the right condyle as a result of repeated trauma to the tympanic temporal bone, the condyle, and the fossa. Note the folding effect of the anterior wall of the tympanic temporal bone posteriorly; increased radiodensity (opacity) of the anterior floor and posterior wall of the tympanic temporal bone; condyle-to-eminentia interference during condylar motions of translation as determined by the osseous destruction of the articular eminence. There is also evidence of destructive osseous changes which causes obliteration of the articular eminence and the fracture of the posterior incline of the glenoid fossa (2 open arrows), and increased radiolucency at the tympanomastoid fissure (2:1 opposing arrows).

With the insertion of the jaw-joint protective appliance, the patient experienced an increase in strength during workouts and a notable decrease in the frequency and intensity of headaches and facial pain after play.

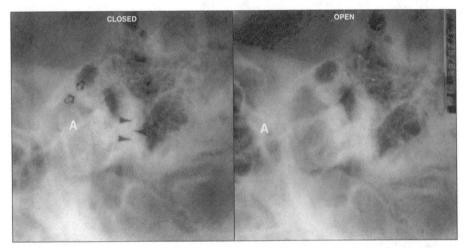

Fig. 4 Left Transcranial

Case 2. A 28-year-old male heavyweight boxer with a ring history of 6 years, presented with symptoms of middle ear pain and undiagnosed severe debilitating headache. The right transcranial radiograph (Fig. 5) shows a tubercle-like extension on the postero-superior surface of the condylar head (A); reshaping of the posterior slope of the glenoid fossa(E); remodelling of the anterior wall of the tympanic temporal bone(O) and the posterior surface of the condylar head due to trauma of the anterior surface, producing an indentation congruent with the posterior surface of the condyle. There is also definite indication of early thinning of the tympanic temporal bone characterized by changes which tend towards concavity (facing the condyle), and loss of osseous integrity of the inferior slope of the articular eminence, indicating interference during condylar translation. Also seen is the fracture(G) of the union between the tympanic temporal and the postglenoid process (2 arrows).

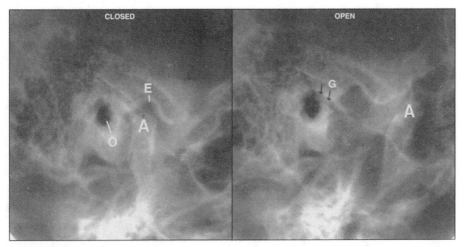

Fig. 5 Right Transcranial

The left transcranial radiograph (Fig. 6) reveals the following: early progressive thinning of the tympanic temporal bone (O); increased radiolucency of the fracture of the union between the tympanic temporal bone and the postglenoid process (G); structural change of the glenoid fossa with the loss in radiographic definition of the posterior slope; functional interference between the postglenoid process and the postero-superior surface of the condyle (open arrows), and loss in the integrity of the inferior slope of the articular eminence. (D).

Here too, the jaw-joint protective appliance proved to be of considerable benefit. All symptoms disappeared upon the insertion and utilization of the appliance.

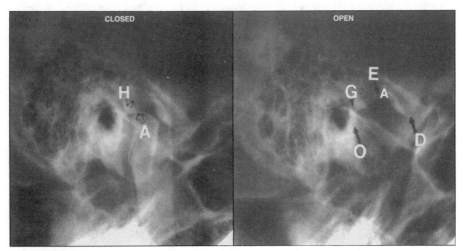

Fig. 6 Left Transcranial

Case 3. This patient, aged 43 years, had a ring history of over 20 years. He was unable to open his mouth more than 22 mm, his speech was soft and slurred, his voice was raspy, he exhibited parkinson-like tremors, and he suffered from impaired balance as evidenced by his "stagger-step" gait. The right transcranial radiograph (Fig. 7) shows a severely thinned anterior wall and floor of the tympanic temporal bone (0-1); loss of definition of the mastoid process; displaced fracture and chronic scarring of the posterior slope of the glenoid fossa (E). In addition, a shallow recess of the fossa and degenerative changes of the articular eminence (2 arrows). There is also a loss of structural definition of the postglenoid process (H).

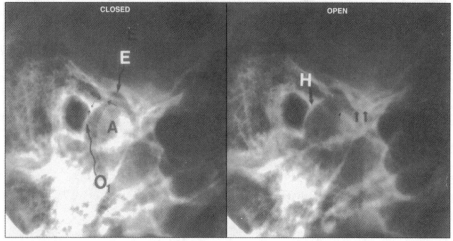

Fig. 7 Right Transcranial

The left transcranial radiograph (Fig. 8) reveals a slender and diminished condylar head with degenerative changes in the neck of the condyle(A); displaced and nondisplaced fractures of the posterior wall; fracture of the surface of the anterior wall(O-1) and inferior surface(O-2) of the

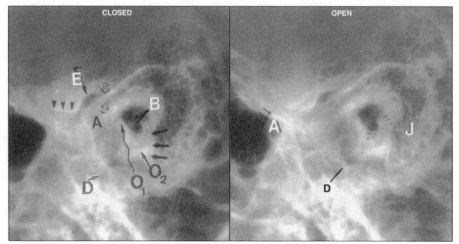

Fig. 8 Left Transcranial

tympanic temporal bone. Also identified are shallow glenoid fossa(E) with a displaced healed fracture of its posterior slope; change in the morphology of the postglenoid process interfering with the posterior surface of the condyle at rest (open arrows); concavity of the anterior wall of the tympanic temporal bone (0-1) facing the condyle (A); increased radiolucency of the tympanomastoid fissure (3 arrows) and increased radiolucency of the posterior wall of the tympanic temporal bone. Present also are changes in the mastoid air cells (J); a severely eroded tympanic temporal bone, sharply exposing to view the underlying petrous temporal bone and the internal carotid canal(D); and a fracture of the posterior wall of the tympanic temporal bone (3 small arrows).

In this case the jaw-joint protective appliance proved to be of limited benefit although the tremors and the stagger-step gait decreased dramatically with its use.

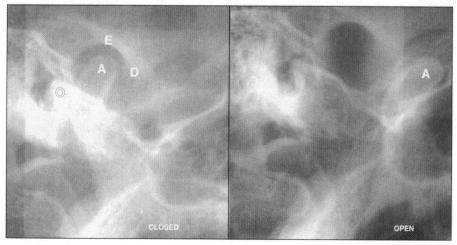

Fig. 9 Right Transcranial

Case 4. A twenty three year-old female soccer player with field play experience of thirteen years, presented with migraine-like headaches, facial pain, deviated jaw movements and a past history of headaches and jaw problems which appeared after games and continued to worsen with time. She had previously undergone a condylectomy with no apparent benefit. The right transcranial radiograph (Fig. 9) reveals the condyle (A) in a higher than usual position in the recess of the fossa (E); feathering of the articular eminence (D), indicating interference during translation. Also visible are green-stick (O) fracture of the anterior wall of the temporal tympanic bone; sclerotic changes in the temporal tympanic bone, indicative of repetitive loading of that bone; and increased opacity of the squamotympanic fissure.

The left transcranial radiograph (Fig. 10) reveals the condylectomy (A) restricted translation during opening; feathering of the articular eminence; a nondisplaced fracture at the postglenoid process; and increased opacity of the temporal tympanic bone and squamotympanic fissure.

With the use of the jaw-joint protection appliance during play and training, the patient volunteered that her headaches diminished in frequency and intensity and that she experienced greater facial comfort after the athletic event.

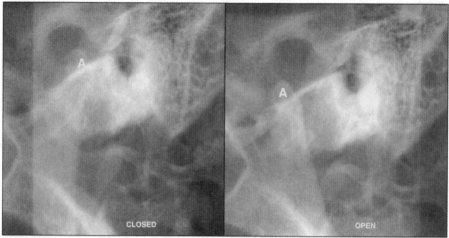

Fig. 10 Left Transcranial

DISCUSSION

Head and facial trauma as the underlying cause of TMD, mandibular and condylar fractures and dislocations, and related bone damage has not been widely reported in the past, possibly because of difficulties encountered in demonstrating TMJ/VCT damage with conventional radiographic techniques. The recent literature [1,3,21-25] reports a significant percentage of patients with internal derangements with a history of facial trauma before the onset of the TMD. The disorders included osseous fractures, disc interference, degenerative joint changes, and condylar dislocations. In our study, we encountered similarly devastating effects of head and facial trauma more often than in a normal population because of the homogeneity of the patient population. All were athletes, either football, soccer players or boxers, who were repeatedly exposed to the punishing effects of head and facial trauma. All had used accepted or mandated types of mouthguards. Much of the damage sustained was radiographically visible.

Among the taller football players, we observed diminished disc space with upward condylar positioning and pyramidal-shaped fossae; tympanic plate fractures resulting in atresia of the external auditory meatus; condylar morphology changes and posterior displacement of the condyle. While condylar damage and dislocations as well as other damage to the TMJ/VCT and surrounding areas have been observed in the general population [1,22-28], atresia of the external auditory meatus per se, has not been reported.

The reports of Akers and co-workers [21] and those of Worthington [22] mention involvement of the external auditory meatus in patients who sustained injuries in automobile accidents. Akers observed posterior dislocation of the condyloid process into the external ear canal, and later, partial stenosis of the external ear canal in the same patient. (Female patients encountered in our practice who were victims of spousal abuse, exhibited similar clinical symptoms and findings). Worthington in his report of a patient with multiple injuries, including a fractured mandible, observed that "...on occasions circumstances may so combine as to allow posterior dislocation with fracture of the bony tympanic plate and disruption of the external auditory meatus." In all contact sports the VCT is repeatedly exposed to potentially injurious forces beyond the tolerable load design of the jaw-joint mechanism. This repetitive impact loading superimposed on already weakened or compromised VCT structure will predispose the athlete to more serious injuries.

In football, damage to the VCT is induced by repeated blows to the chin, faceguard, and helmet. The relative force exerted at the point of impact (considering the body mass of the individuals involved, their combined speed, and the angle of impact) is more than the VCT can reasonably absorb. The four point chin strap contributes to the progression of damage, because its positioning, which secures the helmet to the head, also pulls the mandible superiorly and posteriorly. This antagonistic positioning of the condyles, adversely influences the neurologic and physiologic functions of the delicate structures of the vital cranial triad. This impacts the characteristic potential for injury. Contact against the faceguard also greatly contributes to VCT damage. Furthermore, in this critical area, repetitive load forces are intensified. These forces are directly transmitted from a bone of higher mass and density (the condyle) to bones and tissue of lesser mass and density (the undercarriage of the skull and brain).

Similar destructive changes were noted and identified in boxers. Radiographic studies revealed osseous changes, including bone thinning resulting from microfractures of the tympanic temporal bone and posterior surface of the condyle. The progressive erosion of the anterior and medial walls of the tympanic temporal bone as well as the erosion of the floor and posterior wall are attributable to microfractures induced by the cumulative effects of multiple blows to the jaw forcefully driving the condyle posteriorly and medially. In addition, the thinning of the temporal bones rendered the VCT more vulnerable to fracture of the glenoid fossa, cranial vault and exposure to the cranial vault and blood supply.

Copenhaver and colleagues [3] described a fracture of the glenoid fossa and dislocation of the mandibular condyle into the middle cranial fossa of a young patient who sustained trauma to the chin after falling from a bicycle. After surgery, the patient recovered and showed no signs of neurologic deficit. They stated that although craniofacial structures may serve to prevent violation of the cranial cavity, occasional condylar dislocations occur which may be related to several factors, including the magnitude and direction of the trauma, morphological abnormalities of the condyle and a particularly thin glenoid fossa roof. Orban [2], on the other hand, observed that "...the thinness of the bone in the articular fossa is responsible for fractures if the mandibular head is driven into the fossa by a heavy blow. In such cases injuries of the dura mater (subdural hematomas) and brain have been reported."

These changes may explain the headaches and intracranial pressures experienced in athletes engaged in contact sports. It may also explain, to some degree, symptoms suggestive of encephalopathy as in Case 3, where radiographic evidence pointed to massive damage to the VCT, including the medial encroachment of the condyle on cranial nerve trunks and the internal carotid artery which produce symptoms that mimic brain damage in boxers. The insertion of an appliance which positions the condyle anteriorly and inferiorly to the fossa, unloads the joint and relieves pressure on the vital structures, was used in the boxer with parkinsonian -like tremors. The severity and extent of his tremors decreased and his gait and balance improved. Considering the long professional career of this boxer, it is not at all unlikely that neurologic symptoms may have developed concurrently with, as a result of, or independently of damage to the VCT.

Brain damage and brain atrophy in boxers is discussed elsewhere in the literature [4,29-31]. It should be noted, that in all instances (except for Case 3) the insertion of an appliance which unloads the joint, elicited beneficial responses. Symptoms were ameliorated, impaired neurologic function was improved and significant muscular strength and resistance was restored.

Clinical experience points to an unusually high incidence of VCT damage among soccer players and focuses our attention to the net effects of "heading the ball" while contending with an opponent in the field. As Fig. 11 illustrates, the risk of injury to the VCT in soccer players may be as great as in football, hockey and boxing. Attention must also be focused on the assumption that there are now more women participating in physical sports than ever before. Injuries to the delicate area of the VCT may have a more intensely adverse influence on the physical functions of the female. Further studies in this area are indicated.

The unusual nature of the symptoms reported by the athletes in this communication requires further comment. As can be seen from Table 1 there were a variety of symptoms reported which are not usually associated with TMD, but are unique to athletes with jaw-joint disorders and VCT damage. In all likelihood, these symptoms arose as a result of cranial nerve trunk and blood vessel damage, following traumatic displacement of the condyles (particularly the left condyle because most boxers are right-handed and inflict power blows to the left side of their opponents jaw) from a blow with a

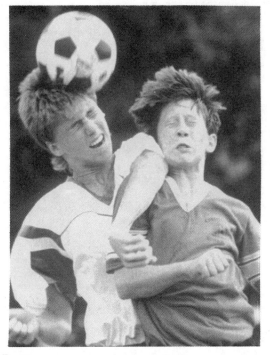

Fig. 11

posterior, medial and superior force vector. Following such a blow, the left condyle moves posteriorly, medially and superiorly into the area of the temporal tympanic bone and the inferior surface of the petrous temporal bone, thus encroaching on the area of the jugular foramen. Porting the jugular foramen directly off the brain stem are three cranial nerve trunks: (1) the glossopharyngeal, which influences the muscles of the pharynx, the stylopharyngeus and muscles of the soft palate and pharynx, which affect gag reflex, taste, swallowing patterns, and tongue sensations; (2) the vagus, which influences the voice box thus affecting speech and speech patterns. The vagus also branches to form the superior laryngeal and recurring pharyngeal nerves which influence changes in voice volume and tone (in boxers this is characterized by low volume conversational tone, rasping voice, etc). The vagus also supplies heart, diaphragm and the gastrointestinal area. The consequent trauma can produce a vagal-vagal response such as nausea and vomiting (the chief symptoms of the boxer previously described). A large portion of the vagus nerve is afferent, sending impulses to reflex centers of the brain affecting many other bodily functions. It should also be noted that the vagus nerve (through its reflex functions) may be the principal cranial nerve involved in the recapture of strength loss experienced by athletes with VCT injuries. (3) the spinal accessory nerves which supply the sternocleidomastoideus and trapezius muscles. These muscles directly affect head and shoulder movement, limit abduction and adduction of the upper appendages and inhibit subscapular rotation, causing painful movements of the upper appendages. This is often misdiagnosed as a rotator-cuff injury. A fourth cranial nerve (the hypoglossal nerve) ports through this area after leaving the hyperglossal canal into the jugular sheath. Injury to this nerve affects tongue movement, causing slurring speech and thick-tongue syndrome. In juxtaposition to the jugular foramen lies the carotid canal which houses the internal carotid artery, one of the principal arteries which supply the brain. Trauma to this area adversely affects the nerve trunks and the internal carotid. Repeated trauma to the artery will produce fissures of the intimal surface, which predisposes this tissue to localized atherosclerotic development. Complicating this development, is the inability of the injured carotid artery (after making a turn into the bony sheath of the internal carotid canal) to accommodate the progressive accumulation of plaque. What follows is the occlusion of the artery and a diminution of the blood and oxygen supply to the brain thereby, predisposing the athlete to stroke and other encephalopathies seen among retired contact-sports' athletes.

Recent developments in the management of jaw-joint injuries in athletes make particularly timely an appraisal of mouthguards in current use. While conventional mouthguards prevent dental damage, they also potentiate damage to the VCT and, as we have observed, the protection they offer to the VCT is far from satisfactory. It is important to recognize that the mouthguard design must provide stabilization of the jaw-joint. Clinical stability of the jaw-joint is defined as the ability of the condyle to limit its patterns of displacement of physiological loads to prevent damage, interference, or irritation to any of the structures of the vital cranial triad. Condylar instability/displacement perpetuates disc disease and degenerative changes of the vital cranial triad. Obviously a compelling need has always existed for an appliance which could effect and sustain adequate protection of the VCT to reduce risk factors during offensive exchanges in the ring or the athletic arena. Lateral loading of the condyle can produce hyperextension of the condylar capsule and impingement of the medial surface of the condyle onto the protective conduit of the bones of the VCT. With repeated injurious lateral forces, the capsular compliance is lost. This increases condylar displacement, producing destruction or fractures of the protective conduit bones and damage to cranial nerves and blood supply.

Our observations of a newly designed Jaw-Joint Protection Appliance, **WIPSS**™, indicate that damage to the VCT can be prevented and risk factors reduced. The WIPSS Appliance is designed to create a buffer or recoil space between the condyle and the VCT by repositioning the condyles (Fig.12,13).

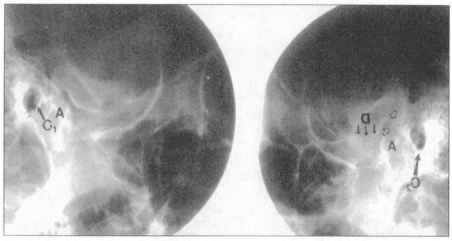

Fig. 12   Condyle Position with Mouthguard

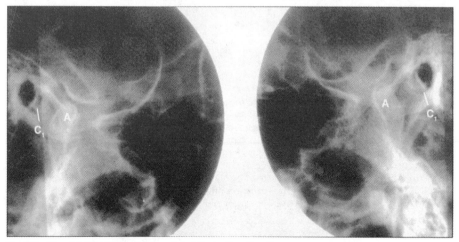

Fig. 13   Condyle Position with Jaw-Joint Protection Appliance

The recoil space created by the insertion of WIPSS, and the WIPSS appliance with the dental arches act in concert to absorb and dissipate the impact of any blow to the head, chin or face. It also reduces traumatic lateral displacement of the lower jaw (Figs.14,15), thus protecting the temporal bone complex, the base of the cranium, the dental arches and the dentition against fractures. Most impor-

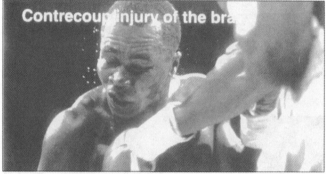

tantly, the repositioning of the condyles, anterior to the injured structures, permits the athlete to function at optimal physical levels (increased muscular strength, resistance and thereby decreased fatigue) thus decreasing the likelihood of cervical and other facial injuries.

Unstable Jaw, Athlete Wearing Mouthguard

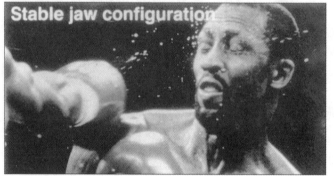

Stable Jaw, Athlete Wearing Jaw Joint Protection Appliance

CONCLUSIONS

Contact sports are hazardous. Protective equipment such as helmets and face shields cannot protect athletes from all injuries to the head, face and jaw-joint. In fact, existing equipment can and does potentiate jaw-joint injuries. In sports, where retention performance of the helmet is based on a chin cup or the faceshield in contact with the chin, impact loading to the helmet or faceshield transmits the load force directly to the jaw-joint. The resultant injuries include bone fractures, damage to the delicate tissue at the base of the skull and repeated bleeding episodes at the base of the brain, i.e. subdural hematoma. After careful study and evaluation of the mechanisms and forces involved in head injuries and recognition of the pervasiveness of jaw-joint injuries, safety specifications for jaw-joint protective equipment are warranted. Consideration must be given to the dentition of the upper and lower arch and related structures, and to the vital cranial triad. The intent is to maximize clincal stability and minimize traumatic jaw displacement, as well as prevent injury to the delicate structures of the VCT, when subjected to load force. The result of utilizing a jaw-joint protective appliance (WIPSS) does indeed dramatically reduce jaw-joint and related head injuries.

REFERENCES

[1] Bessette, R.W., Katzberg, R., Natiella, J.R., and Rose, M.J., "Diagnosis and Reconstruction of the Human Temporomandibular joint after Trauma or Internal Derangement," Plastic and Reconstructive Surgery, Vol. 75, 1984, pp 192-205.

[2] Bhaskar,S.N., Orban's Oral and Embryology, C.V. Mosby Co., St. Louis, 1986.

[3] Copenhaver, R.H., Dennis, M.J., Kloppedal., E., Edwards, D.B., and Scheffer, R.B., "Fracture of the Glenoid Fossa and Dislocation of the Mandibular Condyle into the Middle Cranial Fossa",Journal of Oral and Maxillofacial Surgery Vol. 43, 1985, pp 974-977.

[4] Enzenauer, R.W., Montrey, J.S., Enzenauer, R.J., and Mauldin, W., Boxing-related Injuries in the United States Army through 1985", Journal of the American Medical Association, Vol. 261, 1989. pp 1463-1466.

[5] Harkens, S.J., and Marteney, J.L., "Extrinsic Trauma: A Significant and Precipitating Factor in Temporomandibular Dysfunction", Journal of Prosthetic Dentistry, Vol. 54, 1985, pp 271-272.

[6] Hildebrandt, J.H., "The Importance of Repeated Injurty to the maxillofacial Area USA/ABF Ringside Physicians Cert. Manual, USA Amateur Boxing Federation, Sports Medicine Committee, Colorado Springs 199, pp 22-22.

[7] Hurt, T.L., Fisher, B., Peterson, B.M., and Lynch, F., "Mandibular Fractures in Association with Chim Trauma in Pediatric Patients", Pediatric Emergency Care, Vol 4, 1988, pp 121-123.

[8] Moos, K.F., Leattar, A., "Ten Years of Mandibular Fractures; An Analysis of 2, 137 Cases", Oral Surgery, Vol. 59, 1985, pp 120-129.

[9] Normank, J.F., "Post-traumatic Disorders of the Jaw Joint", Annals of the Royal College of Surgeons (England) Vol. 64, 1982, pp 27-36.

[10] Pavia, N.A., and Lara Fernandezx, J.L., "Sports Dentistry: Report of a Double Mandibular Fracture in a Boxer", Practica Odontologica Vol, 8, 1987, pp 23-24.

[11] Wilkes, C.H., "Arthrography of the Temporomandibular Joint in Patients with TMJ-Pain Dysfunction Syndrome", Minnesota Medicine Vol. 61, 1978, pp 645-653.

[12] Bell, W.E., "Temporomandibular Disorders. Classification, Diagnosis, Management", Yearbook Medical Publishers (3Ed) Chicago, 1986, pp 199-214

[13] Kozeniauskas, J.J., and Ralph, W.J., "Bilateral Arthrographic Evaluation of Unilateral Temporomandibular Joint Pain and Dysfunction", Journal of Prosthetic Dentistry, Vol. 60, 1988, pp 98-105.

[14] Leary, J.M., Johnson, W.T., and Harvey, B.V., "An Evaluation of Temporomandibular Joint Radiographs", Journal of Prosthetic Dentistry Vol, 60, 1988, pp 94-97.

[15] Okeson, J.P., "Management of Temporomadibular Disorders and Occlusion", 2nd Ed. C.V. Mosby Co., Philadelphia, 1989, pp 235-251

[16] Preti, C., and Fava, C., "Lateral Transcranial Radiography of Temporomandibular Joints", Journal of Prosthetic Dentistry, Vol. 59, 1988, pp 85-93.

[17] Christianson, E.L., Moore, R.J., Hasso, A.N., and Hinshaw, D.B. Jr., "RadiationDose in Radiography, CT, and Arthrography of the Temporomandibular Joint", American Journal of Roentgenology, Vol. 148, 1987, pp 107-109.

[18] Lydiatt, D., Kapla, P., Tu, H., and Sledeer P., "Morbiity Associated with Temporamandibular Joint Arthrography in Clinically Normal Joints", Journal of Oral and Maxillofacial Surgery, Vol. 44, 1986, pp 8-10.

[19] Chilvarquar, L., McDavid, W.W.D. Langlais, R.P., Chilvarquar, L.W., and Numikowski P.V., "A New Technique for Imaging the Temporomandibular Joint with a Panoramic X-Ray Machine", Oral Surgery, Oral Medicine, Oral Pathology, Vol. 65, 1988, pp 626-631.

[20] Cohen, H., Ross, S., and Gordon, R., "Computerized Tomography as a Guide in the diagnosis of Temporomandibular Joint Disease", Journal of the American Dental Association, Vol, 110, 1985, pp 57-60.

[21] Akers, J.O., Narang, R., and De Champlain, R.W., "Posterior Dislocation of the Mandibular Condyle into the External Ear Canal", Journal of Maxillofacial Surgery, Vol. 40, No. 6, June 1982, pp 369-370.

[22] Worthington, P., "Dislocation the Mandibular Condyle into the Temporal Fossa", Journal of Maxillofacial Surgery, Vol. 10, 1982, pp 24-27.

[23] Solberg, W.K., "Temporomandibular Disorders: Clinical Significance of TMJ Changes", British Dental Journal, Vol. 160, 1986, pp 231-236.

[24] Bean, L.R., and Thomas, C.A., "Significance of Condylar Positions in Patients with Temporomandibular Disorders", Journal of the American Dental Association, Vol, 114, 1987, pp 76-77.

[25] Pullinger, A.G., "The Significance of Condyle Positioning in Normal and Abnormal Temporomandibular Joint Function", in Clark, G.T., and Solberg, W.K., (Eds.) Perspectives in Temporomandibular Disorders, Quintessence Publishing Co., Chicago, 1987, pp 89-103.

[26] Christiansen, E.L., Thompson, J.R., and Hasso, A.N., "CT Evaluation of Trauma to the Temporomandibular Joint", Journal of Oral and Maxillofacial Surgery, Vol. 45, 1987, pp 920-923.

[27] Leake, D., Koykos, J. III, Habal, M.B., Murray, J.F., "Long-Term Follow-Up of Fractures of the Mandibular Condyle in Children", Plastic and Reconstructive Surgery, Vol. 47, 1971, pp 127-131.

[28] Weinberg, S., and La Pointe, H., "Cervical Extension-Flexion Injury (Whiplash) and Internal Derangement of the Temporomandibular Joint", Journal of Oral Maxillofacial Surgery Vol. 45, 1987, pp 653-656.

[29] Casson, J.R., Siegel, O., Sham, R., Campbell, E.A., Tarlau, M., and DiDomenico, A., "Brain Damage in Modern Boxers", Journal of the American Medical Association, Vol. 251, 1984, pp 2663-2667.

[30] Lampert, P.W., and Hardman, J.M., "Morphological Changes in Brains of Boxers", Journal of the American Medical Association, Vol. 251, 1984, pp 2676-2679.

[31] Morrison, R.G., "Medical and Public Health Aspects of Boxing", Journal of the American Medical Association, Vol. 255, 1986, pp 2475-2480.

Author Index

Subject Index

A

Acceleration, 142
  impact, 177
  rotational, 177
  translational, 177
Achievement motivation, 85
Air bag, 142
American Medical Association, 249
American Red Cross, 77
Aquatic Injury Safety Group, 77
ASTM Standards, 28, 73
  F 1292: 340
Axial compression, 127
Axial compressive loading, 168
Axial loading, 127, 142

B

Baseball, 223
Bending, lateral, 127
Bicycle safety helmets, 321
Boxing, 249, 257
  tempomandibular disorders, 346
Brain swelling, 287
Buckling analysis, 168

C

Cerebral concussion, 116, 249
Collar air bag, 142
Collegiate sports, 13
Coma, lucidity prior to, 287
Committee on Prevention of Spinal Cord Injuries Due to Hockey, 37
Compression, 154, 203
Computer simulation, 142, 168
Concussion, 13
  grading system, 249
Concussion gun, 177
Consumer Product Safety Commission, 47, 340

Contact injuries, 321
Contact velocity, 154
Cortical contusion, 154

D

Deformation depth, 154
Depth minimum, 77
Diving, 57, 77

E

Electromagnetic digitizer, 212
Encephalopathy, chronic, 249
Equestrian sports, 28, 73
ETOH intoxication, 73

F

Fast fourier transform, 304
Field hockey, 13
Flexion, 212
Football, 13
  catastrophic injuries, 3, 20, 239
  helmets, 142
  injury prevention, 3, 20, 142
  spearing, 239
  tempomandibular disorders, 346

H

Hardness, baseball/softball, 223
Hazard patterns, 47
Head Acceleration Device, 177
Headgear, equestrian, 28, 73
Head Injury Criteria, 223
Helmets, 142
  bicycle, 321
  equestrian, 28, 73
  motorcycle, 321
Hematoma, acute subdural, 287

363